Neighborhoods and Health

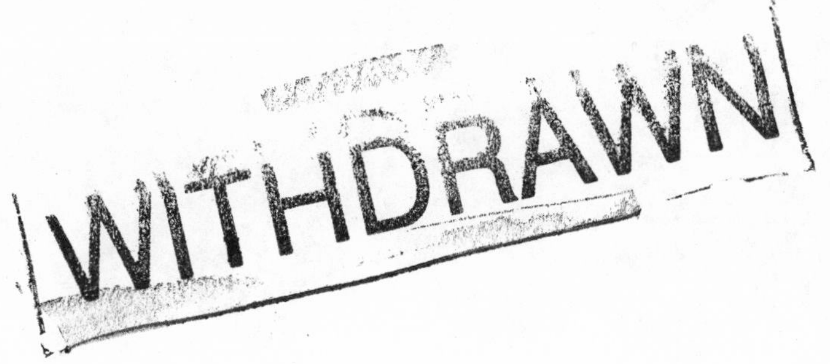

Neighborhoods and Health

SECOND EDITION

Edited by

Dustin T. Duncan

and

Ichiro Kawachi

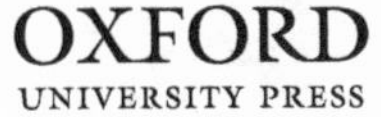

UNIVERSITY PRESS

OXFORD
UNIVERSITY PRESS

Oxford University Press is a department of the University of Oxford. It furthers the University's objective of excellence in research, scholarship, and education by publishing worldwide. Oxford is a registered trade mark of Oxford University Press in the UK and certain other countries.

Published in the United States of America by Oxford University Press
198 Madison Avenue, New York, NY 10016, United States of America.

First Edition published in 2003
Second Edition published in 2018

Library of Congress Cataloging-in-Publication Data
Names: Duncan, Dustin T., editor. | Kawachi, Ichiro, editor.
Title: Neighborhoods and health / [edited by] Dustin T. Duncan, Ichiro Kawachi.
Description: Second edition. | Oxford ; New York : Oxford University Press, [2018] |
Includes bibliographical references and index.
Identifiers: LCCN 2017042776 | ISBN 9780190843496 (hardcover : alk. paper) |
ISBN 9780190843502 (pbk. : alk. paper)
Subjects: | MESH: Health Services Accessibility |
Health Services Research | Community Health Services
Classification: LCC RA427 | NLM W 76.1 | DDC 362.12—dc23
LC record available at https://lccn.loc.gov/2017042776

1 3 5 7 9 8 6 4 2

Paperback printed by Webcom Inc., Canada
Hardback printed by Bridgeport National Bindery, Inc., United States of America

CONTENTS

FOREWORD

Ana V. Diez Roux

Twenty years ago, when the study of "contextual effects" was just emerging as a distinct area of empirical study in public health, I often found myself explaining why on earth one would be interested in "ecologic" variables when trying to explain the causes of disease in individuals. This proved to be a good exercise: It forced us to clearly articulate why (and how) context might be important and, more generally, why multilevel thinking (not just multilevel analysis) was critical not only to fully understand causation but also to identify promising policies to improve health. Fortunately, the argument had a strong conceptual basis, was supported by sociological research, and resonated with practitioners (including physicians) who saw the embodied impact of context in their patients every day. It made total sense: A variety of contexts could directly affect proximal health-related determinants (behaviors and biological processes like the stress response) or could interact with individual-level characteristics to affect health. But of course demonstrating this empirically was no easy task. And then, most important, what could we do about it?

Neighborhoods quickly emerged as a prime example of possible contextual influences on health. It is interesting to think about why this happened, given the multiplicity of "levels" and contexts that we as individuals navigate over our lives (and that might impact heath). Perhaps a prime reason is the long-standing public health focus on "place" as a key correlate of variations in health (remember the epidemiologic triad of person, place, and time!). A second reason may have been the influence of the growing literature in the social sciences arguing for contextual effects of place on a range of behaviors and social processes (child development and educational outcomes, reproductive behaviors, and criminality, among others). And last but not least, a third reason was the simple practicality and ease with which "neighborhood" variables as proxied by various census measures could be attached to existing individual-level data from surveys or epidemiologic studies. The development of multilevel analytical methods and the growing availability of software to fit multilevel models gave the field an aura of methodological sophistication (rightly or wrongly), and the modern study of neighborhood health effects was born.

CONTEXT AND COMPOSITION: IS THERE SOMETHING OUT THERE?

The first empirical studies specifically focused on the impact of neighborhoods on health were largely secondary analyses of existing individual-level studies linked to "neighborhood" data from censuses. Many, many studies have now used this approach in an attempt to estimate whether something about neighborhood context (roughly proxied by census indicators) is associated with health outcomes after controlling for the individual-level characteristics (compositional characteristics) of study participants. Of course, and as repeated in the many discussion sections of papers using this approach, these studies have many limitations in terms of drawing causal conclusions. Although naïve interpretations have assumed that the causal question investigated was about neighborhood composition itself (what is the impact on health of living in a low-income neighborhood?), generally these census measures were used as very rough proxies for a broad set of physical and social attributes correlated with neighborhood composition that could be the real etiologic factors behind any associations observed. It was clear that this approach would not take us very far in unpacking whether and how neighborhood context affected health. All it could do is suggest the question was worth of further investigation, put it on the research map so to speak, and spur the search for greater specificity in the causal hypotheses tested.

THE SEARCH FOR SPECIFICITY: HOW AND WHEN?

The next generation of neighborhood health effects studies focused on the testing of much more specific hypotheses about what neighborhood factors affected specific health-related processes and outcomes. This required more sophisticated theorizing about what neighborhood characteristics might be most important and how they might operate, including the time frames over which one might expect their effects to occur. Testing hypotheses derived from these more specific conceptual models required much more sophisticated measurement. Much work went into improving on the measurement of neighborhood attributes (including more precise specifications of the relevant spatial context) and more specific measures of the attributes presumed to be most important. This led to important advances in measurement tools (many of which are reviewed in this book) and more careful thinking about the possible health impact of spatial context generally (of which "neighborhoods" in the traditional sense are only one example).

BUT IS IT REALLY CAUSAL?

Neighborhood effects research stimulated (and was in turn affected by) renewed interest within epidemiology and public health in the thorny problems inherent in causal inference from observational studies. A number of causal inference problems had been acknowledged by researchers in the field of neighborhood health effects (and neighborhood effects more generally) from the very beginning. These included violations of the exchangeability assumption (or residual confounding by individual-level characteristics related to place of residence), the possibility of off-support inferences (or lack in sufficient overlap in distributions to allow meaningful and reliable adjustment for individual-level characteristics), and reverse causation (individual factors driving selection into neighborhoods and therefore "causing" neighborhood exposures rather than the other way around). New study designs (longitudinal designs in particular), richer data, and novel analytical methods (propensity score matching, marginal structural models, and econometric fixed effects models, among others) have been increasingly used in attempts to address these challenges. Interest also centered on the implications of spatially lagged effects (the role of adjacent or more distant neighborhoods) and the causal inference consequences of spatial dependencies in outcomes remaining after other factors were taken into account. Although the causal inference challenges are certainly not unique to neighborhood health effects research, work in this area became a good example to all those interested in upstream and multilevel causation.

Hard skeptics of observational studies have argued that experimental studies are the only way forward. But for many reasons experiments are not always possible in the study of neighborhoods and health. Although they can provide valuable insights, the experiments that have been possible (like randomizing individuals to move) may not answer the most policy-relevant questions (like the impact of a specific neighborhood improvement policy). And sometimes experiments raise new questions (about mechanisms, for example, or about conditional effects), the answers to which may require returning to observational studies. So-called natural experiments that capitalize on experiment-like conditions occurring in the real world have received increasing attention (although they have their own set of challenges), and as illustrated by this book, experiments can often be mined in multiple ways to answer a broader set of questions. The growing utilization of experimental and quasi-experimental studies in the study of neighborhood health effects has greatly enriched the field.

OH, MY GOD, IT'S (REALLY) COMPLICATED . . .

The increasing theoretical and methodologic sophistication of neighborhood health effects research made it increasingly obvious that complex dynamics were likely involved. These dynamics had been articulated in conceptual papers on neighborhood health effects from the very beginning and include processes like the dynamics of neighborhood choice (individual characteristics driving residential location through choice and external constraints), the reciprocal relation between individuals and neighborhoods (neighborhoods affect people but people also affects neighborhoods), social contagion like processes (e.g., the impact of social norms and relations), neighborhood composition generating differences in neighborhood physical and social environments which in turn reinforces neighborhood segregation, and the bidirectional influences of neighborhoods on each other (neighborhoods themselves as dependent units). But until relatively recently it was difficult to study these processes explicitly or understand their impact on causal inferences and their implications for interventions. The growing interest and familiarity with the concepts and tools of complex systems in public health has made it possible to begin to apply these approaches to questions regarding the drivers of population health. As illustrated in this book, the study of neighborhood health effects has been one area where these tools have begun to be utilized.

THE WAY FORWARD: INTEGRATING MULTIPLE SOURCES OF EVIDENCE

All around us patterns of health differences are created and reinforced by the social and economic systems that we have created. Understanding how these systems are structured, how they work, and how we can best intervene on them to improve health and promote health equity is no easy task. The world is a messy and complicated place. A single approach will not be sufficient to generate the understanding we need to act.

True understanding of the ways in which neighborhoods affect health will require combining evidence from observational studies, experiments (or natural experiments), and systems simulation approaches. These approaches are complementary and feed into each other: Observation drives experiments, which in turn generate questions that need to be answered through new observation; both observation and experiments feed into simulation modeling, which in turn raises new questions that can only be answered through new observations and new experiments. And then of course there is action, which sometimes (for ethical reasons) needs to occur even in the face of incomplete evidence, but we can learn about causes from action, and we can learn about how systems work from evaluating the impact of actions.

It is by integrating what we learn through observation, experimentation, simulation, and action that we will generate richer understanding and more effective actions to achieve our goals. The study of neighborhood health effects over the past 20 years is an excellent example of this. This book will guide you through that history, highlighting successes and challenges, and previewing the path ahead. Today when I say that my research has focused on neighborhoods and health, I no longer have to explain in great detail why this might be important, as I did (oh my gosh!) 20 years ago. This book will show you why.

CONTRIBUTORS

Mariana C. Arcaya, ScD
Assistant Professor
Department of Urban Studies and Planning
Massachusetts Institute of Technology

Jason Block, MD, MPH
Assistant Professor
Department of Population Medicine
Harvard Medical School and Harvard Pilgrim Health Care Institute

Basile Chaix, PhD
Research Director
French National Institute of Health and Medical Research (INSERM)
Institut Pierre Louis d'Epidémiologie et de Santé Publique

Rumi Chunara, PhD
Assistant Professor
College of Global Public Health and Tandon School of Engineering
New York University

Ana V. Diez Roux, MD, PhD
Distinguished University Professor and Dean
Department of Epidemiology
Dornsife School of Public Health
Drexel University

Dustin T. Duncan, ScD
Associate Professor
Spatial Epidemiology Lab
Department of Population Health
New York University School of Medicine

Abdulrahman El-Sayed, MD, DPhil
Health Commissioner
Detroit Health Department
City of Detroit

Sandro Galea, MD, DrPH
Robert A. Knox Professor and Dean
School of Public Health
Boston University

Samson Y. Gebreab, PhD
Research Scientist
National Institutes of Health

William C. Goedel, BA
Program Manager
Spatial Epidemiology Lab
Department of Population Health
New York University School of Medicine

Pedro Gullón, MD, PhD
Postdoctoral Research Fellow
Social and Cardiovascular Epidemiology Research Group
Universidad de Alcalá

Brenda Heaton, PhD, MPH
Assistant Professor
Henry M. Goldman School of Dental Medicine
Boston University

Peter James, ScD, MHS
Assistant Professor
Department of Population Medicine
Harvard Medical School and Harvard Pilgrim Health Care Institute

Ichiro Kawachi, MD, PhD
John L. Loeb and Frances Lehman Loeb Professor of Social Epidemiology and Chair
Department of Social and Behavioral Sciences
Harvard T.H. Chan School of Public Health

Danya E. Keene, PhD
Assistant Professor
Department of Social and Behavioral Sciences
School of Public Health
Yale University

Michael R. Kramer, PhD
Associate Professor
Department of Epidemiology
Rollins School of Public Health
Emory University

Gina S. Lovasi, PhD, MPH
Dornsife Associate Professor of Urban Health
Co-Director, Collaborative Urban Health
Dornsife School of Public Health
Drexel University

Quynh C. Nguyen, PhD, MSPH
Assistant Professor
Department of Epidemiology and Biostatistics
University of Maryland School of Public Health

Theresa L. Osypuk, ScD, ScM
Associate Professor
Division of Epidemiology and Community Health
University of Minnesota

Mark B. Padilla, PhD, MPH
Professor
Department of Global and Sociocultural Studies
Steven J. Green School of International and Public Affairs
Florida International University

Seann D. Regan, MA
Geospatial Analyst
Spatial Epidemiology Lab
Department of Population Health
New York University School of Medicine

Nicole M. Schmidt, PhD, MS
Research Scientist
Minnesota Population Center
University of Minnesota

Michael Seward
Research Assistant
Department of Population Medicine
Harvard Medical School

1

NEIGHBORHOODS AND HEALTH
A PROGRESS REPORT

Dustin T. Duncan and Ichiro Kawachi

Like real estate, health is location, location, location.
—George Kaplan, Professor Emeritus, University of Michigan

The field of neighborhoods and health (sometimes referred to as spatial epidemiology) has grown exponentially in the 15 years since the publication of the first edition of *Neighborhoods and Health*, edited by Ichiro Kawachi and Lisa Berkman in 2003. The purpose of this new edition is to provide an update of the many methodological and substantive advances that have occurred in the field since the original textbook.

What are neighborhoods, and why study them? According to the World Health Organization (2008), the social determinants of health consist of "the conditions in which people are born, grow, learn, work and age." Alongside schools and workplaces, neighborhoods represent one of the major contexts in which people lead a considerable portion of their lives. As every real estate agent knows, place and location (neighborhoods) can determine the quality of schools, access to services, retail stores, jobs, and transport, as well as exposure to noise, crime, air pollution, and multiple other environmental features. It follows that residential location can exert a decisive influence on variations in people's health.

Like the definition of the word *community* (of which more than 50 versions exist) (Berkman & Kawachi, 2000), a universally agreed-upon definition of *neighborhood* is likely to elude the researcher and student. Nonetheless, for the purposes of our book, neighborhoods will be hereafter defined as *geographical places that can have social and cultural meaning to residents and nonresidents alike and are subdivisions of large places*. Neighborhoods themselves are shaped by the broader context. For example, features of the physical environment (such as the presence of bicycle lanes and sidewalks) are reflections of urban planning decisions made at the metropolitan level. Neighborhoods are thus nested within larger entities (cities, states, nations) and influenced by the macroeconomic forces and political decisions operating "upstream."

A (BRIEF) HISTORICAL PERSPECTIVE ON NEIGHBORHOODS RESEARCH

Attempts to link residential location to health outcomes long predate the first edition of this textbook. The study of neighborhood contextual influences on health outcomes has been investigated throughout history, as Macintyre and Ellaway pointed out in the first edition of this book (Chapter 2). In the fifth century BCE, Hippocrates' treatise *On Airs, Waters and Places* laid the foundation for one of the earliest understanding of the relationships between places, health, and disease. John Snow is frequently cited as an early instance of a pioneer who (literally) drew the connection between neighborhoods and health by means of a map in the 19th century. Before his time, cholera was believed to be caused by a miasma (μίασμα, from the Greek word for "pollution")—or literally "bad air" wafting over the metropolis. By developing a precise dot map of cases of and deaths from cholera in 1854, Snow pinpointed the source of cholera to the infamous Broad Street pump in the Soho neighborhood in London.

In the early 19th century as yellow fever raged through Brooklyn, New York, medical professionals debated the etiology of this illness. A popular theory blamed the "filth" of Brooklyn compared to neighboring areas of New York; that is, it was a widely held belief that yellow fever was generated as a consequence of the general "negligence and filth" of the local populace. Again, this miasma theory was dispelled by the detection of a contagion that spread from a foreign ship, *The Concordia*, which had sailed from "The Havanna" and was experiencing its own epidemic. J. D. Gillespie stated:

> The Concordia lay at Sands' lower dock, and I have been at the trouble to procure a reputable surveyor to make a survey, and even a map of that dock and the adjacent neighbourhood, in which the fever prevailed; from the inspection of this map now in the possession of our board of health, it appears, as stated in my official report, that "the disease was, from beginning to end, almost exclusively confined within a circle of two hundred yards diameter from the Concordia." ("The Yellow Fever of Brooklyn in 1809," 1810, pp. 258–259)

Another pioneering investigation of neighborhoods was conducted by Louis-René Villermé in 1826. Villermé, an economist and physician in early industrial France, connected mortality rates with wealth and based them on neighborhoods (*arrondissements*) in Paris (Julia & Valleron, 2011). Across the English Channel during roughly the same period of rapid industrialization, Edwin Chadwick (1842) was documenting the striking contribution of *place* over and above the characteristics of individuals (such as social class) in determining their longevity. Indeed, the life expectancy of "gentry and professionals" living in Liverpool (35 years) was shown to be lower than "laborers and artisans" living in rural Rutland (38 years). Not surprisingly, living conditions (and life expectancy) were the worst of all for the laboring classes living in the crowded basements of the inner city, as documented by Friedrich Engels in his study, *The Condition of the Working Class in England* (1845).

Across the Atlantic, the American sanitary engineer James Cooper Bayles was an early advocate of the notion that sanitation infrastructure must be studied and assessed at a neighborhood level. In his 1877 study, *House Drainage and Water Service in Cities, Villages, and Rural Neighborhoods*, he pointed to neighborhood-level differences in the connections between water service and health, as well as articulating the ways in which social factors, such as class, influence these associations (Bayles, 1878).

RECENT DIRECTIONS IN NEIGHBORHOODS AND HEALTH RESEARCH

Since the 19th century, the focus of public health—at least in the developed world—has shifted from infectious diseases such as cholera and yellow fever. The focus of neighborhood research has also shifted from sanitation ("ditches and drains") toward other concerns, thanks to the development of sewage systems, water sanitation, and municipal garbage collection. Nonetheless, stark disparities persist in health status across neighborhoods.

Contemporary research on neighborhoods and health began by examining how neighborhood disadvantage (variously defined, but often incorporating measures of aggregate poverty) may relate to mortality. For a summary of some research in that area, the reader is referred to Chapter 1 of the first edition of this text. As an exercise in descriptive epidemiology, these studies served the purpose of pointing out that health disparities were patterned not only by personal attributes (such as social class or race/ethnicity) but also by the particular locations where people lived. However, it is an inferential leap to conclude that residential contexts are *causally* linked to people's health. That is, simply observing that residents of neighborhood A exhibit worse health profiles than residents of neighborhood B does not necessarily prove that conditions in neighborhood A caused ill health. One reason is that residents can end up being clustered into different neighborhoods according to their health characteristics. For example, health-conscious people will tend to move into neighborhoods that offer healthy food retail outlets (or conversely, healthy food stores will find it more profitable to open in neighborhoods where there is greater demand for their products). Thus, we should not be surprised if neighborhoods with better access to healthy food options also correlated with more residents with healthy dietary patterns. A major part of the neighborhood research agenda in the past decade has been devoted to shifting from initial descriptive studies (of place-based health disparities) to a deeper understanding of how neighborhood contexts can causally influence people's health. The chapters throughout this new edition reflect this ongoing agenda, especially Chapter 6, which focuses on the use of quasi-experimental designs in neighborhoods and health research.

In the first edition of the textbook, Macintyre and Ellaway proposed a distinction between the *contextual* influences of neighborhoods from *compositional* influences. The former may be defined as the "difference that places make to people," whereas the latter can be defined as the "difference that people make to places." To return to our previous example, if we observe that neighborhood A has worse average health than neighborhood B, it could be because more unhealthy people live in neighborhood A (a compositional effect), or it could be because neighborhood A has worse access to services, retail stores, jobs, and transport, as well as exposure to noise, crime, air pollution, and other adverse environmental conditions (a contextual effect). As Macintyre and Ellaway were careful to point out, the two influences are seldom (or ever) totally separable—that is, "people make places, but places also make people." Nevertheless, a considerable part of the effort in neighborhoods research during the past 15 years has been devoted to measuring specific neighborhood characteristics, including the built environment and the local food environment (as discussed in Chapters 8 and 9, respectively), linking them with specific health outcomes (such as obesity, depression, and substance use) and health behaviors (such as food and dietary choices, engagement in physical activity, as well as alcohol and tobacco consumption). This level of specificity—that is, drilling down to detailed mechanisms—is likely to strengthen causal inference and to yield useful information for public health action. Newer approaches, such as agent-based modeling (further discussed in Chapter 5), are now being applied in the neighborhoods and health literature to identify and evaluate the complex causal effects of neighborhood factors on individual-level outcomes.

WHAT HAVE WE LEARNED SO FAR?

There is a large literature on the influence of place on health to date. Many reviews and technical reports of accumulated neighborhoods and health research have been conducted (e.g., Akinyemiju et al., 2015; Bauermeister, Connochie, Eaton, Demers,

& Stephenson, 2017; Caspi, Sorensen, Subramanian, & Kawachi, 2012; Chaix, 2009; Christian et al., 2015; Ding, Sallis, Kerr, Lee, & Rosenberg, 2011; Kim, 2008; Mair, Roux, & Galea, 2008; Schüle & Bolte, 2015; van Vuuren, Reijneveld, van der Wal, & Verhoeff, 2014; Won, Lee, Forjuoh, & Ory, 2016; Yen, Michael, & Perdue, 2009). Reviews have focused on particular neighborhood characteristics (e.g., the built environment), specific health behaviors or health outcomes (e.g., physical activity), particular geographic locations (e.g., United States), particular populations (e.g., older adults), particular methods (e.g., multilevel statistical methods), and/or particular time periods (e.g., 2000 to 2010). For example, Kim conducted a review on the relationship between the built environment and depression (Kim, 2008); Akinyemiju and colleagues conducted a review on the relationship between neighborhoods and breast cancer incidence and mortality (Akinyemiju et al., 2015); Humpel and colleagues (Humpel, Owen, & Leslie, 2002) conducted a review on environmental factors associated with participation in physical activity; and Bauermeister and colleagues conducted a review on multilevel studies of neighborhoods and HIV prevention and care outcomes among men who have sex with men (Bauermeister et al., 2017). Rather than reviewing all reviews of neighborhoods and health research in this chapter, we highlight one recent comprehensive broad neighborhoods and health review by Arcaya and colleagues (2016), focusing on neighborhoods and health research in the United States.

This systematic review revealed significant patterns in the study characteristics of research assessing neighborhood effects on health in the United States. Studies overwhelmingly used cross-sectional designs (70% of the studies in fact) and pulled from over 100 neighborhoods, sampling at least 1,000 individuals. In terms of neighborhood definition, the majority of studies pulled from census tract boundaries, and in terms of the exposures within those neighborhoods, over 90% used an aspatial variable (e.g., percent poverty) as their sole predictor. Most studies with a primary neighborhood predictor focused on socioeconomic status (such as poverty), or built environment, though approximately 20% of studies had multiple neighborhood predictors or assessed variations in health outcomes by neighborhoods. Studies most commonly examined body mass index (BMI) or obesity as their primary health outcome, followed by mental health and related conditions, as well as pregnancy and birth-related outcomes.

Taken together, we have discerned the following trends in the field since the publication of the first text of *Neighborhoods and Health* in 2003:

1. *After a decade of predominantly cross-sectional studies, the field is moving toward longitudinal studies (including fixed effect designs), as well as natural experiments.* Recent studies—such as the ones from Ana Diez-Roux's group based in the

Multi-Ethnic Study of Atherosclerosis (MESA), as well as studies from Jussi Vahtera and Jaana Halonen's group (Finnish Public Sector Cohort Study) have begun to leverage *residential mobility* as a way to approach causal inference. This is (arguably) stronger than the usual longitudinal analysis approach (i.e., measure exposures at baseline and then follow outcomes over time), because it enables us to examine *change* in residential environment on *change* in health behaviors and outcomes. In theory at least, this type of first-difference (or fixed effects) approach cleans out all of the observed and unobserved time-invariant confounders between neighborhood exposures and individual outcomes. A recent study using MESA data examined change in walking and BMI following residential relocation and found that moving to a neighborhood with increased walkability was associated with increased walking and reduced BMI (Hirsch, Diez Roux, Moore, Evenson, & Rodriguez, 2014). Of course, we need to add that a die-hard skeptic might still remain unconvinced, because fixed effects analysis cannot rule out time-*varying* confounders. For example, among people who changed neighborhoods, some of them might have been motivated by health-related factors (e.g., walkability) because they were initially or became more health conscious between baseline and follow-up—for example, they were told by their physician to shed some weight. There is no way for fixed effects analysis to take account of this kind of "private" (i.e., unobserved) motivation for people's choices, and again a way to address this is to collect data on residential preferences and neighborhood selection factors at each wave (Frank, Saelens, Powell, & Chapman, 2007).

In some instances, performing a fixed effects analysis resulted in a conclusion that neighborhood researchers might not welcome—for example, Markus Jokela's paper in the *American Journal of Epidemiology* (Jokela, 2014) (with accompanying commentary by Michael Oakes) (Oakes, 2014), suggesting that after implementing fixed effects, there is no apparent causal association between neighborhood socio-economic conditions and individual mortality risk; that is, it is all apparently due to unobserved confounding factors. This approach is not without its critics—for example, most fixed effects analyses end up being underpowered due to the short time intervals of observing changes, as well as the limited number of participants who move neighborhoods in a typical epidemiological sample. Lastly, some researchers (e.g., Osypuk and colleagues—see Chapter 6) have been analyzing the result of actual randomized experiments (of residential mobility) to approach the issue of causality.

2. *Increasing methodological sophistication has been accompanied by the maturing of studies that were designed specifically for studying neighborhood effects on health.* Earlier studies of neighborhood effects were often hampered by the fact that

researchers were forced to "piggy back" their hypotheses on cohort studies that were not specifically designed for the purpose of studying neighborhood effects. Consequently, these studies often offered rich and detailed information about the individuals (e.g., health behaviors, medical history) but scant information about the neighborhoods in which they lived.

As interest in neighborhood contexts grew, we have witnessed the launch of several new studies that have been designed explicitly to understand how neighborhoods relate to health, including the Detroit Neighborhood Health Study (Johns et al., 2012); the Project for Human Development in Chicago Neighborhoods (PHDCN) (Jain, Buka, Subramanian, & Molnar, 2010; Molnar, Buka, Brennan, Holton, & Earls, 2003); the Los Angeles Family and Neighborhood Study (LA FANS) (Camacho-Rivera, Kawachi, Bennett, & Subramanian, 2014; Sastry, Ghosh-Dastidar, Adams, & Pebley, 2006); the NYC Low-Income Housing, Neighborhoods and Health Study (Duncan et al., 2014, 2016), and the Residential Environment and Coronary Heart Disease (RECORD) Cohort Study (Chaix et al., 2011, 2014), to name a few examples. Also major contributions are now being made as a result of geocoding cohort studies and/or adding questionnaire components on neighborhood perceptions, effectively turning them into studies of neighborhood effects—for example, the Atherosclerosis Risk in Communities Study (ARIC), the Multi-Ethnic Study of Atherosclerosis (MESA), and the Finnish Public Sector Cohort Study. The latter studies are particularly attractive because they are able to study residential moves over multiple waves (or, alternatively, changes in residential environment over multiple waves)—thereby enabling a fixed effects design that moves us one step closer to causal inference—beyond the conventional prospective, longitudinal analyses. In addition, studies designed specifically to study the impact of neighborhood on health often focus on a single site (often a city). A limitation of this design is generalizability if similar neighborhood characteristics produce different health effects in different places. Turning existing studies, including multisite studies, into a neighborhoods and health database increases generalizability of any effects found.

3. *There is growing specificity in examining neighborhood effects. Increasing specificity has occurred on both the exposure side (characterizing neighborhood exposures) as well as on the outcomes side*. On the exposure side, most first-generation studies focused on some aspect of neighborhood deprivation or poverty. Although these studies were important in pointing out that disparities can occur based on where people live, they do not tell us *why* or through what mechanisms deprivation is thought to be harmful; that is, they yield little in the way of clues for a policy response. On the outcomes side, many early studies focused on total mortality

(very nonspecific). Total mortality can tell us that "something is there," but it does not offer many clues about pathways or mechanisms. For example, excess total mortality could be either due to increased disease incidence (which would nudge policy makers in the direction of primary prevention), or it could be due to worse disease prognosis/survival (which would push policy makers in the direction of providing better treatment services, i.e., secondary prevention).

The second generation of studies (following the focus on total mortality) focused heavily (if you excuse the unintended pun) on obesity as an outcome of interest because (a) we are in the midst of an obesity epidemic, and (b) people entertained a suspicion that neighborhood environments might have contributed to the epidemic. However, as the authors of Chapters 8 and 9 conclude, the more closely we look at obesity as an outcome (using state-of-the-science analytical methods), the more questions are raised. The point is that more specificity is welcome in this field. There is something going on—but we need to be more specific and provide more convincing demonstrations for the evidence to be useful to policy makers. From this focus on obesity, the literature then moved to the study of the environmental determinants of physical activity and dietary behaviors (Caspi et al., 2012; Ding et al., 2011).

4. *Studies have evolved from ecological designs to multilevel designs to spatial designs.* Suppose neighborhood A has a worse average health profile compared to neighborhood B. Ecological studies cannot tell us if neighborhood A has worse health because of the characteristics of people who live in that neighborhood (a compositional effect) or because something about neighborhood A is harmful to health (a contextual effect). If the difference in health between neighborhoods is purely a compositional artifact, then a healthy resident of neighborhood B would not be expected to suffer any health penalty as a result of moving into neighborhood A. On the other hand, if there is something unhealthy about neighborhood A per se (e.g., lack of safety, exposure to crime), even a healthy resident moving from B to A might begin to suffer adverse health effects (a contextual effect). Multilevel analysis, often based on neighborhoods defined as census tracts, can help tease out "where the action is happening"—at the individual level or neighborhood level. However, as Oakes (2014) points out in his review, multilevel studies still do not tell us whether an association between neighborhood context and individual health is causal. In order to address that question, we must move toward quasi-experimental designs. Beyond multilevel designs, spatial designs focus on the specific context of individuals (often using more localized neighborhood definitions) and are more appropriate to examine spillover effects; that is, neighboring neighborhoods have similar qualities such as

health outcomes. As an example, drug use in neighborhood A will be of a similar level in neighborhood B; these neighborhoods are in geographic proximity to each other. By thinking spatially, researchers are beginning to measure people's mobility to understand neighborhood effects (Chaix et al., 2013, 2016; Zenk et al., 2011) (see Chapter 2 on methods to operationalize neighborhood boundaries).

5. *More researchers are advocating the embrace of complexity.* Neighborhoods are dynamic—that is, their characteristics reflect the dynamic interplay between residents and the environment. This is what Macintyre and Ellaway meant when they said "people make places, and places make people." Take gentrification, for example; prior to gentrification, neighborhoods are generally low-income, high-minority and, while they may be close-knit, they often have few resources and may be ridden with crime and other markers of social disorganization—see Lance Freeman's book *There Goes the 'Hood: Views of Gentrification from the Ground Up* (Freeman, 2011). Postgentrification neighborhood residents and characteristics can be the complete opposite than before; for example, the neighborhood residents are generally high-income and nonminority after gentrification has occurred. The development of *conceptual models* is critical to understand the complexity and facilitate causal understanding of how neighborhoods can relate to health (which is briefly discussed in the first edition, including in Chapter 2). These conceptual models and theories also facilitate understanding confounding and effect modification in neighborhoods and health research. They further facilitate understanding of direct neighborhood effect as compared with mediation effects. Not surprisingly, there is no single conceptual model or theory of how neighborhoods may relate to health.

FUTURE DIRECTIONS IN NEIGHBORHOOD HEALTH RESEARCH

To quote Niels Bohr, prediction is difficult, especially about the future. Nevertheless, as we gaze into our crystal ball, we can discern several promising directions for neighborhood health research. With the advent of "big data," and advances in personal recording devices and smartphone applications, we foresee a future that includes much more detailed and comprehensive characterization of people's lived realities—some have referred to this as the "quantified self" movement. See thoughts on smartphone-based digital phenotyping by Jukka-Pekka Onnela and Scott Rauch (2016). The era of big data and data science indeed will likely impact neighborhood health research in terms of the methods used and the analytical approaches employed for geographic big data, including the use of electronic health records in neighborhoods and health research.

We can also see different streams of research beginning to converge. For example, the field is ripe for examining the joint impact of neighborhoods and social networks on health, using rigorous methods for both contexts. We note that there is some research on social networks and neighborhoods (Carpiano, Kelly, Easterbrook, & Parsons, 2011; Egan et al., 2011; Evans, Onnela, Williams, & Subramanian, 2016; Fujimoto et al., 2017; Gibson, Perley, Bailey, Barbour, & Kershaw, 2015; Zelenev, Long, Bazazi, Kamarulzaman, & Altice, 2016) (this topic was covered in Chapter 13 of the first edition and some of the ensuing chapters briefly mention social network effects), but most studies have yet to apply state-of-the-science methods from the two fields and there are networks beyond social networks, such as sexual networks and drug-using networks. Future research will grapple with the issues of modeling spatial (neighborhood) and network data over time—that is, developing and implementing longitudinal models that account for spatial and network autocorrelation. Multiple contexts, beyond social networks, will be a focus of future neighborhoods and health research, including research focusing on integrating neighborhoods with working conditions, such as working hours, and neighborhoods with housing conditions such as housing units with internal water leakage as well as neighborhoods with family factors such as family disruption. These factors are intrinsically linked, but rarely studied in conjunction. For example, work (place of employment) can determine where one lives, in terms of commuting distance, as well as the salary the individual earns. Neighborhood conditions could also amplify (or buffer) stressors in the workplace. For instance, neighborhood traffic patterns and noise levels can disrupt the sleep patterns of nighttime shift workers, thereby amplifying the risk of disease outcomes. Alternatively, it is also possible that neighborhood exposures are confounded by exposures in other (overlapping) contexts. Future studies examining multiple contexts may show that "neighborhood effects" are, in fact, largely "network effects" (captured via school-based networks or social network groups).

In addition, neighborhood research focusing on "downstream" effects, including biological stress processes, will become more mainstream (Park, Verhoeven, Cuijpers, Reynolds, & Penninx, 2015; Theall, Shirtcliff, Dismukes, Wallace, & Drury, 2017; Zilioli, Slatcher, Fritz, Booza, & Cutchin, 2017). A recent cross-sectional study among a sample of 85 children found neighborhood violence and crime rates were associated with stress, as measured by stress biomarkers (Theall et al., 2017). Future research will also continue to examine salient biases in the literature and, increasingly, studies will continue to be designed to bolster causal inference, accounting for residential mobility and residential preferences (neighborhood selection) and seriously considering reverse causation and mechanisms.

Life course neighborhood studies may also be conducted—that is, investigations of the differential impact of neighborhood exposures over different stages in the life course. Neighborhood exposures may be more important at some points in the life course than others. For example, among school-aged children, school environments might matter more. For working adults, work environments might matter more. But for older adults who are "aging in place," residential neighborhood conditions might be particularly salient.

Last but not least, cross-national neighborhoods and health studies are likely to increase in "new" geographic locations, beyond the Unites States, Europe, and Australia (where the bulk of the neighborhoods and health research has been conducted to date), and connecting neighborhoods to health in disaster areas and conflict-ridden local environments (such as war zones). Because there are few examples (Jiao et al., 2016), international comparisons may be complicated. For example, with cross-national research the measurement of neighborhood exposures needs to be consistent for comparability. This may not be the case, and there may be differential quality of the neighborhood data across geographies.

STRUCTURE OF THE BOOK: METHODS AND SUBSTANTIVE AREAS IN NEIGHBORHOOD HEALTH RESEARCH

This book discusses how neighborhoods influence health primarily from a social epidemiology perspective. The book is divided into two sections. In the first section, we focus on methodological topics—covering both standard methods and newer methods in neighborhoods and health research. Methods we will overview include ways to operationalize neighborhood boundaries (Chapter 2), different approaches for quantitative methods for measuring neighborhood characteristics (Chapter 3), different statistical approaches in neighborhoods and health research (Chapter 4), the use of agent-based models to study the impact of neighborhoods on health (Chapter 5), study designs that improve on causal inference to overcome endogenous neighborhood effects—for example, fixed effects approaches in which changes in neighborhood environment (natural experiments) are examined in relation to changes in the health of residents (Chapter 6), as well as qualitative methods in neighborhood health research (Chapter 7).

In the second section, we turn our focus on substantive content areas, including how the built environment and the food environment can impact health (Chapters 8 and 9, respectively). In addition, Chapter 12 focuses on residential segregation and health, which provides an update to the same topic discussed in the first edition—including overviewing newer methods to study residential segregation. These chapters and other substantive chapters rigorously interrogate the literature in the specific areas and highlight the complexity of the topic at hand. For example, as appropriate, each chapter has a strong focus on measurement. We also overview newer substantive areas (i.e., areas on the "contours") in neighborhoods and health research, including research on neighborhood stigma and health (Chapter 10), in addition to evidence on the effects of home foreclosure rates in neighborhoods on health (Chapter 11).

Although this book focuses on two understudied neighborhood factors, we recognize that certainly there are other emerging neighborhood factors that might be salient to population health and health disparities; there is a burgeoning literature, for example, on neighborhood noise levels as they can relate to health outcomes, such as hypertension (Bodin et al., 2009, 2016; Méline, Van Hulst, Thomas, & Chaix, 2015; Tamura et al., 2017). Therefore, the book does not address *all* aspects of neighborhood health research; indeed, it is in no way exhaustive in that way because it is beyond the scope of this book to fully overview every neighborhood characteristic or method applied to the study of neighborhoods and how they can impact health. Although these are important topics, this book intentionally does not focus on neighborhood social capital or collective efficacy, given the large number of books written on those topics, including *Social Capital and Health* by Ichiro Kawachi, S. V. Subramanian, and Daniel Kim and *Global Perspectives on Social Capital* by Ichiro Kawachi, Soshi Takao, and S.V. Subramanian.

We recognize that the natural neighborhood environment (such as air pollution and weather), as well as chemicals in neighborhoods, is a potentially important factor in population health and health disparities. We do not focus on these neighborhood factors because there has been a large amount of research and many books written on this topic and these topics arguably are less related to social epidemiology. In addition, the topic of what places people in neighborhoods versus another neighborhood is not discussed directly, as it relates less to health and more to social structures. We also acknowledge there is a large volume on the sociology of place, which we refer readers to, including New York University sociologist Patrick Sharkey's book *Stuck in Place*. Furthermore, we do not focus on specific populations, such as racial/ethnic minorities, older adults, or lesbian, gay, bisexual, and transgender (LGBT) populations, though many chapters discuss neighborhood effects by subgroups. Finally, unlike the first edition, chapters do not focus on specific health outcomes such as infectious diseases and asthma. Instead, chapters (as applicable) touch on a wide variety of health outcomes and health behaviors, across a range of populations. It is our strong hope that the ensuing chapters in the book will be helpful for further application and development of neighborhoods and health research, including in areas where the research remains scant.

ACKNOWLEDGMENTS

Dr. Dustin Duncan was funded in part by National Institutes of Health grants R01MH112406, R21MH110190, and R03DA039748 and the Centers for Disease Control and Prevention grant U01PS005122. Dr. Ichiro Kawachi was funded in part by the National Institutes of Health (Award: R01AG042463). We thank Dr. Basile Chaix for commenting on an earlier iteration of this chapter. In addition, we thank the following research assistants in NYU's Spatial Epidemiology Lab for their preparation and providing comments on an earlier iteration of this chapter and for conducting background research: Yazan Al-Ajlouni, William Goedel, and Noah Kreski. We are also grateful for the comments on an earlier, spoken version of this chapter from participants at the Neighborhoods and Health Authors Workshop in Boston in April 2017. We thank the Harvard Center for Population and Development Studies for their support in hosting the Neighborhoods and Health Authors Workshop.

REFERENCES

Akinyemiju, T. F., Genkinger, J. M., Farhat, M., Wilson, A., Gary-Webb, T. L., & Tehranifar, P. (2015). Residential environment and breast cancer incidence and mortality: A systematic review and meta-analysis. *BMC Cancer, 15*(1), 191.

Arcaya, M. C., Tucker-Seeley, R. D., Kim, R., Schnake-Mahl, A., So, M., & Subramanian, S. (2016). Research on neighborhood effects on health in the United States: A systematic review of study characteristics. *Social Science & Medicine, 168*, 16–29.

Bauermeister, J. A., Connochie, D., Eaton, L., Demers, M., & Stephenson, R. (2017). Geospatial indicators of space and place: A review of multilevel studies of HIV prevention and care outcomes among young men who have sex with men in the United States. *The Journal of Sex Research, 54*(4–5), 446–464.

Bayles, J. C. (1878). *House drainage and water service in cities, villages and rural neighborhoods: With incidental consideration of causes affecting the healthfulness of dwellings.* New York: David Williams.

Berkman, L., & Kawachi, I. (2000). *Social epidemiology*. New York, NY: Oxford University Press.

Bodin, T., Albin, M., Ardö, J., Stroh, E., Östergren, P.-O., & Björk, J. (2009). Road traffic noise and hypertension: results from a cross-sectional public health survey in southern Sweden. *Environmental Health, 8*(1), 38.

Bodin, T., Björk, J., Mattisson, K., Bottai, M., Rittner, R., Gustavsson, P., Jakobsson, K., Östergren, P. O., & Albin, M. (2016). Road traffic noise, air pollution and myocardial infarction: A prospective cohort study. *International Archives of Occupational and Environmental Health, 89*(5), 793–802.

Camacho-Rivera, M., Kawachi, I., Bennett, G. G., & Subramanian, S. (2014). Perceptions of neighborhood safety and asthma among children and adolescents in Los Angeles: A multilevel analysis. *PLoS One, 9*(1), e87524.

Carpiano, R. M., Kelly, B. C., Easterbrook, A., & Parsons, J. T. (2011). Community and drug use among gay men: The role of neighborhoods and networks. *Journal of Health and Social Behavior, 52*(1), 74–90.

Caspi, C. E., Sorensen, G., Subramanian, S., & Kawachi, I. (2012). The local food environment and diet: A systematic review. *Health & Place, 18*(5), 1172–1187.

Chadwick, E (1842). Report of an Enquiry into the Sanitary Conditions of the Labouring Population in Great Britain. London: Poor Law Commission.

Chaix, B. (2009). Geographic life environments and coronary heart disease: A literature review, theoretical contributions, methodological updates, and a research agenda. *Annual Review of Public Health, 30,* 81–105.

Chaix, B., Kestens, Y., Bean, K., Leal, C., Karusisi, N., Meghiref, K., Burban, J., Fon Sing, M., Perchoux, C., Thomas F., Merlo, J., Pannier, B., & Thomas, F. (2011). Cohort profile: Residential and non-residential environments, individual activity spaces and cardiovascular risk factors and diseases—The RECORD Cohort Study. *International Journal of Epidemiology, 41*(5), 1283–1292.

Chaix, B., Kestens, Y., Duncan, D. T., Brondeel, R., Méline, J., El Aarbaoui, T., Pannier, B., & Merlo, J. (2016). A GPS-based methodology to analyze environment-health associations at the trip level: Case-crossover analyses of built environments and walking. *American Journal of Epidemiology, 184*(8), 579–589.

Chaix, B., Meline, J., Duncan, S., Merrien, C., Karusisi, N., Perchoux, C., Lewin, A., Labadi, K., & Kestens, Y. (2013). GPS tracking in neighborhood and health studies: A step forward for environmental exposure assessment, a step backward for causal inference? *Health & Place, 21,* 46–51.

Chaix, B., Simon, C., Charreire, H., Thomas, F., Kestens, Y., Karusisi, N., Vallée, J., Oppert, J. M., Weber, C., & Pannier, B. (2014). The environmental correlates of overall and neighborhood based recreational walking (a cross-sectional analysis of the RECORD Study). *International Journal of Behavioral Nutrition and Physical Activity, 11*(1), 20.

Christian, H., Zubrick, S. R., Foster, S., Giles-Corti, B., Bull, F., Wood, L., Knuiman, M., Brinkman, S., Houghton, S., & Boruff, B. (2015). The influence of the neighborhood physical environment on early child health and development: A review and call for research. *Health & Place, 33,* 25–36.

Ding, D., Sallis, J. F., Kerr, J., Lee, S., & Rosenberg, D. E. (2011). Neighborhood environment and physical activity among youth: A review. *American Journal of Preventive Medicine, 41*(4), 442–455.

Duncan, D. T., Regan, S. D., Shelley, D., Day, K., Ruff, R. R., Al-Bayan, M., & Elbel, B. (2014). Application of global positioning system methods for the study of obesity and hypertension risk among low-income housing residents in New York City: A spatial feasibility study. *Geospatial Health, 9*(1), 57.

Duncan, D. T., Ruff, R. R., Chaix, B., Regan, S. D., Williams, J. H., Ravenell, J., Bragg, M. A., Ogedegbe G., Elbel, B. (2016). Perceived spatial stigma, body mass index and blood pressure: A global positioning system study among low-income housing residents in New York City. *Geospatial Health, 11*(2), 399.

Egan, J. E., Frye, V., Kurtz, S. P., Latkin, C., Chen, M., Tobin, K., Yang, C., & Koblin, B. A. (2011). Migration, neighborhoods, and networks: Approaches to understanding how urban environmental conditions affect syndemic adverse health outcomes among gay, bisexual and other men who have sex with men. *AIDS and Behavior, 15*(1), 35–50.

Evans, C. R., Onnela, J.-P., Williams, D. R., & Subramanian, S. (2016). Multiple contexts and adolescent body mass index: Schools, neighborhoods, and social networks. *Social Science & Medicine, 162,* 21–31.

Frank, L. D., Saelens, B. E., Powell, K. E., & Chapman, J. E. (2007). Stepping towards causation: Do built environments or neighborhood and travel preferences explain physical activity, driving, and obesity? *Social Science & Medicine*, *65*(9), 1898–1914.

Freeman, L. (2011). *There goes the hood*. Philadelphia, PA: Temple University Press.

Fujimoto, K., Turner, R., Kuhns, L. M., Kim, J. Y., Zhao, J., & Schneider, J. A. (in press). Network centrality and geographical concentration of social and service venues that serve young men who have sex with men. *AIDS and Behavior*.

Gibson, C., Perley, L., Bailey, J., Barbour, R., & Kershaw, T. (2015). Social network and census tract-level influences on substance use among emerging adult males: An activity spaces approach. *Health & Place*, *35*, 28–36.

Hirsch, J. A., Diez Roux, A. V., Moore, K. A., Evenson, K. R., & Rodriguez, D. A. (2014). Change in walking and body mass index following residential relocation: the multi-ethnic study of atherosclerosis. *American Journal of Public Health*, *104*(3), e49–e56.

Humpel, N., Owen, N., & Leslie, E. (2002). Environmental factors associated with adults' participation in physical activity: A review. *American Journal of Preventive Medicine*, *22*(3), 188–199.

Jain, S., Buka, S. L., Subramanian, S., & Molnar, B. E. (2010). Neighborhood predictors of dating violence victimization and perpetration in young adulthood: A multilevel study. *American Journal of Public Health*, *100*(9), 1737–1744.

Jiao, J., Drewnowski, A., Moudon, A. V., Aggarwal, A., Oppert, J.-M., Charreire, H., & Chaix, B. (2016). The impact of area residential property values on self-rated health: A cross-sectional comparative study of Seattle and Paris. *Preventive Medicine Reports*, *4*, 68–74.

Johns, L. E., Aiello, A. E., Cheng, C., Galea, S., Koenen, K. C., & Uddin, M. (2012). Neighborhood social cohesion and posttraumatic stress disorder in a community-based sample: Findings from the Detroit Neighborhood Health Study. *Social Psychiatry and Psychiatric Epidemiology*, *47*(12), 1899–1906.

Jokela, M. (2014). Are neighborhood health associations causal? A 10-year prospective cohort study with repeated measurements. *American Journal of Epidemiology*, *180*(8), 776–784.

Julia, C., & Valleron, A. J. (2011). Louis-Rene Villerme (1782–1863), a pioneer in social epidemiology: Re-analysis of his data on comparative mortality in Paris in the early 19th century. *Journal of Epidemiology and Community Health*, *65*(8), 666–670. doi:10.1136/jech.2009.087957

Kim, D. (2008). Blues from the neighborhood? Neighborhood characteristics and depression. *Epidemiologic Reviews*, *30*(1), 101–117.

Mair, C. F., Roux, A. V. D., & Galea, S. (2008). Are neighborhood characteristics associated with depressive symptoms? A critical review. *Journal of Epidemiology & Community Health*, jech. 2007.066605.

Méline, J., Van Hulst, A., Thomas, F., & Chaix, B. (2015). Road, rail, and air transportation noise in residential and workplace neighborhoods and blood pressure (RECORD Study). *Noise & Health*, *17*(78), 308.

Molnar, B. E., Buka, S. L., Brennan, R. T., Holton, J. K., & Earls, F. (2003). A multilevel study of neighborhoods and parent-to-child physical aggression: Results from the project on human development in Chicago neighborhoods. *Child Maltreatment*, *8*(2), 84–97.

Oakes, J. M. (2014). Invited commentary: repeated measures, selection bias, and effect identification in neighborhood effect studies. *American Journal of Epidemiology*, *180*(8), 785–787. doi:10.1093/aje/kwu231

Onnela, J.-P., & Rauch, S. L. (2016). Harnessing smartphone-based digital phenotyping to enhance behavioral and mental health. *Neuropsychopharmacology, 41*(7), 1691–1696. doi:10.1038/npp.2016.7

Park, M., Verhoeven, J. E., Cuijpers, P., Reynolds, C. F., III, & Penninx, B. W. (2015). Where you live may make you old: The association between perceived poor neighborhood quality and leukocyte telomere length. *PLoS One, 10*(6), e0128460. doi:10.1371/journal.pone.0128460

Sastry, N., Ghosh-Dastidar, B., Adams, J., & Pebley, A. R. (2006). The design of a multilevel survey of children, families, and communities: The Los Angeles Family and Neighborhood Survey. *Social Science Research, 35*(4), 1000–1024.

Schüle, S. A., & Bolte, G. (2015). Interactive and independent associations between the socio-economic and objective built environment on the neighbourhood level and individual health: A systematic review of multilevel studies. *PLoS One, 10*(4), e0123456.

Tamura, K., Elbel, B., Chaix, B., Regan, S. D., Al-Ajlouni, Y. A., Athens, J. K., Meline, J., Duncan, D. T. (in press). Residential and GPS-defined activity space neighborhood noise complaints, body mass index and blood pressure among low-income housing residents in New York City. *Journal of Community Health.*

Theall, K. P., Shirtcliff, E. A., Dismukes, A. R., Wallace, M., & Drury, S. S. (2017). Association between neighborhood violence and biological stress in children. *JAMA Pediatrics, 171*(1), 53–60.

van Vuuren, C. L., Reijneveld, S. A., van der Wal, M. F., & Verhoeff, A. P. (2014). Neighborhood socioeconomic deprivation characteristics in child (0–18 years) health studies: A review. *Health & Place, 29*, 34–42.

Won, J., Lee, C., Forjuoh, S. N., & Ory, M. G. (2016). Neighborhood safety factors associated with older adults' health-related outcomes: A systematic literature review. *Social Science & Medicine, 165*, 177–186.

World Health Organization. (2008). *Social determinants of health*. Retrieved from http://www.who.int/social_determinants/en/:

The Yellow Fever of Brooklyn in 1809. (1810) *Annals of Medicine, Natural History, Agriculture & The Arts. Conducted by a Society of Gentlemen* (pp. 253–283). Ipswich, MA: Historical Periodicals Collection: Series 1.

Yen, I. H., Michael, Y. L., & Perdue, L. (2009). Neighborhood environment in studies of health of older adults: A systematic review. *American Journal of Preventive Medicine, 37*(5), 455–463.

Zelenev, A., Long, E., Bazazi, A. R., Kamarulzaman, A., & Altice, F. L. (2016). The complex interplay of social networks, geography and HIV risk among Malaysian Drug Injectors: Results from respondent-driven sampling. *International Journal of Drug Policy, 37*, 98–106.

Zenk, S. N., Schulz, A. J., Matthews, S. A., Odoms-Young, A., Wilbur, J., Wegrzyn, L., Gibbs, K., Braunschweig, C., & Stokes, C. (2011). Activity space environment and dietary and physical activity behaviors: A pilot study. *Health & Place, 17*(5), 1150–1161.

Zilioli, S., Slatcher, R. B., Fritz, H., Booza, J. C., & Cutchin, M. P. (2017). Brief report: Neighborhood disadvantage and hair cortisol among older urban African Americans. *Psychoneuroendocrinology, 80*, 36–38. doi:10.1016/j.psyneuen.2017.02.026

PART I

Methodological Approaches to Studying Neighborhood Effects on Health

2

OPERATIONALIZING NEIGHBORHOOD DEFINITIONS IN HEALTH RESEARCH

SPATIAL MISCLASSIFICATION AND OTHER ISSUES

Dustin T. Duncan, Seann D. Regan, and Basile Chaix

A starting point for all research on neighborhoods and health is the question: *What is a neighborhood?* That is, how are neighborhoods operationalized in investigations of neighborhood effects on health? Given the massive body of literature on neighborhoods and health, it seems reasonable to assume that a consensus definition of a neighborhood exists. This, however, is far from the case. Hundreds of operational definitions have been proposed. Interestingly, residents of many places, including cities, have an instinctive feel for their neighborhoods (somewhat reminiscent of US Supreme Court Justice Potter Stewart's oft-repeated definition of obscenity: "I know it when I see it"). In Chapter 1, we described neighborhoods as geographical places that can have social and cultural meaning to residents and nonresidents alike and as subdivisions of larger places. In his book, *Great American City: Chicago and the Enduring Neighborhood Effect*, Harvard sociologist Robert Sampson describes neighborhoods as "spatial units with variable organizational features . . . nested within . . . larger communities. Neighborhoods vary in size and complexity depending on the social phenomenon under study and the ecological structure of the larger community" (Sampson, 2012, p. 54). This is a territorial approach to defining neighborhoods that views neighborhoods as independent geographic entities. This approach is most often used in neighborhoods and health research, and it will be the focus of this chapter. Depending on the neighborhood feature of interest, geographies of "neighborhoods" can vary widely—one's food neighborhood may be very different from his or her social neighborhood, for example (these neighborhood features are discussed in other chapters in this book).

Although there have been many proposed definitions of what constitutes a neighborhood, the focus on how these neighborhood definitions can be operationalized in research designs (i.e., how to meaningfully delineate neighborhood boundaries to assess the features contained within them and the implications of their features for the health of those who live, work, and play within these areas) has rarely received a formal and exhaustive assessment (Chaix, Merlo, Evans, Leal, & Havard, 2009). In this chapter, we provide an overview of the different ways neighborhoods have been defined in public health research. In particular, we discuss specific ways to define neighborhoods for exposure assessment, including the use of traditional administrative neighborhood definitions as well as emerging methods for defining neighborhoods, such as the use of global positioning system (GPS) approaches (Kestens, Wasfi, Naud, & Chaix, 2017; Perchoux, Chaix, Cummins, & Kestens, 2013). Following each overview of methods used to operationalize a neighborhood, we discuss the various strengths and limitations of each approach and some theoretical and methodological considerations for using each type of neighborhood definition.

In addition, we provide direction on how to choose one approach over another when formulating a particular research question as well as examples from the literature, when applicable. Given the lack of theoretical and practical guidance on choosing an appropriate neighborhood definition, it is not surprising that neighborhoods have been defined in various ways across studies on neighborhoods and health research. This, therefore, has generated potentially avoidable heterogeneity between studies that precludes comparability of their findings. This is not an issue unique solely to spatial epidemiology per say, but it remains a concern across many social science fields such as geography, sociology, demography, and criminology. Commenting on neighborhood definitions, sociologist Roderick D. McKenzie in 1921 (reprinted in 1923) stated, "Probably no other term is used so loosely or with such changing content as the term 'neighborhood,' and very few concepts are more difficult to define" (pp. 344–345). It is also critical to highlight that across disciplines, the selection of the neighborhood definition is oftentimes not explicit and, thus, it is unclear how and why a specific approach to delineating neighborhood boundaries is applicable to the research question and outcome being studied. This represents a significant problem for comparative analysis in neighborhoods and health research, but perhaps, more important, it shines light on the various theoretical underpinnings on which analysis are undertaken.

KEY CONCEPTUAL CONSIDERATIONS IN DEFINING NEIGHBORHOODS

One overarching issue we highlight in this chapter is that of "spatial misclassification"—a concept that refers to the incorrect characterization of a neighborhood-level exposure based on the neighborhood definition used (Duncan et al., 2013;

Duncan, Tamura, et al., 2017). For instance, certain neighborhood boundaries may not reflect how residents live and what they are affected by throughout their daily lives. Emphasis is placed on spatial misclassification because, as a critical source of measurement error, we believe it to be a major issue in the field of neighborhoods and health research. The "residential trap," which refers to the exclusive focus on the residential environment as a source of exposure to neighborhood characteristics (Chaix, 2009; Perchoux et al., 2013), is a critical component of spatial misclassification. It implies that researchers need to consider that individuals may spend equivalent (if not more) time outside of this residential environment and be exposed to multiple other neighborhood environments (a concept termed "spatial polygamy") (Matthews, 2011).

Spatial Polygamy and the Residential Trap

Matthews (2011) defines spatial polygamy as the simultaneous belonging or exposure to multiple nested and non-nested, social and geographic, real, virtual, and fictional, and past and present contexts. The concept addresses the so-called residential trap and explicitly acknowledges that individuals are exposed to various neighborhood contexts throughout the course of their daily lives. However, similar to the vast majority of neighborhoods and health research, Leal and Chaix (2011) observed that 90% of studies on environmental influences on cardiometabolic risk factors used the residential neighborhood as the sole neighborhood unit of analysis.

In addition to residential neighborhoods, there are multiple nonresidential neighborhoods that individuals may visit, including those where they work, go to school, socialize, worship, and shop in, among others. All of these neighborhoods have features that may have implications for the enactment of health behaviors or the development of health outcomes. Beyond theoretical and qualitative work, emerging quantitative research demonstrates that spatial polygamy should be considered in neighborhood and health analyses. In assessing the potential influence of factors at the neighborhood-level on violence victimization among a sample of 55 youth (aged 15 to 19 years old) in Philadelphia, Basta and colleagues (Basta, Richmond, & Wiebe, 2010) observed that half of the respondents spent 91.5% or more of their time during a single day outside of the census tract (see Table 2-1 of administrative neighborhood definitions) where their home was located. Using data on 1,000 locations referred to in ethnographic field notes from 34 families participating in the Welfare, Children and Families Study in Boston, Massachusetts and San Antonio, Texas, Matthews, Detwiler and Burton (Matthews, Detwiler, & Burton, 2005) showed that more than 90% of locations relating to child care and other daily life activities (e.g., parks, full-day preschools, after-school programs) were outside of the census tract where the home was located. In a recent study conducted among 598 young gay, bisexual, and other men who have sex with men (MSM) in New York City, Duncan and colleagues (Duncan, Kapadia, & Halkitis, 2014) found that 75% of participants reported that they resided, socialized, and engaged in sexual encounters in three different neighborhoods (defined as each of the five boroughs that constitute New York City).

In geography, including neighborhood health research, the modifiable areal unit problem and the uncertain geographic context problem are often discussed and recognized as issues, especially the former, but arguably the latter is more important.

Uncertain Geographic Context Problem

Related to the aforementioned issues, the uncertain geographic context problem (UGCoP), as articulated by Kwan (2012), highlights two principal concerns in assessing the influence of a geographic context on a given outcome: spatial uncertainty and temporal uncertainty. The first dimension of UGCoP addresses spatial uncertainty—the actual areas that exert contextual influences to each environmental factor of interest on the individuals' behaviors and outcomes being studied are unknown. The second dimension of UGCoP discusses temporal uncertainty—the timing and duration in which individuals experience contextual influences are unknown. Addressing the UGCoP or correctly defining personal exposure areas involves more accurately measuring and estimating the "true causally relevant" geographic context. Failing to correctly assess the personal exposure area of study participants leads to spatial (and spatiotemporal) misclassification.

Modifiable Areal Unit Problem

In 1979, Openshaw and Taylor worked with the election data of the 99 counties in Iowa and first coined the term the "modifiable areal unit problem" (MAUP)—the fact that area boundaries can be arbitrary and can be redrawn (Stan & Neil, 1984; Wong, 2009). These different neighborhood definitions can be implicated in different results. MAUP has a *scale* component and a *zone* component. The scale effect is that different scales may produce different results. The zone effect is that regrouping zones at a given scale may produce different results. MAUP has implications for misclassification, especially exposure misclassification, and there is no substantive solution to MAUP—other than utilizing multiple neighborhood definitions in neighborhoods and health analyses.

Given these challenges, this chapter will focus on appropriate neighborhood definitions as necessary prerequisites for a rigorous and accurate exposure assessment. The goal of this chapter is to highlight the different methods to capture the areas in which neighborhood environmental factors effectively affect the populations exposed to these factors with the aim of estimating neighborhood effects with greater precision. We provide examples from different geographic settings throughout, including New York City, Boston, Chicago, and Paris, as much of the neighborhoods and health literature has focused on Western countries. In the next section, we discuss these operationalizing neighborhood definitions in health research.

OPERATIONALIZING NEIGHBORHOOD DEFINITIONS IN HEALTH RESEARCH

One of the first methods to define neighborhoods is based on perceived neighborhood boundaries, which are based on how individuals define their neighborhoods themselves, including using survey and participatory mapping methods. In the following section, we describe this first approach to defining a neighborhood, its strengths and limitations, and implications for our understanding of neighborhood effects on health.

Defining Neighborhoods With Perceived Boundaries

Perceived neighborhood boundaries are most often assessed via survey items (for more information on the use of surveys to measure neighborhood characteristics, see Chapter 3). For example, a sample of 706 MSM in New York City were asked, "When you think about your home neighborhood, what area do you usually think of?" In response to this item, participants selected one of four response options ("The block you live on"; "The area within 5 blocks around the place you live"; "The area within 10 blocks around the place you live"; and "An area larger than 10 blocks around the place you live") (Koblin et al., 2013). This study found no consistent neighborhood definition was shared by participants: 21.8% of the sample perceived their neighborhood to encompass only the block they lived in, 27.2% reported that their neighborhood included the area within 5 blocks around the place they live, 25.2% reported that their neighborhood included the area within 10 blocks around the place they live, and 25.8% considered their neighborhood to be an area larger than 10 blocks around the place they live. This research demonstrates that people even within the same "neighborhood" perceive the boundaries to be different. This assessment of perceived neighborhood boundaries was based on a standard, non-map-based survey question, and it is consistent with similar studies that we have conducted in New York City with other samples of MSM and low-income populations as well as research in the Los Angeles Family and Neighborhood Study (LA FANS), a study of neighborhoods and health among a representative sample of all households in 65 census tracts in Los Angeles County (Sastry, Pebley, & Zonta, 2002).

Generally speaking, research questions related to the influence of a neighborhood characteristic are rarely grounded in a set of defined neighborhood boundaries. Put differently, when questions are asked about a participant's perception of a neighborhood characteristic (such as neighborhood safety), their interpretation relies implicitly on the participant's perception of what constitutes their neighborhood unless the question explicitly provides a consistent definition of a neighborhood to all participants. For example, the following item was used among a sample of low-income adults in Boston (Bennett et al., 2007) and MSM in Paris (Duncan, Park, et al., 2017) to assess the association between perceived neighborhood safety and physical activity and sleep health, respectively: "In general, how safe do you feel walking alone in your neighborhood at night?" (Bennett et al., 2007; Duncan, Park, et al., 2017). Because this item does not specify a particular spatial scope for all participants to use as a reference point, participants who reside on the same block may provide different responses when presented with this item because they may perceive their neighborhood to start and end in different places.

These types of items, however, can be phrased to include a specific neighborhood definition. For example, Caspi and colleagues (Caspi, Kawachi, Subramanian, Adamkiewicz, & Sorensen, 2012) assessed perceived access to supermarkets among a sample of 828 low-income housing residents in Boston by asking respondents if they had a supermarket "within walking distance" of their home. If "walking distance" is not defined, this presents a similar challenge to survey items without a specified neighborhood definitions—two individuals in the same home, for example, may have different perceptions as to how far they can reasonably walk to get somewhere. "Walking distance" can further be defined as "a 20-minute walk or about a mile" from the participants' homes to generate a shared interpretation of the survey item that is grounded within a particular spatial scope.

For some research questions, it may be useful to constrain participants to focus their answer on a prespecified area radius (for example, when comparing perceived and objective measures of access to resources within a given area around the participants' homes), but for other applications, the ideal scenario would be to let participants freely choose the definition of their neighborhood and then to assess how they defined their neighborhood (for example, when seeking to understand how perceived neighborhood characteristics and boundaries may differ based on participant characteristics, such as race/ethnicity or body mass index [BMI]).

In addition to the use of survey items, participatory mapping is a methodology for participants to self-report their neighborhood definition or to report it with the support of a research assistant (Dongus et al., 2007). In this approach, participants map the boundaries of their neighborhood and often identify where commonly used amenities (e.g., parks, supermarkets) or problem areas (e.g., areas with high rates of violent crime or involvement in illicit activities) are. Because this method allows community members to generate maps that reflect their experiences, the neighborhoods delineated in this process are likely socially meaningful. From a territorial perspective, socially meaningful neighborhoods can be created with input from community leaders and community residents together or separately through an in-person meeting or via an online platform. Bostonography (www.bostonography.com), for example, does the latter; they routinely ask Boston residents to draw neighborhood boundaries as they see them for Boston's named neighborhood to collect a large volume of these crowd-submitted shapes to quantify neighborhood boundaries for different neighborhoods in Boston. In addition, online electronic mapping questionnaires have been developed that allow researchers to survey how participants perceive the boundaries of their own neighborhood, such as the VERITAS (Visualization and Evaluation of Route Itineraries, Travel Destinations, and Activity Space) application that has been used in the French RECORD (Residential Environment and Coronary Heart Disease) Study to collect precise information on perceived neighborhood boundaries and resources for over 6,000 individuals in the Paris metropolitan area (Chaix et al., 2012). These boundaries can be integrated into a geographic information system (GIS) to determine exposure to a neighborhood characteristic (Perchoux, Chaix, Brondeel, & Kestens, 2016) (for more information on GIS approaches to studying neighborhood characteristics, see Chapter 3).

Strengths and Limitations

There are strengths and limitations of this approach that uses perceived neighborhood boundaries for defining neighborhoods. A strength is that "perception is reality," which means that the perception of a boundary may be more meaningful to people and their behavior than actual boundaries defined using other approaches (Orstad, McDonough, Stapleton, Altincekic, & Troped, 2016). As an example, the study we previously discussed by Caspi and her colleagues found that measures of distance to supermarkets derived from GIS-based approaches were *not* associated with fruit and vegetable intake among the sample (Caspi et al., 2012), whereas the survey item measuring perceived supermarket access was strongly and significantly associated with increased fruit and vegetable intake. It is usually easy to evaluate perceived neighborhood definitions when asking a general survey question about a specific neighborhood characteristic or a survey item about a neighborhood characteristic grounded in a neighborhood boundary.

A major limitation of using perceived neighborhood definitions in neighborhoods and health research is that they highly individualized. As such, perceived neighborhood definitions, when created by surveying participants individually rather than through consensus via participatory mapping, might not be policy relevant. This is because policy decisions are often made at the level of an administrative area; therefore, administratively defined neighborhoods (discussed in the next section of the chapter) are more policy relevant than perceived individually designed neighborhoods. Perceptions of neighborhood boundaries are also related to the characteristics of the individuals who report them. For example, environmental psychologists have emphasized that resident-perceived delimitations are a cognitive construct and are a component of the process of self-definition. That is, where we live is part of who we are (Lalli, 1992; Proshansky, Fabian, & Kaminoff, 1983; Uzzell, Pol, & Badenas, 2002). Consequently, individuals may perceive their neighborhoods differently based on their individual characteristics. For example, in mapping the area one considers to be his or her neighborhood, a person of low socioeconomic status may exclude a nearby very high-poverty block from the definition of his or her neighborhood, even if exposed to it on a daily basis, to derive a more socially desirable definition of self. Therefore, resident-perceived boundaries (what individuals want them to be) may not reflect true exposure areas.

In this next part of the chapter, we focus on objective approaches for defining neighborhood boundaries for exposure assessment. We discuss these objective methods in terms of successive eras when they were first widely adopted: (1) first-generation, (2) current-generation, and (3) emerging-generation measures. This classification is based on the chronological era when they were first introduced. "Traditional" methods were commonly used before 2003 (when the first edition of this text was published), "current" methods refer to methods that emerged between 2003 and the time of publication, and emerging methods emerged in the last couple of years preceding publication of this edition. The first edition was largely confined to administrative definitions—for example, the chapter by Nancy Krieger on geocoding and the chapter by David Gordon on area-based deprivation measures. First-generation measures include administrative neighborhood definitions, for example, counties, zone improvement plan (ZIP) codes, and census tracts as a neighborhood definition. Current-generation measures include GIS-spatial buffers, and emerging-generation measures include activity spaces, including those defined via mobility surveys and global positioning system (GPS) data. We will discuss, compare, and provide examples of each generation of objective neighborhood definitions.

Administrative Neighborhood Definitions

Geographically defined administrative neighborhood boundaries represent the earliest approach applied in the definition of neighborhoods and still remain current today. As discussed in Chapter 1, use of administrative boundaries was first used to define neighborhoods because neighborhood-level data were and remain readily available for administrative geographies, including the census tract. Many early studies of neighborhood effects on health focused on neighborhood-level socioeconomic status, such as census tract median income or census tract percent poverty.

This approach of the adoption of existing administrative boundaries as proxies for neighborhoods tends to lump individuals into broad swaths of geography defined for administrative purposes. For example, all individuals who live in the same census tract are assigned the same exposure measure (e.g., fast food restaurant count for that area). As such, it is assumed that everyone—even in a relatively large geographic area—has the same access to food resources. As an example, Figure 2-1 uses

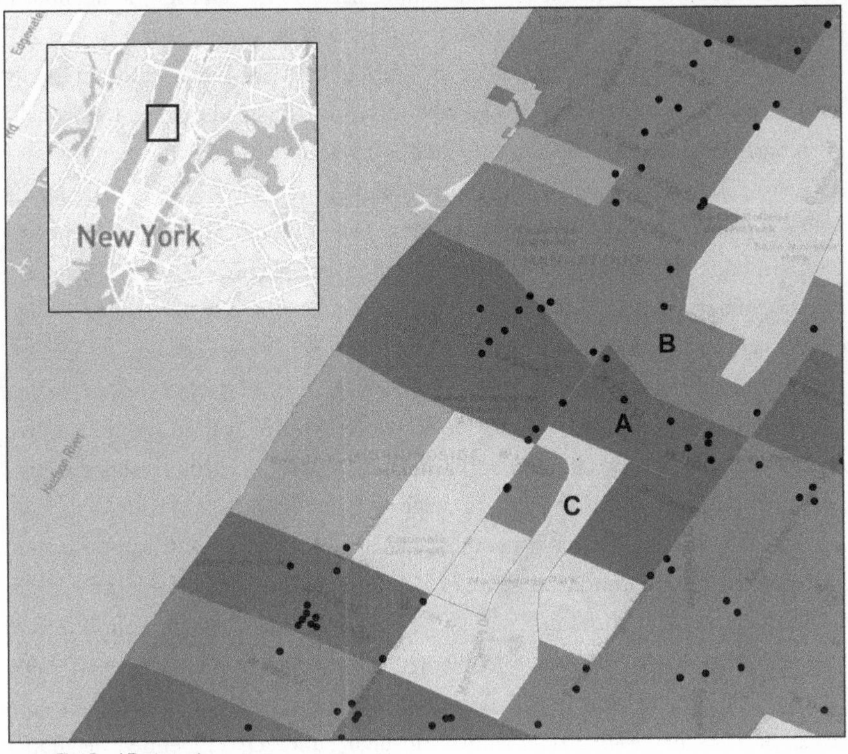

• Fast Food Restaurants

Fast Food Restaurants per Census Tract

- 0
- 1
- 2
- 3 or more

FIGURE 2-1 **Map of fast food outlets in New York, illustrating spatial misclassification.**

ESRI Business location data from InfoUSA to examine geographically the location and density of national chain fast food restaurants situated in census tracts in Upper Manhattan in New York City.

It is important to note that there are many different types of administrative neighborhood definitions. Census tracts are traditionally the most common neighborhood definition in neighborhoods and health research in the United States. These areas are "designed to be relatively homogenous units with respect to population characteristics, economic status, and living conditions" and "average about 4,000 inhabitants." Sometimes researchers combine two or three adjacent census tracts as a single unit known as a census cluster, particularly in urban areas where a single census tract may represent a very small land area. In the Project for Human Development in Chicago Neighborhoods (PHDCN), a large-scale neighborhoods and health study in Chicago, Sampson and colleagues "validated" their definition of neighborhoods (clusters of census tracts) by holding a series of focus groups and public meetings in which they sought the opinions and perceptions of local residents (Sampson, 2003; Sampson, Morenoff, & Earls, 1999; Sampson, Raudenbush, & Earls, 1997). In addition, census block groups (subsets of census tracts) and ZIP codes (administrative geographies for the efficient delivery of mail) are commonly used. Census block groups are nested within census tracts and represent the smallest geographical unit for which the United States Census Bureau publishes sample data. ZIP codes were created by the United States Postal Service in 1963 to designate points along common delivery routes. In other fields different administrative neighborhood units are common; for example, police precincts (districts) are common in criminology, schools districts are common in education research, congressional districts are common in political science, and designated marketing areas (DMAs) are common in media studies.

For illustrative purposes, we provide an overview of the various administrative neighborhood definitions in New York City as an example to demonstrate the multitude of options with this category of neighborhood definitions used in neighborhood health research in this geographic location. In New York City, researchers have defined neighborhoods as census block groups (Barr, Diez-Roux, Knirsch, & Pablos-Méndez, 2001; Gordon et al., 2011; Kwate & Lee, 2007; Kwate, Loh, White, & Saldana, 2013; Kwate, Yau, Loh, & Williams, 2009), census tracts (Beard et al., 2009; Janevic, Borrell, Savitz, Herring, & Rundle, 2010; Neckerman et al., 2009; A. Rundle et al., 2007; Weiss et al., 2011), United Hospital Fund (UHF)–defined neighborhoods (Black & Macinko, 2010; Cooper et al., 2012; Czarnecki et al., 2010; Frank, Hong, Subramanian, & Wang, 2013; White et al., 2011), community districts (Ahern et al., 2013; Cerdá et al., 2013; Galea, Ahern, Rudenstine, Wallace, & Vlahov, 2005; Huynh & Maroko, 2014; Karpati, Bassett, & McCord, 2006), ZIP codes (Brouse,

Hillyer, Basch, & Neugut, 2011; Duncan, Kapadia, et al., 2014; Jack et al., 2013; Lim & Harris, 2015; Lovasi et al., 2013; Villanueva & Aggarwal, 2013), and boroughs/counties (Caravanos, Weiss, Blaise, & Jaeger, 2006; Dragowski, Halkitis, Moeller, & Siconolfi, 2013; Duncan, Kapadia, et al., 2014; Frick & Castro, 2013; Nair, Torian, Forgione, & Begier, 2011; Terzian et al., 2012). (See Table 2-1, which includes these units and their definitions, and Figure 2-2, which shows how these definitions relate to one another.) Many of the aforementioned neighborhoods can be used in different US localities. However, UHF-defined neighborhoods and community districts are unique to the New York City geographic location. Like New York, other locations have their own local administrative definitions. For example, Boston has defined neighborhoods by the Boston Public Health Commission (Chen et al., 2006) and the Boston Redevelopment Authority (Li, Kelsey, et al., 2009; Li, Land, Zhang, Keithly, & Kelsey, 2009).

Strengths and Limitations

There are strengths and limitations of the approach of using administrative neighborhood definitions to define neighborhoods. A major strength is that these boundaries (especially those created by the United States Census Bureau) can be policy-relevant boundaries, where funding may be allocated and policy interventions may occur, and data are routinely organized and collected at these geographies. This is less so the case for ZIP codes, because these boundaries often do not correspond to residents' perceptions of their neighborhoods' boundaries or politically meaningful divisions. However, ZIP codes are often used because they are frequently the only geographic information available in electronic health record systems that provides a source of information on health behaviors and outcomes on an entire patient population and they are very easy to obtain. Although ZIP code data are widely used, they are often updated by the United States Postal Service (USPS), and this can represent an issue in comparing data across multiple years. Policy relevance is a major strength because any analyses using boundaries defined by government agencies provide information that directly pertains to the geographic units of relevance for policymakers. For example, if a study finds that living in a neighborhood (defined as a community district) in New York with more supermarkets is associated with reductions in diabetes, then community boards and their city council representatives can advocate for a greater number of supermarkets to be built in their area. As another example, if a study finds associations between low rates of unemployment in neighborhoods (defined as census tracts) with reductions in violent crimes, then employment initiatives could be targeted to census tracts with high unemployment rates. Sometimes (but not always) administrative

Table 2-1 Summary of Different Neighborhood Units in New York City

Unit	*Definition and Explanation*
Borough/county	*A county is a subdivision of a state. A borough is a municipal corporation. The five boroughs of NYC are each a consolidated county. The boroughs/counties are Bronx [Bronx County], Brooklyn [Kings County], Manhattan [New York County], Queens [Queens County], and Staten Island [Richmond County].*
ZIP code	*The term ZIP is an acronym for Zone Improvement Plan. ZIP codes are defined by the United States Postal Service (USPS), since 1963, for efficient mail delivery and include upward of 30,000 people. The basic format consists of five decimal numerical digits. In 1983, the USPS introduced the ZIP + 4 code, with a hyphen and four digits added to the existing 5-digit ZIP code. Sometimes ZIP Code Tabulation Areas (ZCTAs) are used, which were created by the US Census Bureau based on census blocks and for the most part coincides with ZIP codes.*
Census tract	*Used by the US Census Bureau, census tracts in the United States have an average of approximately 4,000 people (generally they have a population size between 1,200 and 8,000 people) and are "designated to be homogenous spatial units with respect to population characteristics, economic status, and living conditions." Census tracts are small subdivisions of a county. Several tracts commonly exist within a county.*
Census block group	*A statistical subdivision of a census tract. A census block group is the smallest geographic unit for which the US Census Bureau publishes sample data, representing a cluster of census blocks within the same census tract. Typically, census block groups have a population of 600 to 3,000 people (average population = 1,000 residents).*
United Hospital Fund (UHF) defined neighborhood	*UHF neighborhoods were created by nongovernmental organization (NGOs) to facilitate their healthy policy research by aggregating adjoining ZIP codes to approximate the representation of New York City Community Planning Districts. These 42 neighborhoods were later consolidated into 34 neighborhoods to increase statistical power of a sample size in the NYC Community Health Survey conducted by New York City government. However, it is important to note that there are actually three sets of UHF neighborhoods: 42, 33 and 34. 42 and 34 are the most common by far.*
Community district	*Established by local law in 1975, community districts play an active role in neighborhood-level municipal governance in New York City, particularly in matters related to zoning and land use. These are well-defined units, each headed by an administrative community board that, as such, has political and social relevance for the residents. There are 59 community districts as defined by the New York City Office of City Planning through the residents' own descriptions. Community involvement was critical in their development.*

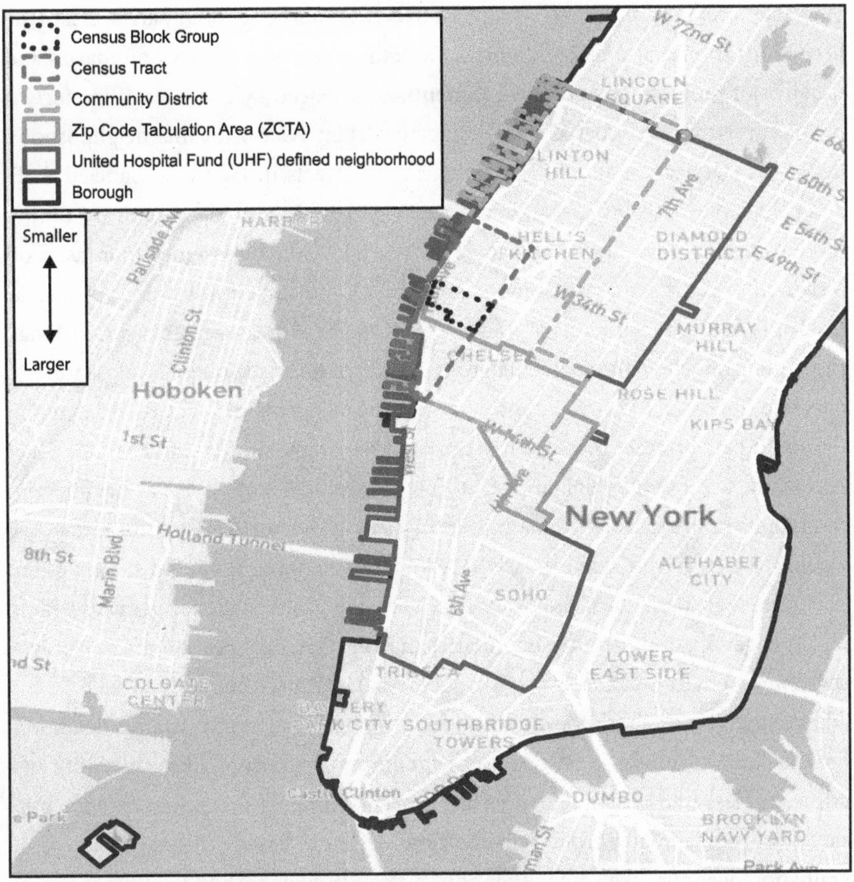

FIGURE 2-2 **Map of six different administrative boundaries in New York City.**

boundaries may be recognized by community leaders, which can also be viewed as a strength because it can build academic, governmental, and community partnerships to tackle social problems. Also worth reiterating is that maps of these neighborhood units are usually widely available and that neighborhood-level data are often available at this spatial scope. For example, census data (capturing a variety of population characteristics, such as racial/ethnic composition and median household income) are available at the census tract and census block group level. The convenience of using these neighborhood boundaries should be not undervalued as we discuss how using more advanced neighborhood boundaries can require substantial technical work and participant engagement. It should be emphasized that certain determinants of health behavior and health, perhaps HIV testing patterns, are optimally captured within administrative areas when they are related to administrative authorities (e.g., social services, schools, police, and health services) operating at the level of these areas.

While strengths of using administrative neighborhood boundaries exist, the limitations should also be highlighted. First, these can be arbitrary boundaries and usually not representative of environments experienced by residents. Therefore, it is not surprising that spatial misclassification is an issue with this neighborhood definition (Duncan et al., 2013). Comparing the tracts in Figure 2-1 labeled A, B, and C illustrates this broader measurement problem. In a model simply examining food resource availability at the tract level, Tract A would be assigned four fast food restaurants, Tract B two restaurants, and Tract C no restaurants at all. As is clear from this figure, the amount of noise present in these measurements is nontrivial. Depending on where the individual lived in tract A, he or she might be close to zero, one, two, three, or four restaurants; similar with residents in Tract B. Residents in the south part of Tract B are clearly close to restaurants on the north end of Tract A. Finally, while individuals living in Tract C would be observed as having zero restaurants in the traditional analysis, if they live in the north end of this tract, they would, in fact, have relatively easy access to two or three restaurants. This figure illustrates that spatial misclassification is especially problematic for people residing on the edges of administrative boundaries. Indeed, residents near boundaries might share more environmental exposures than residents more centrally located in the administrative neighborhood. It is important to note that administrative neighborhood definitions might be relevant for neighborhood exposures like walkability and crime, but less relevant for activities like grocery shopping that might be done outside of the home neighborhood. In addition, while US-based census tracts are generally homogenous, like some other administrative neighborhood definitions, they have huge spatial heterogeneity in their area size despite relevant consistency in the size of population contained within their boundaries. For example, in urban areas, a population of 4,000 people may be contained with a relatively small area, whereas a rural area of 4,000 people may include a larger swath of land.

Given the static nature of these boundaries and the dynamic nature of human mobility, administrative neighborhood definitions make isotropic assumptions regarding one's experience of neighborhood characteristics within one of these areas (i.e., that people equally spent time in all areas of administrative boundaries). This assumption may not be warranted. The isotropic assumption is likely not correct for most people because these administrative definitions are not likely to be relevant to people's social realities and travel patterns. As such, the uncertain geographic context problem is also a concern with this neighborhood definition. Beyond the potential for people to not spend time in all parts of a given administrative area, people move beyond their administrative residential neighborhood. Data from the Los Angeles Family and Neighborhood Study (LA FANS) demonstrate that only 22% of participants shopped for groceries within their own census tract; 42% shopped in adjacent census tracts; and 37% shopped in areas beyond the surrounding census tracts (Inagami, Cohen, Finch, & Asch, 2006; Jones & Pebley, 2014). There is probably systematic heterogeneity in the range of activity space by important residential characteristics such as socioeconomic status (do you own a car, or are you forced to walk or take public transport to reach common destinations?), employment status (e.g., whether one is employed vs. homemaker vs. retired), as well as stage of the life course (e.g., children vs. working adults).

Additionally, it is well known that there are spatiotemporal changes in administrative boundaries. In political science, gerrymandering has been extensively discussed, which is the manipulation of boundaries of an electoral constituency so as to favor one political party over another. In a study by Krieger and colleagues, it was shown that ZIP code boundaries change over time (Krieger et al., 2002). In addition, Logan and colleagues show that census tract boundaries can also change; among other changes, they can be consolidated or split over time (Logan, Xu, & Stults, 2014). For example, between the 2000 and 2010 decennial censuses, 31.1% of census tracts changed: 1.4% merged, 17.2% spilt, and 12.5% underwent other changes (Logan, Stults, & Xu, 2016). If one were conducting longitudinal analyses on the impact of neighborhoods and health, these issues can affect the findings, if not properly addressed when designing the study database. Lastly, evidence also shows that administrative boundaries may be different from perceived neighborhood boundaries (Coulton, Jennings, & Chan, 2013; Robinson & Oreskovic, 2013). One study among a sample of 140 residents of Cleveland, Ohio, found that the typical map of a neighborhood drawn by participants included portions of at least two census tracts and at least three census block groups (Coulton, Korbin, Chan, & Su, 2001). This study noted, in particular, that "discrepancies between researcher and resident-defined neighborhoods are a possible source of bias in studies on neighborhood effects" (p. 371).

Some of the limitations with the use of administrative neighborhood definitions used in the neighborhoods and health literature can be overcome with using GIS-based buffer neighborhood definitions.

GIS-Based Buffer Neighborhood Definitions

GIS-based buffers define a neighborhood as a radius around a particular location, such as a home (which would then be known as a home-based buffer). For instance, the area within a 400-meter radius (roughly a quarter of a mile) of an individual's residential address may be considered the individual's residential "neighborhood." The neighborhood environment, defined by this approach, is specific to each address (see Figure 2-3). In addition to being egocentric (meaning that they are focused on

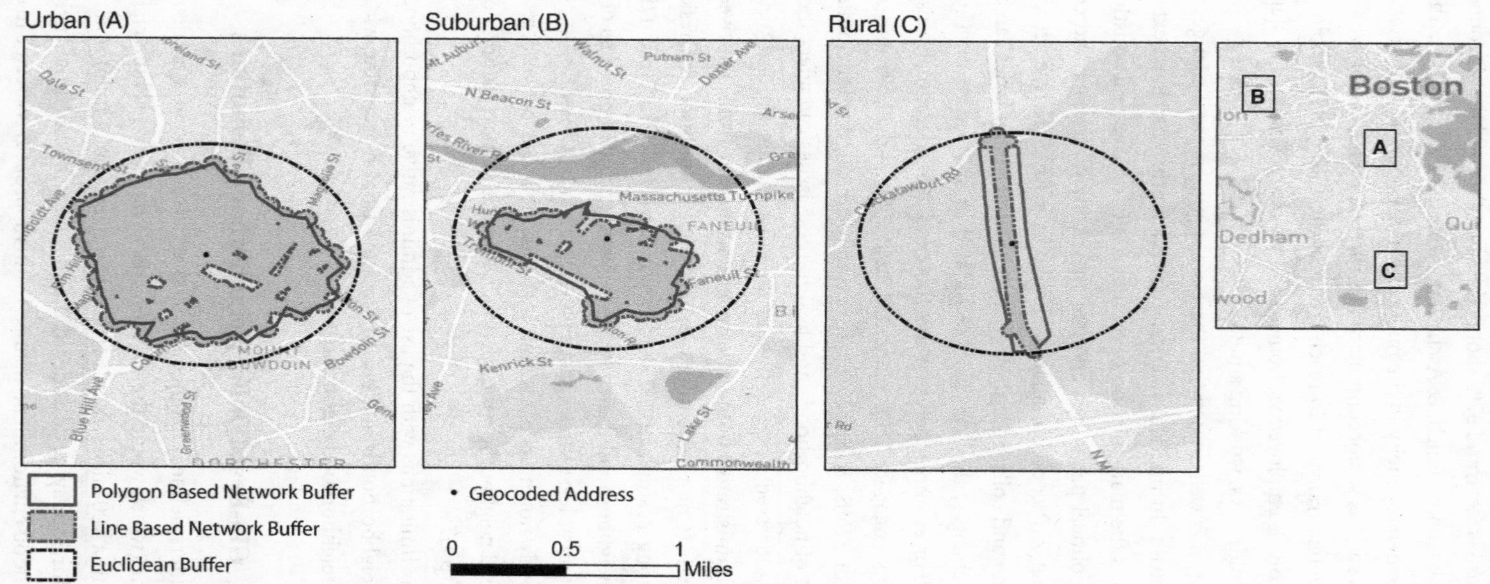

FIGURE 2-3 **Comparison of geographic information system (GIS) buffer-based neighborhood definitions.**

a single location in reference to a single individual), these spatial buffers are static and do not account for individual mobility patterns. To assess these types of neighborhoods, researchers often ask for the participants' home address, which they later geocode, meaning that they determine the latitudinal and longitudinal coordinates corresponding to that location, which is most often computed using GIS software (Duncan, Castro, Blossom, Bennett, & Gortmaker, 2011; Lovasi et al., 2007; McElroy, Remington, Trentham-Dietz, Robert, & Newcomb, 2003).

Various approaches are used for defining and operationalizing the buffers, contributing to between-study heterogeneity. Traditionally, circular-based buffers (also known as Euclidian buffers or straight-line buffers) have been used, although network approaches, or street line-based approaches, are becoming increasingly more common in the literature (refer to Figure 2-3). The organizing geography for circular buffers is a circle radius around a location or address, whereas street network buffers use the street network as the organizing geography (that is, street network buffers use a radius around a location but are confined to the areas within that radius around the streets). It is also important to highlight that there are different variants of street network buffers, including polygon-based network buffer and line-based network buffers. Polygon-based street network buffers are likely created over line-based network buffers because of technical ease. Polygon-based street network buffers follow the street network geography for the distance as threshold selected and then are connected to form a polygon using the outer buffer edges. In the polygon-based network it could be hypothesized that people experience exposure in this total area (for example, if there is a park, this would be captured in the polygon but might be omitted from the street network approach), or people might "cut corners" while walking where the road network does not exist. On the other hand, as connected to a different hypothesis of exposure (e.g., direct sight), line-based network buffers follow the street network for the size selected, creating buffers around the streets. The line-based approach may more realistically follow actual exposure, especially when traveling via the road network (in a car), but may omit areas where there is no road network, in either rural places or in parks or open spaces.

Overall, network approaches are probably more realistic for capturing people's movements than circular approaches, as these are often constrained by the availability of roadways and sidewalks for transportation between destinations. Although the two approaches have been rarely compared in a formal way, a few studies have shown that network buffers may allow researchers to better capture the associations of interest than circular buffers. For example, an increased proportion of commercial land use was associated with significantly decreased odds of walking for errands less than 1 hour per week for both circular and line-based street network buffers in one study (Oliver, Schuurman, & Hall, 2007). However, results showed that a greater proportion of residential land use measured in line-based street network buffers was significantly associated with increased odds of walking for errands less than 1 hour per week, and there were no significant associations reported between this outcome and the proportion of residential land use that contained circular buffers (Oliver et al., 2007).

Buffers can also vary in size and this is common in the neighborhoods and health research literature. Studies (even studies that examine the same association) can use buffer size of 400 meters, 800 meters, 1,600 meters, 10 miles, or anything else, really. For example, a study that examined the relationship between the built environment (including park density) and body mass index (BMI) among adolescents in urban Boston used 400- and 800-meter street network buffers (Duncan et al., 2012). Significant associations, interestingly, were found only for the 800-meter buffer. In another study conducted among rural adolescents, a circular 10-mile buffer was created around each address to examine the relationships between park density and weight (Armstrong, Lim, & Janicke, 2015). Results from that study revealed that increased park density was associated with decreases in BMI *z*-score over time for youth.

Sometimes, these network-defined buffers represent a distance based on time, for example, how far participants could easily walk in 10 minutes and 30 minutes. Radius sizes should depend on the exposure–outcome association that is being assessed. Whereas no standardization is possible in defining neighborhoods using buffers, at a minimum, researchers should provide a strong rationale related to their choice of exposure for the radius selected and discuss it against alternative choices used in the literature. For example, when studying the influence of amenities in the walkable area around a participant's home address and health outcomes such as BMI, the distance threshold should be representative of areas people are willing to reasonably walk, and often this is limited to approximately 10 minutes or approximately 0.5 miles. However, if the metric of analysis is exposure to noise, a threshold of about 100 meters might be more appropriate because noise has been shown to dissipate rapidly.

Strengths and Limitations

Multiple strengths and limitations of this approach to defining neighborhoods exist. From a methodological perspective, a strength of using this approach is that they are often relatively easy to apply in terms of computation, although GIS expertise is required. A caveat is that network-based buffer approaches can be computationally and technically more difficult to create than circular-based approaches. Because GIS buffers are objective, in some ways, this is a strength. Another important strength is that this more personalized neighborhood unit is well suited for the assessment of personal exposure areas, and thus spatial misclassification is minimized as compared to administrative neighborhood definitions.

The uncertain geographic context problem and spatial misclassification remains an issue with this neighborhood definition (Duncan et al., 2013) though, due in part to the aforementioned isotropic assumption of movement within a buffer area and of exposure to all features contained within a buffer. In addition, neighborhoods most frequently are defined by one's residential location, thereby contributing to the residential trap. However, sometimes researchers ascertain, for example, a child's school location and an adult's work location, which are geocoded to create a buffer. Geocoding errors can be a concern as well when using GIS-based buffers (Burgoine & Monsivais, 2013; Carroll-Scott et al., 2015; Davis & Carpenter, 2009; Jeffery, Baxter, McGuire, & Linde, 2006; Lewin et al., 2014; Moore et al., 2013; Simon, Kwan, Angelescu, Shih, & Fielding, 2008). If the location used to create the buffer is "off," then the buffer would be created inaccurately. Some existing research shows that different geocoding methods and parameters can influence the geographic coordinate location assigned to an address (Duncan et al., 2011). However, if the buffer is relatively large and if the exposure of interest shows strong spatial autocorrelation (for further discussion of spatial autocorrelation, see Chapter 4), the resulting error should be of limited magnitude. Small geocoding errors indeed would likely lead to only small errors in buffer-based measures. It is also worth noting that analyses comparing perceived neighborhood boundaries and GIS-based buffer boundaries suggest little overlap (Vallée, Le Roux, Chaix, Kestens, & Chauvin, 2015).

As discussed, multiple strengths as well as limitations exist with GIS-based buffer definitions of neighborhoods. Some of the limitations with the use of GIS-based buffers can be overcome with activity space neighborhood definitions.

Activity Space Neighborhood Definitions

An "activity space" has been defined as a "set of spatial locations visited by an individual over a given period, corresponding to his/her exhaustive spatial footprint; the regular activity space is the subset of locations regularly visited over that period" (Chaix et al., 2012). Conceptually, an activity space has been defined as the combination of locations visited and the routes connecting them (Golledge, 1997). Activity spaces include a variety of common destinations, for example, workplaces, grocery stores, doctor's offices, or places of worship, in addition to one's home. Analysis of activity spaces enables researchers to answer the following questions: Where do you spend more of your time, besides home, work, school, or sleeping? What proportion of time? At which frequency do you visit these locations? A visual of an activity space, compared to the aforementioned neighborhood definitions we previously discussed, is shown in Figure 2-4.

Assessment of self-reported locations is a method to examine and create activity space neighborhoods adapted from transportation geography. This approach was used in LA FANS (Jones & Pebley, 2014) and in the Space-Time Adolescent Risk Study in Philadelphia, Pennsylvania (Wiebe et al., 2016). Without geolocating places, researchers ask participants about daily life activities, such as grocery shopping and socializing with friends, and then ask: "Do you do this inside or outside your neighborhood?" (Kestens et al., 2012; Vallée, Cadot, Grillo, Parizot, & Chauvin, 2010; Vallée, Cadot, Roustit, Parizot, & Chauvin, 2011; Vallée & Chauvin, 2012; Vaughan, Kramer, Cooper, Rosenberg, & Sullivan, 2017). Others have asked participants to self-report detailed paths of the routes they traveled from one location

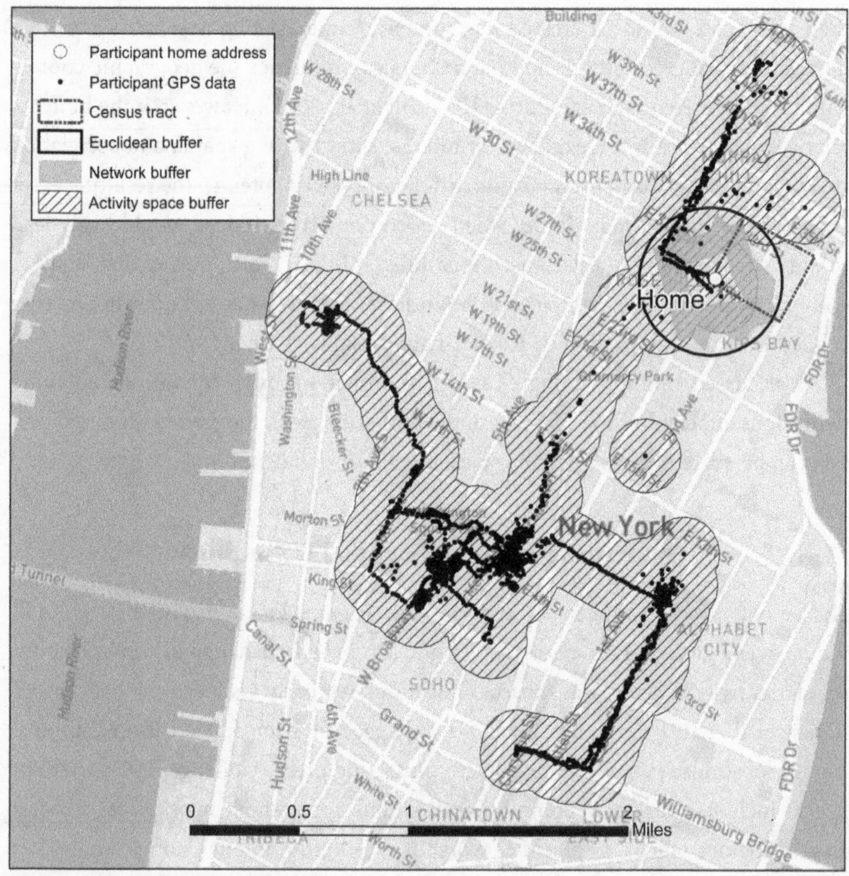

FIGURE 2-4 **An example activity space neighborhood, along with geographic information system (GIS) buffer and administrative neighborhood definitions.**

to the next over a certain period of time such as over the course of one full day (Basta et al., 2010). As another approach, the previously mentioned VERITAS application (Chaix et al., 2012; Stewart et al., 2015) is a specific tool to study activity space neighborhoods. It allows researchers and participants to geocode visited locations (as points), commonly used routes (as polylines), or specific neighborhood boundaries as polygons (Perchoux et al., 2014; Stewart et al., 2015). A novel aspect of tools investigating activity spaces is asking the "why" question or the decision-making process in mobility patterns (Kestens et al., 2017). By asking why people are going to certain locations or why they chose one destination over another, the causal understanding of the effect of neighborhoods on health is improved, that is, that the exposure preceded the outcome. Notably, tools, like VERITAS, that examine activity spaces are starting to also assess social networks within geographic contexts, which represent a new direction of research in spatial epidemiology (Kestens et al., 2017). These networks may be a reason for people's mobility across neighborhoods and may enable their access to resources outside of the home neighborhood (Duncan, Kapadia, et al., 2014).

Activity space neighborhoods can also be defined using global positioning system (GPS) technology. GPS devices can measure activity spaces because they track location in real time, providing more objective location data than the methodologies based on self-report, but often over a restricted period (discussed next). The use of GPS technology is a state-of-the-science approach to defining neighborhoods and exposure areas, which will be discussed further in this section.

Using Global Positioning System Technology for Neighborhood Health Research

A GPS device uses a satellite and ground-based system to identify latitude and longitude coordinates on Earth as well as direction, elevation, and speed. GPS devices do this by measuring the time it takes for a radio signal to reach the receiver from a constellation of 24 satellites using a mathematical technique called trilateration. GPS devices require "line of sight" to at least three satellites (ideally four) to determine a device's location. GPS devices, therefore, enable one to track exact location in real time. When measuring location over time, the GPS devices allow for the measurement of the mobility patterns of individuals through their environment or activity space. GPS devices are pervasive and common, but there are different types—dedicated car GPS devices, hiking GPS devices, and sailing GPS devices as well as GPS-enabled smartphones. Most neighborhoods and health studies using GPS devices to date use a dedicated GPS device—that is, a device whose sole purpose is to collect GPS data. Dedicated GPS devices are highly accurate, to within a 3-meter accuracy, when compared to a known geodetic point (Kerr, Duncan, & Schipperjin, 2011; Schipperijn et al., 2014). However, accuracy of a dedicated GPS device is dependent on many factors, such as how many satellites a GPS receiver can communicate with, cloud cover, and interference from both trees and tall buildings. In addition, the accuracy in determining location will be better in places with low interference and worse in areas with lots of interference. For example, a study conducted in a large urban center with many tall buildings may have more issues with loss of signal than a rural study in an open area. This can also raise issues when comparing data across populations or studies from different locations. GPS devices may also use data triangulation techniques to obtain higher accuracy when signals between satellites and devices are lost; these include Wi-Fi positioning, cell tower triangulation, and use of internal device accelerometers. GPS devices can be worn on a study-provided belt and/or in a participant's pocket or bag. To check and increase compliance to a GPS protocol, we have given participants a travel dairy, including asking participants the following two questions, "Did you charge the GPS monitor today?" and "Did you carry the GPS monitor with you today?" In addition, text-message reminders can be sent to participants encouraging them to charge and wear the device. A handful of neighborhoods and health studies have used GPS-enabled smartphones (Wiehe et al., 2008), and a few studies have utilized GPS-enabled watches (Webber & Porter, 2009). Especially in GPS research using cell phones, ecological momentary assessment and in particular, geographically explicit ecological momentary assessment (GEMA), can be conducted (Epstein et al., 2014; Kirchner & Shiffman, 2016). We describe GEMA in greater detail in Chapter 3, but we briefly note here that this method allows for capturing real-time location data in tandem with real-time data about neighborhood conditions and health behaviors.

Although GPS data have been used to define areas where activity occurs, these data sets may contain thousands or even hundreds of thousands of geolocated points depending on the length of the tracking period and the time interval of data collection selected. To simplify these complex datasets, several methods have been used to transform these data into more easily usable metrics for further analysis (Boruff, Nathan, & Nijënstein, 2012; Hirsch, Winters, Clarke, & McKay, 2014) (see Figure 2-5). One approach is a standard deviational ellipse, which takes the set of latitudinal and longitudinal points and calculates the distances between the coordinates in the data set. The mean center of the data set is used to define the axes of the resultant ellipse. Another technique often used is the creation of a convex hull. While algorithmically complex, a convex hull approach can be thought of as an envelope of geolocated data in which the most external points make up the bounding geometry. In the case

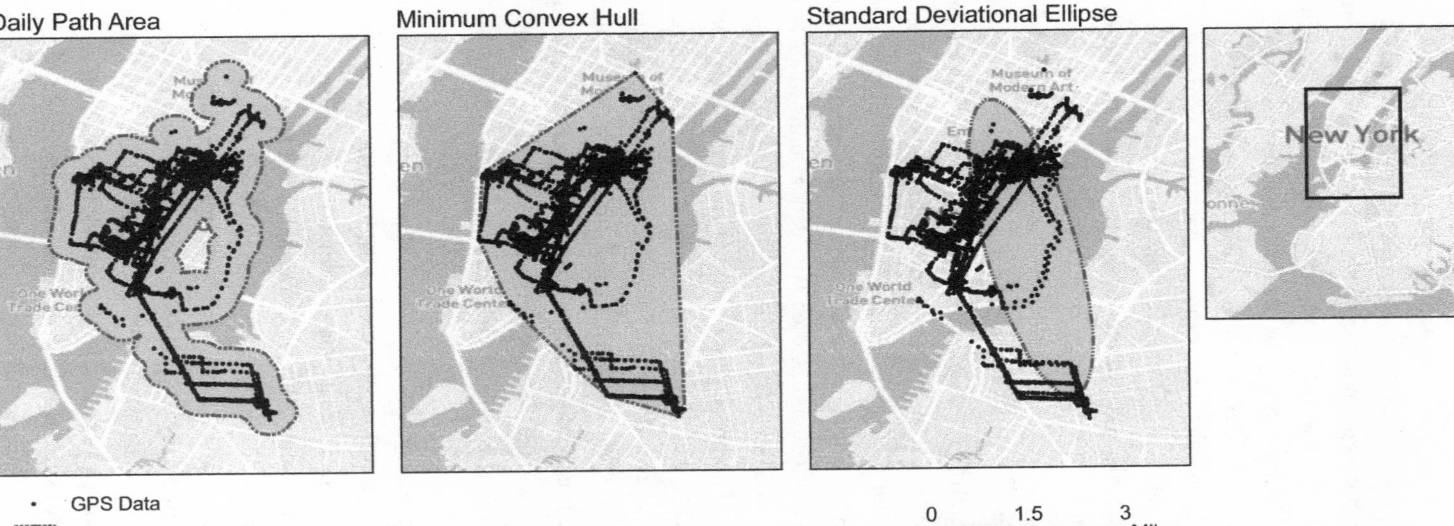

FIGURE 2-5 **Examples of global positioning system (GPS)-derived activity space metrics often used in behavioral geography research.**

of GPS data, a convex hull would be a polygon shape derived from the most exterior points in the data set that contains all points in the data set. Another strategy is to create a daily path area. A daily path area is a buffering zone drawn around the GPS tracks, which is a common method in behavioral geography research used to understand where participants spend the majority of their time and exposure to environments while accounting for commuting corridors (Hirsch et al., 2014; Sherman, Spencer, Preisser, Gesler, & Arcury, 2005; Tamura et al., 2017). Yet another approach, probably more relevant to exposure assessment, is to examine clustering of GPS point data, including approaches based on kernel density estimation. This latter approach disregards large portions of the GPS track. To date, this daily path area method to capture GPS data is most often used in the literature on neighborhoods and health.

We also note that GPS data can be used to define one's residential neighborhood (Rundle et al., 2016). For example, a study by Rundle and colleagues defined actual areas utilized by participants as a minimum convex polygon around the GPS points falling within 1 kilometer of their home. Emerging research has been focused on analyzing trip-level data and assessing environmental factors at each trip origin and trip destination based on GPS data as units in analysis of neighborhoods and health (Chaix et al., 2016; Duncan et al., 2016). This approach is grounded on the use of preprocessing algorithms (Kestens, Thierry, & Chaix, 2016; Paz-Soldan et al., 2014), and then on this basis on the use of a GPS-based mobility survey, that is, on an electronic mobility survey conducted on the basis of the GPS tracks (Chaix et al., 2014; Wolf, Schönfelder, Samaga, Oliveira, & Axhausen, 2004). With this approach, it is possible to confirm or collect information on activities performed in each place and on transport modes used in each trip, which represents a substantial enrichment of GPS data for neighborhood health analysis (Chaix et al., 2016).

There is emerging neighborhood health literature using GPS to define neighborhood boundaries, which will be discussed with the aid of an example. One study based in Chicago examined activity space neighborhood environments and dietary and physical activity behaviors. This study found that fast food outlet density in the residential neighborhood (0.5 mile street network buffer) and GPS-based standard deviation ellipse was *not* associated with dietary intakes. However, fast food outlet density in the GPS-based daily path area was positively associated with saturated fat intake and negatively associated with intake of whole grains (Zenk et al., 2011). In this study, GPS tracking was conducted for a week (seven days). As also noted by the authors, a reason why the association was only documented with the GPS-based measure can be due to the selective daily mobility bias discussed in detail later (Chaix et al., 2013).

Strengths and Limitations

There are strengths and limitations of the activity space method to defining neighborhoods. One strength is overcoming spatial misclassification because these approaches measure someone's actual travel patterns rather than making assumptions about exposure to a neighborhood (Duncan, Tamura, et al., 2017; Harrison, Burgoine, Corder, van Sluijs, & Jones, 2014; Hurvitz & Moudon, 2012; Perchoux et al., 2016), as opposed to other "fixed" neighborhood definitions that are unable to capture travel patterns. This approach also addresses the uncertain geographic context problem and accounts for spatial polygamy. GPS-defined neighborhoods, in particular, are useful at addressing these issues, and we believe they are the best methods in defining neighborhood contexts in a more realistic manner because these methods measure human mobility between neighborhood contexts. Given people's mobility patterns within and across neighborhoods as well as across larger geographic areas such as cities, assessments of residential neighborhoods are clearly not enough. In the Chicago study we discussed earlier, the residential neighborhood as defined by a GIS-spatial buffer around the participant's home and GPS activity space at most *only* shared 12% of the variance in the environmental features being studied (Zenk et al., 2011). This suggests that environmental features of the residential neighborhood are a very poor proxy for people's daily neighborhood exposures because most people's day-to-day activities are conducted outside of their residential neighborhood. As discussed earlier, research has provided evidence for spatial polygamy, showing that people visit destinations outside of their home neighborhood within different neighborhoods that also have implications for health. Previous GPS data that we collected in New York City showed significant mobility outside of the home neighborhood (Duncan et al., 2016; Duncan, Regan, et al., 2014; Goedel et al., 2017).

Recall bias remains an issue with self-reported activity spaces (Dasgupta, Vaughan, Kramer, Sanchez, & Sullivan, 2014; Vaughan, Kramer, Cooper, Rosenberg, & Sullivan, 2016). For example, a Web-based mapping study in men who have sex with men in Atlanta found locational errors when participants identified locations, including when they mapped their homes (the median home location error across participants was 0.65 miles) (Dasgupta et al., 2014). Privacy can be a concern with the analysis and mapping of GPS data. In addition, another limitation is the lack of standardization in collecting, coding, and classifying GPS data, including with respect to neighborhood boundaries. Most GPS research collects data for a 1-week period at a single time point. Some studies collect GPS data for a shorter time period (e.g., a few days) and other collect GPS data for longer periods such as 2 weeks. Compared to 1 week, 2 weeks may better typify one's typical spatial mobility patterns; however, GPS data over 1 or 2 weeks is likely not *regular* mobility, and multiwave assessment is recommended to reach a clear view of regular mobility from GPS data. Rarely are longitudinal GPS studies conducted, although our group has several ongoing longitudinal GPS studies in the field. Consequently, very little work has empirically examined the temporal stability of activity spaces derived from GPS data. In addition, GPS receivers are often used together with accelerometers. When the two devices are linked, for example, fixed on the same belt, accelerometers, apart from physical activity data, can provide information on the wear time of devices, allowing researchers to define "valid days" corresponding to a minimum number of hours of wear time (Choi, Ward, Schnelle, & Buchowski, 2012). In addition, different time intervals have been used for collecting GPS data, with many studies using 30-second intervals for collecting location information. Instead, our ongoing studies propose a novel 2-week protocol using a 10-second time interval with multiple waves of assessment, including assessments every 6 months over a 2-year period. Furthermore, many studies code all days of GPS data when analyses could be conducted by date, or weekday versus weekend day (Duncan & Regan, 2016). It should be noted that neither standard deviational ellipse nor convex hulls are particularly relevant for exposure assessment because they include, by definition, large segments of the territory where the participant did not travel. On the other hand, the daily path area is better to assess places where the participant goes. Regardless of the method selected to define a GPS-based neighborhood, these are large complex data sets, which require specialized training to code and calculate.

GPS data can also have quality issues (Mooney et al., 2016), due to multipath reflectance. Multipath reflectance is the process by which signals between GPS satellites and GPS receiver "bounce" or reflect off tall buildings. When the signal connects with the GPS device, this reflectance causes errors in the location calculation. A review of GPS studies of the built environment and physical activity found that data loss varied from 2.5% to 92% (Krenn, Titze, Oja, Jones, & Ogilvie, 2011), which perhaps can be remedied with use of cell-phone-based GPS measures. Selection bias is an issue regarding samples of individuals in GPS studies, and there can be issues regarding participants' adherence to (advanced) GPS protocols; the latter may be remedied through strong incentives as well as highlighting the altruistic motivations of the research and/or using low-burden methods of collecting spatial data (e.g., using a geolocation tool of the participant's smartphone to collect data on his or her location in the background of his or her daily activities). It is also possible for participants to change their spatial patterns while wearing the GPS device, leading to potential reactivity bias. However, surveys can allow researchers to assess this bias. Importantly, our past work suggests that this issue will be minimal (Duncan et al., 2016; Duncan, Regan, et al., 2014). For example, in the post-GPS protocol survey of data from our pilot work assessing GPS feasibility in a sample of young men who have sex with men in New York City (n = 75), we asked the question, "Did using the GPS device cause you to alter your behavior?" and 99% of the sample answered "No" (Duncan et al., 2016). Therefore, we do not believe that the GPS devices will alter most participants' behavior (thus the resulting definition of their activity space neighborhood)—at least not in substantial ways. Other issues with the use of GPS device include battery life, memory, and cost (Kerr et al., 2011). Further research is needed on the amount of data able to be stored on GPS devices for different time intervals, especially when collecting GPS data from a smartphone, which may matter less if the data are automatically uploaded to the cloud. The effect of continuous GPS tracking features on battery drain and cellular data use of commonly used smartphones in particular needs to be researched.

A concern with classical GPS studies is that they assess exposures on the basis of the observed GPS tracks, which biases the relationship between the exposure and the outcome due to the so-called selective daily mobility bias (Chaix et al., 2013). That is, participants were not "exposed" to neighborhood features per se; they just went to a place where they would not have gone otherwise due to their preferences and to their willingness to conduct the behavior of interest. This serves as a source of confounding (Chaix et al., 2012, 2013), due to the fact that measures of accessibility to resources are also determined from the locations visited to use the corresponding resources (Chaix et al., 2012). For example, regarding fast food restaurants and green spaces, people with strong preferences for high fat food or outdoor exercise will visit fast food restaurants or parks during the GPS assessment period that would otherwise not have been on their way. If we do not consider the fact that these places visited were due to intentions to eat or to exercise when calculating the spatial accessibility to fast food restaurants or parks, we will spuriously conclude that the participants had access to or were exposed to these features (Chaix et al., 2013). The association between the exposure and the behavior will be spuriously increased because it is confounded by preferences. Selective mobility bias is particularly a concern when investigating the effects of accessibility to environmental resources on behaviors. Conversely, there would be no major selective daily mobility bias in a study assessing the relationship between GPS-based exposures and health status (Burgoine, Jones, Brouwer, & Neelon, 2015) (e.g., between the GPS-assessed use of food stores or restaurants and body mass index or between the GPS-based exposure to air pollutants or noise and blood pressure). Although there is no agreement on how to tackle the selective mobility bias, studies are beginning to consider this issue, including a GPS study of 94 schoolchildren in Mebane and Mount Airy, North Carolina (Burgoine, Jones, Brouwer, & Neelon, 2015), and a French GPS study of built environment determinants of walking analyzed at the trip level (Chaix et al.,

2016). A GPS-based mobility survey can identify when the participant intentionally visited a fast food restaurant and whether he or she deviated from her or his otherwise normal behavior, for example, and derive corrected measures of exposure for behavioral studies on the basis of this information. One possibility is to remove these places that were specifically visited to perform the behavior when calculating the spatial accessibility or exposure, or to replace the trip to this destination by a calculated shortest street-network trip from the previous destination to the next one.

SUMMARY AND CONCLUSION

Defining neighborhoods continues to be surprisingly challenging in neighborhoods and health research, as in many other fields. As discussed, there is no single way to define neighborhood boundaries. There are in fact multiple ways to define neighborhoods both empirically and conceptually. This chapter discussed different methods to examine neighborhood boundaries, including self-report, administrative definitions, GIS-based spatial buffers, and activity spaces, including mobility survey-based activity spaces and GPS-defined activity spaces. We also discussed the strengths and limitations of each method of examining neighborhood boundaries (e.g., spatial misclassification, technical difficulty) and provided examples of each neighborhood boundary applied in the neighborhood health literature.

Often colleagues and students ask: *Is it possible to select the "wrong" neighborhood definition?* The search for the ideal operational definition of a neighborhood is probably misplaced. To paraphrase British statistician George Box: All definitions of neighborhoods (models) are wrong, but some are useful (Box & Draper, 1987). Diez Roux and Mair stated: It is important to recognize that "the search for the 'perfect' definition of a neighborhood [that would fit all research questions] is likely to be futile" (2010, p. 134). Researchers should align their neighborhood definition needs with the exposure and outcome of interest as well as the specific research question. Researchers should also be explicit and justify the selected neighborhood definition or set of definitions, which could be driven by theory and previous research taking into account the particular population. As a rule, for estimating an individual's exposure, localized neighborhood definitions (i.e., GIS-based buffers and GPS activity spaces) make the most sense. While administrative boundaries do not always represent real-world experiences, administrative boundaries may be the correct unit for analyzing some processes; for example, for institutional exposures, access to administrative services that depend on living in a certain administrative area are relevant. Importantly, administrative neighborhood definitions are often the metric by which funds for public health are administered and where policy is enacted for better or for worse. Consequently, for policy-level decision making, administrative boundaries may make the most sense because these boundaries can relate to allocation resources. As we discussed, most neighborhood studies focus exclusively on the residential neighborhood, which limits the assessment of the full scope of contexts and exposures one may experience in daily life. Further studies need to examine nonresidential neighborhoods and activity space neighborhoods. Selection of the most appropriate neighborhood definition will increase the study's internal validity and reduce spurious and counterintuitive results.

Research should, when possible, conduct a sensitivity analysis, using multiple neighborhood definitions—addressing the modifiable areal unit problem. O'Campo (2003) stated: "Given that the debate regarding the appropriate size of spatially defined neighborhoods will not be resolved easily and, more likely, that no single unit of neighborhood will simultaneously satisfy the needs for measuring multiple neighborhood processes, one possible solution is to promote use of multiple definitions of neighborhood within the same study" (p. 11). The problem, however, is that—in the absence of strong theory—we have no way of adjudicating what is the truth if we obtain different results depending on different definitions. In addition, while analyses conducted using different neighborhood definitions test the robustness of spatial relationships, the potential risk of generating false findings through multiple testing should also be kept in mind.

ACKNOWLEDGMENTS

Dr. Dustin Duncan was funded in part by National Institutes of Health grants R01MH112406, R21MH110190, and R03DA039748 and the Centers for Disease Control and Prevention grant U01PS005122. Dr. Basile Chaix was supported by Inserm and by the European Research Council. We thank Drs. Peter James and Kosuke Tamura for commenting on an earlier iteration of this chapter. In addition, we thank the following research assistants in NYU's Spatial Epidemiology Lab for their preparation and providing comments on an earlier iteration of this chapter and for conducting background research: Yazan Al-Ajlouni and William Goedel. We are also grateful for the comments on an earlier, spoken version of this chapter from participants at the Neighborhoods and Health Authors Workshop in Boston in April 2017. We thank the Harvard Center for Population and Development Studies for their support in hosting the Neighborhoods and Health Authors Workshop.

REFERENCES

Ahern, J., Cerdá, M., Lippman, S. A., Tardiff, K. J., Vlahov, D., & Galea, S. (2013). Navigating non-positivity in neighbourhood studies: An analysis of collective efficacy and violence. *Journal of Epidemiol Community Health*, *67*(2), 159–165.

Armstrong, B., Lim, C. S., & Janicke, D. M. (2015). Park density impacts weight change in a behavioral intervention for overweight rural youth. *Behavioral Medicine, 41*(3), 123–130.

Barr, R. G., Diez-Roux, A. V., Knirsch, C. A., & Pablos-Méndez, A. (2001). Neighborhood poverty and the resurgence of tuberculosis in New York City, 1984–1992. *American Journal of Public Health, 91*(9), 1487–1493.

Basta, L. A., Richmond, T. S., & Wiebe, D. J. (2010). Neighborhoods, daily activities, and measuring health risks experienced in urban environments. *Social Science & Medicine, 71*(11), 1943–1950.

Beard, J. R., Cerdá, M., Blaney, S., Ahern, J., Vlahov, D., & Galea, S. (2009). Neighborhood characteristics and change in depressive symptoms among older residents of New York City. *American Journal of Public Health, 99*(7), 1308–1314.

Bennett, G. G., McNeill, L. H., Wolin, K. Y., Duncan, D. T., Puleo, E., & Emmons, K. M. (2007). Safe to walk? Neighborhood safety and physical activity among public housing residents. *PLoS Medicine, 4*(10), e306.

Black, J. L., & Macinko, J. (2010). The changing distribution and determinants of obesity in the neighborhoods of New York City, 2003–2007. *American Journal of Epidemiology, 171*(7), 765–775.

Boruff, B. J., Nathan, A., & Nijënstein, S. (2012). Using GPS technology to (re)-examine operational definitions of "neighbourhood" in place-based health research. *International Journal of Health Geographics, 11*(1), 22.

Box, G. E., & Draper, N. R. (1987). *Empirical model-building and response surfaces* (Vol. 424). New York, NY: Wiley.

Brouse, C. H., Hillyer, G. C., Basch, C. E., & Neugut, A. I. (2011). Geography, facilities, and promotional strategies used to encourage indoor tanning in New York City. *Journal of Community Health, 36*(4), 635–639.

Burgoine, T., Jones, A. P., Brouwer, R. J. N., & Neelon, S. E. B. (2015). Associations between BMI and home, school and route environmental exposures estimated using GPS and GIS: Do we see evidence of selective daily mobility bias in children? *International Journal of Health Geographics, 14*(1), 8.

Burgoine, T., & Monsivais, P. (2013). Characterising food environment exposure at home, at work, and along commuting journeys using data on adults in the UK. *International Journal of Behavioral Nutrition and Physical Activity, 10*(1), 85.

Caravanos, J., Weiss, A. L., Blaise, M. J., & Jaeger, R. J. (2006). A survey of spatially distributed exterior dust lead loadings in New York City. *Environmental Research, 100*(2), 165–172.

Carroll-Scott, A., Gilstad-Hayden, K., Rosenthal, L., Eldahan, A., McCaslin, C., Peters, S. M., & Ickovics, J. R. (2015). Associations of neighborhood and school socioeconomic and social contexts with body mass index among urban preadolescent students. *American Journal of Public Health, 105*(12), 2496–2502.

Caspi, C. E., Kawachi, I., Subramanian, S., Adamkiewicz, G., & Sorensen, G. (2012). The relationship between diet and perceived and objective access to supermarkets among low-income housing residents. *Social Science & Medicine, 75*(7), 1254–1262.

Cerdá, M., Ransome, Y., Keyes, K. M., Koenen, K. C., Tardiff, K., Vlahov, D., & Galea, S. (2013). Revisiting the role of the urban environment in substance use: the case of analgesic overdose fatalities. *American Journal of Public Health, 103*(12), 2252–2260.

Chaix, B. (2009). Geographic life environments and coronary heart disease: A literature review, theoretical contributions, methodological updates, and a research agenda. *Annual Review of Public Health, 30*, 81–105.

Chaix, B., Kestens, Y., Duncan, D. T., Brondeel, R., Méline, J., El Aarbaoui, T., Pannier, B., & Merlo, J. (2016). A GPS-based methodology to analyze environment-health associations at the trip level: Case-crossover analyses of built environments and walking. *American Journal of Epidemiology, 184*(8), 579–589.

Chaix, B., Kestens, Y., Duncan, S., Merrien, C., Thierry, B., Pannier, B., Brondeel, R., Lewin, A., Karusisi, N., Perchoux, C., Thomas, F., & Méline J. (2014). Active transportation and public transportation use to achieve physical activity recommendations? A combined GPS, accelerometer, and mobility survey study. *International Journal of Behavioral Nutrition and Physical Activity, 11*(1), 124.

Chaix, B., Kestens, Y., Perchoux, C., Karusisi, N., Merlo, J., & Labadi, K. (2012). An interactive mapping tool to assess individual mobility patterns in neighborhood studies. *American Journal of Preventive Medicine, 43*(4), 440–450.

Chaix, B., Meline, J., Duncan, S., Merrien, C., Karusisi, N., Perchoux, C., Lewin, A., Labadi, K., & Kestens, Y. (2013). GPS tracking in neighborhood and health studies: A step forward for environmental exposure assessment, a step backward for causal inference? *Health & Place, 21*, 46–51.

Chaix, B., Merlo, J., Evans, D., Leal, C., & Havard, S. (2009). Neighbourhoods in eco-epidemiologic research: delimiting personal exposure areas. A response to Riva, Gauvin, Apparicio and Brodeur. *Social Science & Medicine, 69*(9), 1306–1310.

Chen, J. T., Rehkopf, D. H., Waterman, P. D., Subramanian, S., Coull, B. A., Cohen, B., Ostrem, M., & Krieger, N. (2006). Mapping and measuring social disparities in premature mortality: The impact of census tract poverty within and across Boston neighborhoods, 1999–2001. *Journal of Urban Health, 83*(6), 1063–1084.

Choi, L., Ward, S. C., Schnelle, J. F., & Buchowski, M. S. (2012). Assessment of wear/nonwear time classification algorithms for triaxial accelerometer. *Medicine and Science in Sports and Exercise, 44*(10), 2009.

Cooper, H., Des Jarlais, D., Ross, Z., Tempalski, B., Bossak, B. H., & Friedman, S. R. (2012). Spatial access to sterile syringes and the odds of injecting with an unsterile syringe among injectors: A longitudinal multilevel study. *Journal of Urban Health, 89*(4), 678–696.

Coulton, C. J., Jennings, M. Z., & Chan, T. (2013). How big is my neighborhood? Individual and contextual effects on perceptions of neighborhood scale. *American Journal of Community Psychology, 51*(1–2), 140–150.

Coulton, C. J., Korbin, J., Chan, T., & Su, M. (2001). Mapping residents' perceptions of neighborhood boundaries: A methodological note. *American Journal of Community Psychology, 29*(2), 371–383.

Czarnecki, K. D., Goranson, C., Ellis, J. A., Vichinsky, L. E., Coady, M. H., & Perl, S. B. (2010). Using geographic information system analyses to monitor large-scale distribution of nicotine replacement therapy in New York City. *Preventive Medicine, 50*(5), 288–296.

Dasgupta, S., Vaughan, A. S., Kramer, M. R., Sanchez, T. H., & Sullivan, P. S. (2014). Use of a Google Map tool embedded in an internet survey instrument: Is it a valid and reliable alternative to geocoded address data? *JMIR Research Protocols, 3*(2).

Davis, B., & Carpenter, C. (2009). Proximity of fast-food restaurants to schools and adolescent obesity. *American Journal of Public Health, 99*(3), 505–510.

Diez Roux, A. V., & Mair, C. (2010). Neighborhoods and health. *Annals of the New York Academy of Sciences, 1186*(1), 134.

Dongus, S., Nyika, D., Kannady, K., Mtasiwa, D., Mshinda, H., Fillinger, U., . . . Killeen, G. F. (2007). Participatory mapping of target areas to enable operational larval source management to suppress malaria vector mosquitoes in Dar es Salaam, Tanzania. *International Journal of Health Geographics*, *6*(1), 37.

Dragowski, E. A., Halkitis, P. N., Moeller, R. W., & Siconolfi, D. E. (2013). Social and sexual contexts explain sexual risk taking in young gay, bisexual, and other young men who have sex with men, ages 13–29 years. *Journal of HIV/AIDS & Social Services*, *12*(2), 236–255.

Duncan, D. T., Castro, M. C., Blossom, J. C., Bennett, G. G., & Gortmaker, S. L. (2011). Evaluation of the positional difference between two common geocoding methods. *Geospatial Health*, *5*(2), 265–273.

Duncan, D. T., Castro, M. C., Gortmaker, S. L., Aldstadt, J., Melly, S. J., & Bennett, G. G. (2012). Racial differences in the built environment—body mass index relationship? A geospatial analysis of adolescents in urban neighborhoods. *International Journal of Health Geographics*, *11*(1), 11.

Duncan, D. T., Kapadia, F., & Halkitis, P. N. (2014). Examination of spatial polygamy among young gay, bisexual, and other men who have sex with men in New York City: The p18 cohort study. *International Journal of Environmental Research and Public Health*, *11*(9), 8962–8983.

Duncan, D. T., Kapadia, F., Regan, S. D., Goedel, W. C., Levy, M. D., Barton, S. C., Friedman, S. R., & Halkitis, P. N. (2016). Feasibility and acceptability of global positioning system (GPS) methods to study the spatial contexts of substance use and sexual risk behaviors among young men who have sex with men in New York City: A p18 cohort sub-study. *PloS One*, *11*(2), e0147520.

Duncan, D. T., Kawachi, I., Subramanian, S., Aldstadt, J., Melly, S. J., & Williams, D. R. (2013). Examination of how neighborhood definition influences measurements of youths' access to tobacco retailers: A methodological note on spatial misclassification. *American Journal of Epidemiology*, *179*(3), 373–381.

Duncan, D. T., Park, S. H., Goedel, W. C., Kreski, N. T., Morganstein, J. G., Hambrick, H. R., Jean-Louis, G., & Chaix, B. (2017). Perceived neighborhood safety is associated with poor sleep health among gay, bisexual, and other men who have sex with men in Paris, France. *Journal of Urban Health*, *94*(3), 399–407.

Duncan, D. T., & Regan, S. D. (2016). Mapping multi-day GPS data: A cartographic study in NYC. *Journal of Maps*, *12*(4), 668–670.

Duncan, D. T., Regan, S. D., Shelley, D., Day, K., Ruff, R. R., Al-Bayan, M., & Elbel, B. (2014). Application of global positioning system methods for the study of obesity and hypertension risk among low-income housing residents in New York City: A spatial feasibility study. *Geospatial Health*, *9*(1), 57.

Duncan, D. T., Tamura, K., Regan, S. D., Athens, J., Elbel, B., Meline, J., .Al-Ajlouni, Y. A., & Chaix, B. (2017). Quantifying spatial misclassification in exposure to noise complaints among low-income housing residents across New York City neighborhoods: A Global Positioning System (GPS) study. *Annals of Epidemiology*, *27*(1), 67–75.

Epstein, D. H., Tyburski, M., Craig, I. M., Phillips, K. A., Jobes, M. L., Vahabzadeh, M., Vahabzadeh, M., Mezghanni, M., Lin, J. L., Furr-Holden, C. D. M., & Preston, K. L. (2014). Real-time tracking of neighborhood surroundings and mood in urban drug misusers: Application of a new method to study behavior in its geographical context. *Drug and Alcohol Dependence*, *134*, 22–29.

Frank, J. W., Hong, C. S., Subramanian, S., & Wang, E. A. (2013). Neighborhood incarceration rate and asthma prevalence in New York City: A multilevel approach. *American Journal of Public Health*, *103*(5), e38–e44.

Frick, M., & Castro, M. C. (2013). Tobacco retail clustering around schools in New York City: Examining "place" and "space." *Health & Place, 19*, 15–24.

Galea, S., Ahern, J., Rudenstine, S., Wallace, Z., & Vlahov, D. (2005). Urban built environment and depression: A multilevel analysis. *Journal of Epidemiology & Community Health, 59*(10), 822–827.

Goedel, W. C., Reisner, S. L., Janssen, A. C., Poteat, T. C., Regan, S. D., Kreski, N. T., Confident, G., & Duncan, D. T. (2017). Acceptability and feasibility of using a novel geospatial method to measure neighborhood contexts and mobility among transgender women in New York City. *Transgender Health, 2*(1), 96–106.

Golledge, R. G. (1997). *Spatial behavior: A geographic perspective.* New York, NY: Guilford Press.

Gordon, C., Purciel-Hill, M., Ghai, N. R., Kaufman, L., Graham, R., & Van Wye, G. (2011). Measuring food deserts in New York City's low-income neighborhoods. *Health & Place, 17*(2), 696–700.

Harrison, F., Burgoine, T., Corder, K., van Sluijs, E. M., & Jones, A. (2014). How well do modelled routes to school record the environments children are exposed to? A cross-sectional comparison of GIS-modelled and GPS-measured routes to school. *International Journal of Health Geographics, 13*(1), 5.

Hirsch, J. A., Winters, M., Clarke, P., & McKay, H. (2014). Generating GPS activity spaces that shed light upon the mobility habits of older adults: A descriptive analysis. *International Journal of Health Geographics, 13*(1), 51.

Hurvitz, P. M., & Moudon, A. V. (2012). Home versus nonhome neighborhood: Quantifying differences in exposure to the built environment. *American Journal of Preventive Medicine, 42*(4), 411–417.

Huynh, M., & Maroko, A. (2014). Gentrification and preterm birth in New York City, 2008–2010. *Journal of Urban Health, 91*(1), 211–220.

Inagami, S., Cohen, D. A., Finch, B. K., & Asch, S. M. (2006). You are where you shop: grocery store locations, weight, and neighborhoods. *American Journal of Preventive Medicine, 31*(1), 10–17.

Jack, D., Neckerman, K., Schwartz-Soicher, O., Lovasi, G. S., Quinn, J., Richards, C., Bader, M., Weiss, C., Konty, K., Arno, P., Viola, D., Kerker, B., & Rundle, A. (2013). Socio-economic status, neighbourhood food environments and consumption of fruits and vegetables in New York City. *Public Health Nutrition, 16*(7), 1197–1205.

Janevic, T., Borrell, L. N., Savitz, D. A., Herring, A. H., & Rundle, A. (2010). Neighbourhood food environment and gestational diabetes in New York City. *Paediatric and Perinatal Epidemiology, 24*(3), 249–254.

Jeffery, R. W., Baxter, J., McGuire, M., & Linde, J. (2006). Are fast food restaurants an environmental risk factor for obesity? *International Journal of Behavioral Nutrition and Physical Activity, 3*(1), 2.

Jones, M., & Pebley, A. R. (2014). Redefining neighborhoods using common destinations: Social characteristics of activity spaces and home census tracts compared. *Demography, 51*(3), 727–752.

Karpati, A. M., Bassett, M. T., & McCord, C. (2006). Neighbourhood mortality inequalities in New York City, 1989–1991 and 1999–2001. *Journal of Epidemiology & Community Health, 60*(12), 1060–1064.

Kerr, J., Duncan, S., & Schipperjin, J. (2011). Using global positioning systems in health research: A practical approach to data collection and processing. *American Journal of Preventive Medicine, 41*(5), 532–540.

Kestens, Y., Lebel, A., Chaix, B., Clary, C., Daniel, M., Pampalon, R., Theriault, M., & Subramanian, S. (2012). Association between activity space exposure to food establishments and individual risk of overweight. *PloS One, 7*(8), e41418.

Kestens, Y., Thierry, B., & Chaix, B. (2016). Re-creating daily mobility histories for health research from raw GPS tracks: Validation of a kernel-based algorithm using real-life data. *Health & Place, 40*, 29–33.

Kestens, Y., Wasfi, R., Naud, A., & Chaix, B. (2017). "Contextualizing context": Reconciling environmental exposures, social networks, and location preferences in health research. *Current Environmental Health Reports, 4*(1), 51–60.

Kirchner, T. R., & Shiffman, S. (2016). Spatio-temporal determinants of mental health and well-being: Advances in geographically-explicit ecological momentary assessment (GEMA). *Social Psychiatry and Psychiatric Epidemiology, 51*(9), 1211–1223.

Koblin, B. A., Egan, J. E., Rundle, A., Quinn, J., Tieu, H.-V., Cerdá, M., Ompad, D. C., Greene, E., Hoover, D. R., & Frye, V. (2013). Methods to measure the impact of home, social, and sexual neighborhoods of urban gay, bisexual, and other men who have sex with men. *PloS One, 8*(10), e75878.

Krenn, P. J., Titze, S., Oja, P., Jones, A., & Ogilvie, D. (2011). Use of global positioning systems to study physical activity and the environment: A systematic review. *American Journal of Preventive Medicine, 41*(5), 508–515.

Krieger, N., Waterman, P., Chen, J. T., Soobader, M.-J., Subramanian, S. V., & Carson, R. (2002). Zip code caveat: Bias due to spatiotemporal mismatches between zip codes and us census–defined geographic areas—the public health disparities geocoding project. *American Journal of Public Health, 92*(7), 1100–1102.

Kwan, M.-P. (2012). How GIS can help address the uncertain geographic context problem in social science research. *Annals of GIS, 18*(4), 245–255.

Kwate, N. O. A., & Lee, T. H. (2007). Ghettoizing outdoor advertising: Disadvantage and ad panel density in black neighborhoods. *Journal of Urban Health, 84*(1), 21–31.

Kwate, N. O. A., Loh, J. M., White, K., & Saldana, N. (2013). Retail redlining in New York City: Racialized access to day-to-day retail resources. *Journal of Urban Health, 90*(4), 632–652.

Kwate, N. O. A., Yau, C.-Y., Loh, J.-M., & Williams, D. (2009). Inequality in obesigenic environments: Fast food density in New York City. *Health & Place, 15*(1), 364–373.

Lalli, M. (1992). Urban-related identity: Theory, measurement, and empirical findings. *Journal of Environmental Psychology, 12*(4), 285–303.

Leal, C., & Chaix, B. (2011). The influence of geographic life environments on cardiometabolic risk factors: A systematic review, a methodological assessment and a research agenda. *Obesity Reviews, 12*(3), 217–230.

Lewin, A., Pannier, B., Méline, J., Karusisi, N., Thomas, F., & Chaix, B. (2014). Residential neighborhood, geographic work environment, and work economic sector: Associations with body fat measured by bioelectrical impedance in the RECORD Study. *Annals of Epidemiology, 24*(3), 180–186.

Li, W., Kelsey, J. L., Zhang, Z., Lemon, S. C., Mezgebu, S., Boddie-Willis, C., & Reed, G. W. (2009). Small-area estimation and prioritizing communities for obesity control in Massachusetts. *American Journal of Public Health, 99*(3), 511–519.

Li, W., Land, T., Zhang, Z., Keithly, L., & Kelsey, J. L. (2009). Small-area estimation and prioritizing communities for tobacco control efforts in Massachusetts. *American Journal of Public Health, 99*(3), 470–479.

Lim, S., & Harris, T. G. (2015). Neighborhood contributions to racial and ethnic disparities in obesity among New York city adults. *American Journal of Public Health, 105*(1), 159–165.

Logan, J. R., Stults, B. J., & Xu, Z. (2016). Validating population estimates for harmonized census tract data, 2000–2010. *Annals of the American Association of Geographers, 106*(5), 1013–1029.

Logan, J. R., Xu, Z., & Stults, B. J. (2014). Interpolating US decennial census tract data from as early as 1970 to 2010: A longitudinal tract database. *The Professional Geographer, 66*(3), 412–420.

Lovasi, G. S., Schwartz-Soicher, O., Neckerman, K. M., Konty, K., Kerker, B., Quinn, J., & Rundle, A. (2013). Aesthetic amenities and safety hazards associated with walking and bicycling for transportation in New York City. *Annals of Behavioral Medicine, 45*(1), 76–85.

Lovasi, G. S., Weiss, J. C., Hoskins, R., Whitsel, E. A., Rice, K., Erickson, C. F., & Psaty, B. M. (2007). Comparing a single-stage geocoding method to a multi-stage geocoding method: How much and where do they disagree? *International Journal of Health Geographics, 6*(1), 12.

Matthews, S. A. (2011). Spatial polygamy and the heterogeneity of place: Studying people and place via egocentric methods, In *Communities, neighborhoods, and health* (pp. 35–55). New York, NY: Springer.

Matthews, S. A., Detwiler, J. E., & Burton, L. M. (2005). Geo-ethnography: Coupling geographic information analysis techniques with ethnographic methods in urban research. *Cartographica: The International Journal for Geographic Information and Geovisualization, 40*(4), 75–90.

McElroy, J. A., Remington, P. L., Trentham-Dietz, A., Robert, S. A., & Newcomb, P. A. (2003). Geocoding addresses from a large population-based study: Lessons learned. *Epidemiology, 14*(4), 399–407.

McKenzie, R. (1923). *The Neighborhood: A Study of Local Life in the City of Columbus, Ohio.* Chicago, IL: The University of Chicago Press.

Mooney, S. J., Sheehan, D. M., Zulaika, G., Rundle, A. G., McGill, K., Behrooz, M. R., & Lovasi, G. S. (2016). Quantifying distance overestimation from Global Positioning System in urban spaces. *Journal Information, 106*(4).

Moore, K., Roux, A. V. D., Auchincloss, A., Evenson, K. R., Kaufman, J., Mujahid, M., & Williams, K. (2013). Home and work neighbourhood environments in relation to body mass index: The Multi-Ethnic Study of Atherosclerosis (MESA). *Journal of Epidemiology and Community Health, 67*(10), 846–853.

Nair, H. P., Torian, L. V., Forgione, L., & Begier, E. M. (2011). Evaluation of HIV incidence surveillance in New York City, 2006. *Public Health Reports, 126*(1), 28–38.

Neckerman, K. M., Lovasi, G. S., Davies, S., Purciel, M., Quinn, J., Feder, E., Raghunath, N., Wasserman, B., & Rundle, A. (2009). Disparities in urban neighborhood conditions: Evidence from GIS measures and field observation in New York City. *Journal of Public Health Policy, 30*(1), S264–S285.

O'Campo, P. (2003). Invited commentary: Advancing theory and methods for multilevel models of residential neighborhoods and health. *American Journal of Epidemiology, 157*(1), 9–13.

Oliver, L. N., Schuurman, N., & Hall, A. W. (2007). Comparing circular and network buffers to examine the influence of land use on walking for leisure and errands. *International Journal of Health Geographics, 6*(1), 41.

Orstad, S. L., McDonough, M. H., Stapleton, S., Altincekic, C., & Troped, P. J. (2016). A systematic review of agreement between perceived and objective neighborhood environment measures and associations with physical activity outcomes. *Environment and Behavior*, 0013916516670982.

Paz-Soldan, V. A., Reiner R. C., Jr, Morrison, A. C., Stoddard, S. T., Kitron, U., Scott, T. W., Elder, J. P., Halsey, E. S., Kochel, T. J., Astete, H., & Vazquez-Prokopec, G. M. (2014). Strengths and weaknesses of Global Positioning System (GPS) data-loggers and semi-structured interviews for capturing fine-scale human mobility: Findings from Iquitos, Peru. *PLoS Neglected Tropical Diseases, 8*(6), e2888.

Perchoux, C., Chaix, B., Brondeel, R., & Kestens, Y. (2016). Residential buffer, perceived neighborhood, and individual activity space: New refinements in the definition of exposure areas—The RECORD Cohort Study. *Health & Place, 40*, 116–122.

Perchoux, C., Chaix, B., Cummins, S., & Kestens, Y. (2013). Conceptualization and measurement of environmental exposure in epidemiology: Accounting for activity space related to daily mobility. *Health & Place, 21*, 86–93.

Perchoux, C., Kestens, Y., Thomas, F., Van Hulst, A., Thierry, B., & Chaix, B. (2014). Assessing patterns of spatial behavior in health studies: Their socio-demographic determinants and associations with transportation modes (the RECORD Cohort Study). *Social Science & Medicine, 119*, 64–73.

Proshansky, H. M., Fabian, A. K., & Kaminoff, R. (1983). Place-identity: Physical world socialization of the self. *Journal of Environmental Psychology, 3*(1), 57–83.

Robinson, A. I., & Oreskovic, N. M. (2013). Comparing self-identified and census-defined neighborhoods among adolescents using GPS and accelerometer. *International Journal of Health Geographics, 12*(1), 57.

Rundle, A., Roux, A. V. D., Freeman, L. M., Miller, D., Neckerman, K. M., & Weiss, C. C. (2007). The urban built environment and obesity in New York City: A multilevel analysis. *American Journal of Health Promotion, 21*(4 Suppl), 326–334.

Rundle, A. G., Sheehan, D. M., Quinn, J. W., Bartley, K., Eisenhower, D., Bader, M. M. D., Lovasi, G., & Neckerman, K. M. (2016). Using GPS data to study neighborhood walkability and physical activity. *American Journal of Preventive Medicine, 50*(3), e65–e72.

Sampson, R. J. (2003). The neighborhood context of well-being. *Perspectives in Biology and Medicine, 46*(3), S53–S64.

Sampson, R. J. (2012). *Great American city: Chicago and the enduring neighborhood effect*. Chicago, IL: University of Chicago Press.

Sampson, R. J., Morenoff, J. D., & Earls, F. (1999). Beyond social capital: Spatial dynamics of collective efficacy for children. *American Sociological Review, 64*(5), 633–660.

Sampson, R. J., Raudenbush, S. W., & Earls, F. (1997). Neighborhoods and violent crime: A multilevel study of collective efficacy. *Science, 277*(5328), 918–924.

Sastry, N., Pebley, A. R., & Zonta, M. (2002). Neighborhood definitions and the spatial dimension of daily life in Los Angeles. *California Center for Population Research*. Retrieved from https://www.rand.org/pubs/drafts/DRU2400z8.readonline.html

Schipperijn, J., Kerr, J., Duncan, S., Madsen, T., Klinker, C. D., & Troelsen, J. (2014). Dynamic accuracy of GPS receivers for use in health research: A novel method to assess GPS accuracy in real-world settings. *Frontiers in Public Health, 2*, 21.

Sherman, J. E., Spencer, J., Preisser, J. S., Gesler, W. M., & Arcury, T. A. (2005). A suite of methods for representing activity space in a healthcare accessibility study. *International Journal of Health Geographics, 4*(1), 24.

Simon, P. A., Kwan, D., Angelescu, A., Shih, M., & Fielding, J. E. (2008). Proximity of fast food restaurants to schools: Do neighborhood income and type of school matter? *Preventive Medicine, 47*(3), 284–288.

Stan, O., & Neil, W. (1984). *The modifiable areal unit problem.* Norwich, UK: Geo Books.

Stewart, T., Duncan, S., Chaix, B., Kestens, Y., Schipperijn, J., & Schofield, G. (2015). A novel assessment of adolescent mobility: A pilot study. *International Journal of Behavioral Nutrition and Physical Activity, 12*(1), 18.

Tamura, K., Elbel, B., Chaix, B., Regan, S. D., Al-Ajlouni, Y. A., Athens, J. K., Meline, J., & Duncan, D. T. (in press). Residential and GPS-defined activity space neighborhood noise complaints, body mass index and blood pressure among low-income housing residents in New York City. *Journal of Community Health.*

Terzian, A. S., Bodach, S. D., Wiewel, E. W., Sepkowitz, K., Bernard, M.-A., Braunstein, S. L., & Shepard, C. W. (2012). Novel use of surveillance data to detect HIV-infected persons with sustained high viral load and durable virologic suppression in New York City. *PloS One, 7*(1), e29679.

Uzzell, D., Pol, E., & Badenas, D. (2002). Place identification, social cohesion, and environmental sustainability. *Environment and Behavior, 34*(1), 26–53.

Vallée, J., Cadot, E., Grillo, F., Parizot, I., & Chauvin, P. (2010). The combined effects of activity space and neighbourhood of residence on participation in preventive health-care activities: The case of cervical screening in the Paris metropolitan area (France). *Health & Place, 16*(5), 838–852.

Vallée, J., Cadot, E., Roustit, C., Parizot, I., & Chauvin, P. (2011). The role of daily mobility in mental health inequalities: The interactive influence of activity space and neighbourhood of residence on depression. *Social Science & Medicine, 73*(8), 1133–1144.

Vallée, J., & Chauvin, P. (2012). Investigating the effects of medical density on health-seeking behaviours using a multiscale approach to residential and activity spaces: Results from a prospective cohort study in the Paris metropolitan area, France. *International Journal of Health Geographics, 11*(1), 54.

Vallée, J., Le Roux, G., Chaix, B., Kestens, Y., & Chauvin, P. (2015). The "constant size neighbourhood trap" in accessibility and health studies. *Urban Studies, 52*(2), 338–357.

Vaughan, A. S., Kramer, M. R., Cooper, H. L., Rosenberg, E. S., & Sullivan, P. S. (2016). Completeness and reliability of location data collected on the web: Assessing the quality of self-reported locations in an internet sample of men who have sex with men. *Journal of Medical Internet Research, 18*(6).

Vaughan, A. S., Kramer, M. R., Cooper, H. L., Rosenberg, E. S., & Sullivan, P. S. (2017). Activity spaces of men who have sex with men: An initial exploration of geographic variation in locations of routine, potential sexual risk, and prevention behaviors. *Social Science & Medicine, 175*, 1–10.

Villanueva, C., & Aggarwal, B. (2013). The association between neighborhood socioeconomic status and clinical outcomes among patients 1 year after hospitalization for cardiovascular disease. *Journal of Community Health, 38*(4), 690–697.

Webber, S. C., & Porter, M. M. (2009). Monitoring mobility in older adults using global positioning system (GPS) watches and accelerometers: A feasibility study. *Journal of Aging and Physical Activity, 17*(4), 455–467.

Weiss, C. C., Purciel, M., Bader, M., Quinn, J. W., Lovasi, G., Neckerman, K. M., & Rundle, A. G. (2011). Reconsidering access: Park facilities and neighborhood disamenities in New York City. *Journal of Urban Health, 88*(2), 297–310.

White, K., Borrell, L. N., Wong, D. W., Galea, S., Ogedegbe, G., & Glymour, M. M. (2011). Racial/ethnic residential segregation and self-reported hypertension among US- and foreign-born blacks in New York City. *American Journal of Hypertension*, *24*(8), 904–910.

Wiebe, D. J., Richmond, T. S., Guo, W., Allison, P. D., Hollander, J. E., Nance, M. L., & Branas, C. C. (2016). Mapping activity patterns to quantify risk of violent assault in urban environments. *Epidemiology (Cambridge, Mass.)*, *27*(1), 32.

Wiehe, S. E., Carroll, A. E., Liu, G. C., Haberkorn, K. L., Hoch, S. C., Wilson, J. S., & Fortenberry, J. (2008). Using GPS-enabled cell phones to track the travel patterns of adolescents. *International Journal of Health Geographics*, *7*(1), 22.

Wolf, J., Schönfelder, S., Samaga, U., Oliveira, M., & Axhausen, K. (2004). Eighty weeks of global positioning system traces: Approaches to enriching trip information. *Transportation Research Record: Journal of the Transportation Research Board* (1870), 46–54.

Wong, D. (2009). The modifiable areal unit problem (MAUP). In *The SAGE handbook of spatial analysis* (pp. 105–123). Thousand Oaks, CA: Sage.

Zenk, S. N., Schulz, A. J., Matthews, S. A., Odoms-Young, A., Wilbur, J., Wegrzyn, L., Gibbs, K., Braunschweig, C., & Stokes, C. (2011). Activity space environment and dietary and physical activity behaviors: A pilot study. *Health & Place*, *17*(5), 1150–1161.

3

QUANTITATIVE METHODS FOR MEASURING NEIGHBORHOOD CHARACTERISTICS IN NEIGHBORHOOD HEALTH RESEARCH

Dustin T. Duncan, William C. Goedel, and Rumi Chunara

If you can't measure it, it doesn't exist.
—Unknown

Decades of research have investigated the role of a range of neighborhood characteristics (e.g., neighborhood walkability, neighborhood disorder) on health outcomes and health behaviors. These characteristics were discussed in detail in the first edition of *Neighborhoods and Health* by Ichiro Kawachi and Lisa Berkman in 2003, as well as in the introductory chapter of this second edition. Neighborhood-level characteristics are often of substantive interest as primary predictors in spatial epidemiological studies, and at other times, they are considered as confounding variables or sources of effect modification in these investigations. Regardless, there are few resources that provide an overview of the range of methods one can use to measure neighborhood characteristics, especially with regard to the measurement of these characteristics as they relate to health. Methods used to assess neighborhood characteristics vary considerably from study to study. This is not a problem per se, but it is important to note the strengths and limitations of each. In some circumstances, one methodological approach might be more appropriate than another, but the reasons for selecting one method over another have not been a major discussion point in the literature on neighborhoods and health.

Although some methods of studying neighborhood characteristics were discussed in the first edition 15 years ago, new methods exist for the measurement of neighborhood characteristics. This chapter will provide an overview of a range of established and emerging quantitative methods used in neighborhoods and health research, including emerging methodological approaches deriving measures of neighborhood environments from postings on social media platforms and crowd-sourced Web-based data. We provide examples from the literature, alongside the strengths and limitations of each methodological approach. Overall, we have classified the methodological approaches into three different approaches: (1) traditional, (2) current, and (3) emerging methods (Table 3-1). This classification is based on the chronological era when they were first introduced. "Traditional" methods were commonly used before 2003 (when the first edition was published), "current" methods refer to methods that emerged between 2003 and the time of publication, and emerging methods emerged in the last couple of years preceding publication of this edition. We do not focus on qualitative methods in neighborhood health research (e.g., PhotoVoice) or mixed-methods approaches (which combine qualitative and quantitative methods) because these are discussed in Chapter 7.

TRADITIONAL METHODS FOR MEASURING NEIGHBORHOOD CHARACTERISTICS

Traditional methods for measuring neighborhood characteristics have included self-report surveys and systematic field observation (SFOs). In this section, we discuss these first two approaches and present examples of their application from the literature.

Self-Report Measures

A study using self-report measures includes a survey or questionnaire, in which respondents read a question and select a response option. This method is frequently applied in neighborhoods and health research to assess perceived neighborhood characteristics (such as aesthetic quality, amenities available for walking and exercise, safety from crime, violence, access to healthy foods, and social cohesion) via direct reports from residents. There have been many tools developed to collect self-report measures to assess neighborhood conditions across studies. A prime example of such a tool is the Neighborhood Environment Walkability Scale (NEWS) (Cerin, Saelens, Sallis, & Frank, 2006; Rosenberg et al., 2009; Saelens, Sallis, Black, & Chen, 2003), a self-report scale measuring several neighborhood characteristics relevant to physical activity, including residential density, street connectivity, aesthetics, traffic, and safety from crime. An example question from NEWS is: "About how long would it take to get from your home to the nearest businesses or facilities listed below if you walked to them?" In completing this scale, respondents are presented with amenities common to most neighborhoods (e.g., a bus or train stop, a fast food restaurant, a post office) and asked to select one of six answer choices ("1–5 minutes," "6–10

Table 3-1 Approaches to Quantitative Data Collection

Approach	*Examples from Neighborhoods and Health Literature*
	Traditional methods
Self-report	Duncan, D. T., Park, S. H., Goedel, W. C., Kreski, N. T., Morganstein, J. G., Hambrick, H. R., Jean-Louis, G., & Chaix, B. (2017). Perceived neighborhood safety is associated with poor sleep health among gay, bisexual, and other men who have sex with men in Paris, France. *Journal of Urban Health, 94*(3), 399–407.
Systematic field observation	Sampson, R. J., & Raudenbush, S. W. (1999). Systematic social observation of public spaces: a new look at disorder in urban neighborhoods. *American Journal of Sociology, 105*(3), 603–651.
	Current methods
Geographic information systems	Duncan, D. T., Sharifi, M., Melly, S. J., Marshall, R., Sequist, T. D., Rifas-Shiman, S. L., & Taveras, E. M. (2014). Characteristics of walkable built environments and BMI z-scores in children: evidence from a large electronic health record database. *Environmental Health Perspectives, 122*(12), 1359–1365.
Web-based geospatial data	Hirsch, J. A., Moore, K. A., Evenson, K. R., Rodriguez, D. A., Diez Roux, A. V. (2013). Walk score and transit score and walking in the multi-ethic study of atherosclerosis. *American Jounral of Preventive Medicine, 45*(2), 158–166.
	Emerging methods
Wearable geospatial monitors	Oliver, M., Doherty, A. R., Kelly, P., Badland, H. M., Mavoa, S., Shepherd, J., Kerr, J., Marshall, S., Hamilton, A., & Foster, C. (2013). Utility of passive photography to objectively audit built environment features of active transport journeys: An observational study. *International Journal of Health Geographics, 12*, 20.
Crowd-sourced data	Cawkwell, P. B., Lee, L., Weizman, M., & Sherman, S. E. (2015). Tracking Hookah Bars in New York: Utilizing yelp as a powerful public health tool. *JMIR Public Health and Surveillance, 1*(2), e19.
Social media and other Internet-sourced data	Chae, D. H., Clouston, S., Hatzenbuehler, M. L., & Kramer, M. R., Cooper, H. L., Wilson, S. M., Stephens-Davidowitz, S. I., Gold, R. S., & Link, B. G. (2015). Association between an Internet-Based Measure of Area Racism and Black Mortality. *PLoS One, 10*(4), e0122963.

minutes," "11–20 minutes," "20–30 minutes," "30+ minutes," and "Don't know") to reflect their perceptions of how close these amenities are by foot to their home.

In addition to measuring perceived access to the built environment, self-report measures can also be used to assess the social environment and social processes within communities. For example, participants in the NYC Low-Income Housing, Neighborhoods, and Health Study were presented with the following item to measure the reputation of their neighborhood, a component of spatial stigma (discussed in detail in Chapter 10): "Overall, what is the reputation of your neighborhood?" For this item, participants were presented with four response options ("Good," "Moderate," "Bad," and "Don't know/Not sure") to reflect how they felt their neighborhood is perceived by other people (Duncan, Ruff, et al., 2016; Ruff et al., 2016). In measuring community-level norms regarding condom use, participants in HIV Prevention Trials Network (HPTN) Protocol #063 (Goedel, Safren, Mayer, & Duncan, 2017; Safren et al., 2016) were presented with the following statement: "In my community, asking to use a condom suggests that you distrust your partner." Respondents selected an answer choice on a four-point Likert scale (ranging from "Disagree strongly" to "Agree strongly") to indicate to what extent the statement reflects the beliefs held by members of their community. Another example is from the Project on Human Development in Chicago Neighborhoods (PHDCN), a population-based study of residents of Chicago's neighborhoods aimed at understanding the causes and pathways of juvenile delinquency, adult crime, substance abuse, and violence. This study examined neighborhood collective efficacy, including "informal social control" and "social cohesion and trust" (Sampson, Raudenbush, & Earls, 1997). "Informal social control," defined as the reactions of individuals and groups that bring about conformity to norms and laws, was measured with a five-item Likert-type scale, asking residents about the likelihood that their neighbors could be counted on to intervene in various ways if (1) children were skipping school and hanging out on a street corner, (2) children were spray-painting graffiti on a local building, (3) children were showing disrespect to an adult, (4) a fight broke out in front of their house, and (5) the fire station closest to their home was threatened with budget cuts.

Methods to Capture Self-Report Data

Traditional methods of administrating questionnaires to collect self-reported information are based on "pen and paper" surveys, along with tablets, surveys administered via telephone, and audio computer-assisted self-interviews (ACASI) delivered on desktop computers. Newer methods exist to survey participants using online platforms (such as Facebook) and mobile technologies, including smartphones and smartphone applications (hereby referred to as "apps"). To illustrate, researchers have implemented surveys through geosocial-networking smartphone applications—those that utilize the geolocation features of smartphones to connect users with other users based on their physical proximity. Grindr, for example, is a commonly and widely used app for gay, bisexual, and other men who have sex with men (MSM) that is often used to arrange sexual encounters. Recent studies on the health and health behaviors of MSM have utilized broadcast advertisements (i.e., pop-up advertisements presented to users when they log in to the app) targeted to users in specific geographic areas on Grindr and similar applications. These types of advertisements have been used to recruit users into research studies in numerous locations, including—but not limited to—Atlanta, New York City, Los Angeles, London, and Paris (Duncan, Goedel, et al., 2016; Duncan et al., 2017; Gibbs & Rice, 2016; Goedel & Duncan, 2015; Goedel, Hagen, et al., 2017; Goedel, Halkitis, Greene, & Duncan, 2016; Goedel, Schneider, Hagen, & Duncan, 2017; Huang, Marlin, Young, Medline, & Klausner, 2016). For example, in a study of Grindr users recruited in Paris, perceived neighborhood safety and self-reported sleep quality and duration as well as self-reported sleep problems were measured in a Web-based survey delivered to users via a broadcast advertisement (Duncan et al., 2017).

Survey-based assessments of neighborhood conditions can also be delivered via text messages. These approaches can function as a form of ecological momentary assessment (EMA) (Shiffman, 2013; Shiffman, Stone, & Hufford, 2008; Stone & Shiffman, 1994). EMA methods can captures data on neighborhood environments and health behaviors and outcomes in real time from participants as they experience their daily lives (Dunton, Kawabata, Intille, Wolch, & Pentz, 2012; Liao, Intille, & Dunton, 2015; Zenk et al., 2017, 2014). Studies utilizing EMA methods often involve repeated measures over varying durations, affording the temporal resolution needed to assess the dynamics of within-subject changes in behavior and experience over time and across context (Shiffman, 2013; Shiffman et al., 2008; Stone & Shiffman, 1994). EMA methods are effective in contextualizing the environments in which health behaviors occur, as they can provide insight into where they occur. In particular, reports collected using EMA protocols can be integrated with data collected via global positioning system (GPS) devices and geolocation features of smartphones in an approach sometimes referred to as "geographically explicit ecological momentary assessment" (GEMA) (Epstein et al., 2014; Kirchner & Shiffman, 2016). This type of approach can measure both health behaviors and their contexts simultaneously in real time, overcoming traditional limitations associated with retrospective recall in research settings. In a recent study, Mitchell and colleagues (2014) piloted a protocol in which adults with attention-deficit/hyperactivity disorder (ADHD) carried a dedicated GPS device for 7 days while using an electronic diary to record smoking behaviors and ADHD symptoms in real time (Mitchell et al., 2014). This approach allowed researchers to understand the spatial distribution of smoking episodes and ADHD symptoms and begin to understand what contexts may "trigger" certain behaviors, like smoking.

Analysis of Survey Data at the Neighborhood Level

As discussed, researchers resort to analyzing individual perceptions of neighborhood conditions. However, other approaches can be applied to survey data to extend its applications beyond the level of the individual respondents. As discussed in detail later, a good first step is to establish a scale's "ecometric" properties (e.g., reliability of responses from individuals in the same neighborhood) to allow researchers to shift from individual-level research to neighborhood-level research. Then, researchers can use a process known as spatial aggregation, whereby responses from community residents are combined at the neighborhood level to create measures of neighborhood exposures for study participants from the same neighborhoods (Rothman et al., 2011; Sampson et al., 1997). For example, Rothman and colleagues (Rothman et al., 2011) surveyed adult residents of Boston about collective efficacy, social cohesion, and social control along with neighborhood disorder as part of the Boston Neighborhood Survey in 2008 and aggregated results from adults living in the same neighborhoods to create neighborhood-level measures of these variables. These variables were then paired with data from youth residing in these neighborhoods who were surveyed on their experiences with physical violence involving dating partners as part of the Boston Youth Survey in 2008 to assess the potential influence of neighborhood context on adolescent dating violence.

Researchers have analyzed aggregated survey responses for various reasons, including minimizing same-source bias—when the health outcome is also self-reported (Roux, 2007). Same-source bias can induce spurious association between self-reported neighborhood conditions and self-reported health outcomes, due to correlated measurement error. When there are few individuals per neighborhood unit, spatial aggregation may not be possible. The reason is because the sample does not have more than one individual per neighborhood and therefore aggregation is not possible. The major drawback of aggregation is that the response could be contaminated by individual biases—for example, people who do not exercise outdoors will tend to underreport the presence of exercise facilities in the neighborhood. Aggregating many residents' responses has the advantage, however, of improving the validity and reliability of the survey responses.

In addition, geospatial statistical methods, such as spatial interpolation, can be applied to neighborhood survey data, although such an approach is rarely employed

(Auchincloss, Roux, Brown, Raghunathan, & Erdmann, 2007). Interpolation is the generic name for a family of techniques used for mapping of surfaces from limited sample data to estimate values at nonsampled locations. Spatial interpolation, for example, can be used to estimate the value of a neighborhood-level variable for all points in a neighborhood based on the available data for areas surrounding those points, even for places where there are no data or where data are missing, either because residents of a given area did not respond to certain survey items, and/or because residents of these areas were not surveyed. This method operates under the principle of Waldo Tobler's First Law of Geography: "Everything is related to everything else, but near things are more related than distant things." There are many methods of interpolation; kriging and inverse distance weighted (IDW) interpolation are the two most widely used (we do not discuss these further in this chapter, but note that spatial statistics and, in particular, geostatistics books cover this information). Some research has compared different approaches, including a study that examined associations between features of neighborhoods (such as better walkability and availability of healthy foods) and hypertension (Mujahid et al., 2008). They systematically compared different aggregation and geospatial statistical methods, including using simple aggregation (crude means) and empirical Bayes estimation (unconditional, conditional, and spatial) (Mujahid et al., 2008). In general, associations between neighborhood characteristics and hypertension were slightly stronger for the empirical Bayes estimation methods.

Reliability and Validity

The reliability and validity of self-report survey items is dependent on their interpretation by respondents, and these may be influenced by recall bias (Stone & Shiffman, 2002). Survey items can and likely should be tailored to the local geographical context in which they are administered to generate meaningful results. For example, working in collaboration with the International Physical Activity and the Environment Network (IPEN), Oyeyemi et al. (2013) brought together the creators of the original NEWS questionnaire with public health scientists in Nigeria to create a version that retained comparability with the original instrument while generating information relevant to the local context of Nigeria's cities. In this process, the final adaptation of the NEWS included all items of the original instruments in their original or slightly modified form, with 18 additional items describing features of the environment relevant to Sub-Saharan Africa. The test-retest reliability values reported for the subscales of this adapted version of the NEWS were comparable to those reported for the original version in the United States as well as versions used in Australia and China. Like many other studies using the NEWS, the subscales of the adapted version used in Nigeria relating to land use mix diversity and traffic safety were significantly associated with measures of physical activity.

Sometimes self-report surveys of neighborhood conditions must be developed for specific contexts. For example, we recently created a neighborhood scale for the UAE (United Arab Emirates) Healthy Futures Study (previously known as the Abu Dhabi Cohort Study), a prospective cohort study of 20,000 UAE nationals to study the determinants of diabetes, cardiovascular disease, and other health conditions common in Abu Dhabi, the capital of the United Arab Emirates. This survey was developed through scanning the literature on potential salient neighborhood-level determinants of health (especially in the Middle East), modifying previously used questions to better measure the unique neighborhood environment of Abu Dhabi as well as through discussions with the investigative team of the UAE Healthy Futures Study—many of whom live and work in Abu Dhabi. The survey was developed to include three sections, each measuring a different aspect of neighborhoods: (1) the built environment, (2) the food environment, and (3) other environmental characteristics. As an example, one survey item for assessing fresh fruit and vegetable availability in local environments (from the "food environment" section) reads: "The fruits and vegetables available at the baqala are usually fresh. Would you say that you . . ." *Baqala* is an Arabic word that literally translates to convenience store in English; these local convenience stores are frequented by UAE nationals. In response to this item assessing food quality at a baqala, participants responded on a four-point Likert scale (ranging from "Strongly disagree" to "Strongly agree") to reflect the concordance of the statement with their perceptions. Another item, aimed at measuring access to hookah and shisha lounges, reads: "Within a 10-minute drive, it is easy to find a hookah or shisha lounge. Would you say that you . . ." Similar to the previous item, participants respond on a four-point Likert scale to indicate their perceived access to this common feature of many neighborhoods in Abu Dhabi.

Some research on the reliability of self-reported neighborhood characteristics has been conducted. Echeverria, Diez-Roux, and Link (2004), for instance, conducted repeated face-to-face and telephone-administered interviews, including a questionnaire on perceived neighborhood characteristics, with 48 participants in New York City over a 2-week period. The Cronbach's alpha for the scales ranged from .77 to .94 for the scales, with test-retest correlations ranging from .78 to .91. This suggests strong reliability of these perceived neighborhood measures. "Ecometric" assessments (discussed in detail in Chapter 5 of the first edition of *Neighborhoods and Health*) of surveys have been conducted, with early work in this area conducted by Raudenbush and Sampson (1999) in the Project for Human Development in Chicago Neighborhoods (PHDCN). Ecometric assessments seek to quantify how consistently respondents (or field researchers) in the same neighborhood rate neighborhood characteristics similarly on the same measures. Ecometric assessments include evaluating the intraclass or intraneighborhood correlation (ICC) and neighborhood reliabilities. The ICC ranges from 0 to 1, with a higher value indicating greater agreement between respondents within a neighborhood; values closer to 1 also indicate that a higher neighborhood reliability. Recent research, including by Mujahid and her colleagues, show many scales of self-reported neighborhood characteristics have strong ecometric properties (Mujahid, Diez Roux, Morenoff, & Raghunathan, 2007).

Strengths and Limitations

There are both strengths and limitations related to using self-reported measures of neighborhood characteristics. A notable strength of self-reported survey data is that perceptions are often relevant to the lived realities of participants. In a cross-sectional study, Caspi and her colleagues (Caspi, Kawachi, Subramanian, Adamkiewicz, & Sorensen, 2012), for example, examined how access to supermarkets influenced diet among low-income housing residents in the Greater Boston area and found strong and significant associations when using the survey measures of supermarket access as predictor variables, but no association of diet with an objective measure of access to local supermarkets (Caspi et al., 2012) derived from geographic information systems (GIS) data. Another example is from criminology—that is, the difference between perceived crime in a neighborhood versus objective crime (e.g., via police reports). Psychologists have shown that people's behavior (e.g., seniors being afraid to venture outdoors) is more closely tied to their perceptions than to objective reality. Thus, what really matters in this instance is the subjective perception, not the objective reality. Additionally, self-reported measures are easy to administer and can be cost effective. The use of ACASI as a method of survey administration in particular can also reduce potential for bias, including socially desirability bias, as participants can report on sensitive topics (e.g., exposure to community violence, involvement in or knowledge of illegal activities) in private. EMA methods have the benefit of overcoming biases associated with retrospective recall because these methods collect data in real time.

General limitations of using survey data are related to reliability and validity, especially perhaps for newer constructs and certain populations, where psychometric (and ecometric) properties of the items have not been evaluated. As previously discussed, self-reported measures of neighborhood measures can be implicated in same-source bias (Roux, 2007). To overcome this bias, researchers can randomly sample community residents residing in the same neighborhood as study participants to create measures of neighborhood exposures and then link that to health outcomes derived from a separate individual-level data source. Low response rates and a biased sample are also concerns with survey data; this is the case with different sampling designs, especially with nonprobability samples. For example, in the aforementioned study of geosocial-networking smartphone application users in Paris, while the final sample included 580 participants, this represents only 11% of the users who clicked on the advertisement (Duncan et al., 2017). The use of probability sampling methods to generate representative samples can increase the generalizability of survey-based results. Self-report bias (including recall bias) can be an issue with survey measurements as well.

Additionally, there are strengths and limitations specific to the use of spatial interpolation with survey data. Strengths include this being an innovative method of transforming self-reported data to data applicable to a level wider than the individual and it being a cost-effective method (since the data being aggregated or interpolated have already been collected, resulting in no additional expenditures). A key limitation is that the choice of method to interpolate can influence estimates of neighborhood features. General caveats with the approach of spatial interpolation are if the data have few clusters with large gaps in between them, one can obtain unreliable estimates when interpolating. Almost all interpolation methods will underestimate the highs and overestimate the lows, as this is a limitation inherent to averaging.

Systematic Field Observation

Systematic field observation (SFO), also known as environmental auditing, is another well-established method to study neighborhood characteristics.

Methods to Capture Systematic Field Observation

Two approaches to SFO include (1) sending trained auditors into neighborhoods with a pen and clipboard and (2) capturing data from video-mounted vehicles. The first method of SFO, including a series of in-person assessments of neighborhood environments conducted by trained neighborhood raters, has been frequently implemented. A team of neighborhood raters are trained, which can include them participating in a workshop to review the survey and then having the raters rate the same neighborhood characteristics in the same neighborhood at a similar time point to ensure features being rated consistently and reliably across raters. It is best to have raters audit neighborhoods during the same time to control for "time-of-day" effects because neighborhood conditions are likely to vary by the time of the day. However, it also can be useful to conduct statistical adjustment to further control for time-of-day differences. SFO has been applied in many studies available in the literature, including in the Project on Human Development in Chicago Neighborhoods (PHDCN). In a study conducted between June and October 1995, observers trained at the National Opinion Research Center (NORC) drove a sport utility vehicle (SUV) at a rate of 5 miles per hour down every street in 196 Chicago census tracts and videotaped the block faces. These videotaped assessments were used to create measures of neighborhood-level features, such as neighborhood disorder, which later were linked to health outcomes and health behaviors (Molnar, Gortmaker, Bull, & Buka, 2004; Sampson & Raudenbush, 1999).

Photographic assessments of neighborhoods from vehicle-mounted cameras traveling through the neighborhoods, such as those used to create Google Street View photographs, are beginning to be used in studies to measure neighborhood features, including features of the built environment and neighborhood disorder (Marco, Gracia, Martín-Fernández, & López-Quílez, 2017; Odgers, Caspi, Bates, Sampson, & Moffitt, 2012; Rundle, Bader, Richards, Neckerman, & Teitler, 2011). This approach can be used to quantify neighborhood characteristics completely without needing to visit each neighborhood being studied and document their features in person.

Across methods of SFO, different instruments can be applied to collect information systematically across neighborhoods, including the Environmental Assessment of Public Recreation Spaces (EAPRS) Tool (Saelens et al., 2006; Van Dyck et al., 2013). The EAPRS Tool is used to assess the physical environments of parks and playgrounds, with a specific focus on evaluating physical elements and qualities of these spaces with respect to their functionality (or potential functionality) when used by adults and children. The survey has sections designated to review trails, paths, general areas (such as meadows and open areas), water areas, eating/drinking areas, facilities, educational or historic components, non-trail sitting and resting spots, landscaping, general aesthetics, accessibility, information-related features, safety features, play sets, other play components that are not part of the play set, and athletic/recreation fields that often comprise a public recreation space. This tool requires comprehensive observation tactics that include, but are not limited to, walking all paths, paved trails, and unpaved trails at their full length; driving on all roads within the park or that border the park; walking around and through all parking lots; trying all playground equipment; sitting on any resting features in a given area; and walking around the available perimeter of the park. This tool, for example, asks an observer to rate the flatness of paved trails as either "completely flat," "some incline or decline," or "significant incline or decline" as a measure of ease of use of the trails. Importantly, the EAPRS tool could likely not be implemented with a moving vehicle; trained auditors need to walk the actual locations, so the particular SFO method may depend on the instrument used.

Reliability and Validity

As discussed, an important step of SFO involves the training of the raters, so that they develop adequate interrater reliability. Studies have been conducted to examine the reliability and validity of SFO in neighborhoods and health research. Using data from the Project on Human Development in Chicago Neighborhoods (PHDCN), Raudenbush and Sampson (1999), for example, conducted an ecometric analysis, where the authors studied bias and random error in the assessment of neighborhoods. In particular, the authors sought to assess the reliability and validity of measures derived from SFO as compared to relevant measures obtained from the US Census and a citywide survey of neighborhood residents in Chicago. First, it was found that the highest levels of reliability for measures of physical disorder within a neighborhood cluster were reached when between 80 and 100 block faces were sampled, but that higher numbers of block faces would need to be sampled to attain comparable levels of reliability for measures of social disorder. Measures of physical disorder derived from SFO correlated highly with relevant constructs measured in the community survey and other independent sources (i.e., police records, census data). Similar correlations were found for measures of social disorder, but the magnitudes of these associations were smaller. Taken together, this suggests that reliable and valid measures of physical disorder and social disorder can be derived from SFO.

Strengths and Limitations

SFO has several strengths, including the ability to measure actual neighborhood conditions and measuring the social dimensions of neighborhood environments. A study conducted by the Built Environment and Health Research Group at Columbia University found that Google Street View was a useful tool to measure pedestrian safety, motor vehicle traffic, parking, and infrastructure for active travel remotely for neighborhoods in New York City. These measures derived from Google Street View had relatively high levels of concordance with measures derived from in-person SFOs (Rundle et al., 2011).

Despite this strength, traditional in-person SFOs are well known to be time intensive and have several logistical constraints, including the burden of physically traveling to and examining multiple neighborhoods within a given study area. Another limitation is that SFO requires specialized training of raters so that all neighborhoods are observed with the same rigor and attention. In addition, SFO can be very costly when raters must travel to the neighborhoods they are assessing (this is less so the case when using Google Street View for this purpose but still labor intensive).

Use of SFO can potentially be perceived by local residents as intrusive and, therefore, there can be safety issues for research staff, particularly in neighborhoods with high rates of violent crime or in neighborhoods with unsafe infrastructure. An additional limitation of SFO is the need to account for seasonality and neighborhood change as these assessments are usually only conducted at one time point. Take Google Street View as an example; it provides a single picture for each location being assessed, and it may not be current.

In the aforementioned study in New York City, Rundle and colleagues (2011) found that Google Street View–derived measures had low levels or concordance with in-person SFO when the features were small (e.g., litter) or often exhibited temporal variability (e.g., social and commercial activity) (Rundle et al., 2011). An additional caveat is that Google Street View cannot evaluate dynamic features of neighborhoods, such as noise levels, unpleasant odors or pollution, or traffic speeds, among other features, which may be salient to health and well-being, as this resource only provides still images of block faces. Overall, although there are unique strengths and limitations of in-person SFO as compared with virtual assessments via Google Street View, the latter is likely to be faster, easier, cheaper, and safer in many cases.

As discussed, multiple strengths and limitations exist with traditional methods for measuring neighborhood characteristics. Some of the limitations with the use of traditional methods can be overcome with current methods used in the neighborhoods and health literature.

CURRENT METHODS FOR MEASURING NEIGHBORHOOD CHARACTERISTICS

More recently, the most common approach for quantifying neighborhood characteristics is the use of geographic information systems (GIS). At the time of this publication, Web-based geospatial tools are being used extensively in quantitative neighborhoods and health research.

Geographic Information Systems

Geographic information systems (GIS), increasingly, are being used to evaluate neighborhood characteristics. GIS technologies facilitate the storage, management, analysis, and presentation of data that are linked to a location. These databases can be linked to participant health data, after geocoding participant addresses, to measure associations between features of neighborhoods and health outcomes among their residents. After this, researchers can load a single GIS layer or a set of GIS layers of interest (e.g., those with locations of parks and local supermarkets) and create GIS-based variables to quantify different features of neighborhoods (e.g., density of parks in neighborhood, intersection density, distance to the nearest tobacco retailer). GIS metrics can include both distance metrics and density metrics, and these are the most commonly applied approaches in neighborhood health research. For example, a distance metric can be operationalized as the distance from the participant's home address to the nearest park and/or the mean distance from the participant's home address to the nearest five parks. A density metric can be defined as the density of parkland within a given spatial buffer or administrative region (for further discussion of methodological concerns related to neighborhood boundary definition, see Chapter 2). Advanced GIS metrics also exist, including applying a distance decay function to GIS variables, such as calculating the density of parkland within a spatial buffer of a participants' homes and applying higher weights to park density that is closer in proximity to participants' homes.

In a study conducted in Massachusetts, we examined the association between the built environment (discussed in detail in Chapter 8) and childhood body mass index among a sample of children in a healthcare system ($n = 49{,}770$) using multiple GIS-based measures, such as proximity to recreational open spaces, residential density, and traffic density (Duncan, Sharifi, et al., 2014). Increasingly, studies are using multiple GIS methods in the same study to examine a single latent construct (such as the food environment, discussed in detail in Chapter 9). For example, a study examining associations between the food environment and body mass index in the Framingham Heart Study Offspring Cohort living in four Massachusetts towns had the following primary exposure variables: (1) the driving distance between each subject's residential address and the nearest restaurant or food store, divided into specific categories of establishments (fast food restaurants, full-service restaurants, bakeries/coffee shops, chain supermarkets, grocery stores, and convenience stores), and (2) the mean driving distance to the five closest restaurants or food stores, divided by these categories to measure the overall construct of access to healthy and unhealthy foods (Block, Christakis, O'Malley, & Subramanian, 2011). Both of these studies obtained the built and food environment data from several sources, including files of open and closed food establishments maintained by local boards of health, historical local telephone book yellow and white pages, and previously compiled commercial databases.

In addition to features of the built environment and the food environment, a range of other GIS neighborhood measures can be created to measure the social environment, including measures of neighborhood crime rates using data from local police departments. Using data on lesbian, gay, bisexual, and transgender (LGBT) hate crime incidents from the Boston Police Department Community Disorders

Unit, we examined whether LGBT hate crime rates were associated with the physical and mental health of sexual minority youth (i.e., those who identify as lesbian, gay, or bisexual, among other nonheterosexual identities) (Duncan & Hatzenbuehler, 2014; Duncan, Hatzenbuehler, & Johnson, 2014). This specific measure of neighborhood-level LGBT hate crime rates, unlike rates of other types of crime (e.g., violent and property crime), was associated with self-reported suicidal ideation and suicide attempts self-reported marijuana use among sexual minority youth (Duncan & Hatzenbuehler, 2014; Duncan, Hatzenbuehler, et al., 2014).

Data obtained from other government agencies, including the US Census Bureau (such as the decennial US Census or annual American Community Survey), can also be used to create a range of neighborhood demographic characteristics. Several variables from these data sources can be combined to create indexes to represent a single construct. To illustrate, Messer and colleagues (2006) created an index of neighborhood deprivation at the census tract level using data on the following variables from the US Census: (1) percent of males in management and professional occupations, (2) percent of crowded housing (defined as housing in which there is more than one person in the household per room in the housing unit), (3) percent of households in poverty, (4) percent of female-headed households with dependents, (5) percent of households on public assistance, (6) percent of households earning <$30,000 per year, (7) percent earning less than a high school education, and (8) the percent unemployed. The index was then associated with the unadjusted prevalence of preterm birth and low birthweight across census tracts in 19 cities (Messer et al., 2006).

Another (less often) used data source in neighborhoods and health research is data collected through remote sensing, which is often integrated with GIS software. Remote sensing is the acquisition of information by scanning the Earth via satellite or high-flying aircraft to obtain information about areas of interest. For example, tree canopy density derived from remote sensing can be used to measure access to urban trees (e.g., Heynen, Perkins, & Roy, 2006; Landry & Chakraborty, 2009; Schwarz et al., 2015). In a GIS study, Duncan and colleagues (Duncan, Kawachi, et al., 2014) used high-resolution aerial photos taken by the City of Boston's Department of Innovation and Technology to estimate the spatial distribution of trees within the city and to assess demographic differences in exposure to trees across the city. Using the data derived from these photos, a census-level measurement of tree density (defined as the number of trees per square kilometer for each census tract) was calculated. A similar study by Frey (2016) created similar measures for Washington, DC. In both studies, no significant disparities in exposure to trees were found by demographic characteristics after accounting for spatial autocorrelation (for more on spatial autocorrelation, see Chapter 4).

Reliability and Validity

GIS data have reliability and validity concerns. For example, GIS data can have errors, including positional errors and errors of omission (Boone, Gordon-Larsen, Stewart, & Popkin, 2008; Lebel et al., 2017). For example, a study of the validity of commercially available business data on food establishments found high variation in data quality (Lebel et al., 2017). In addition, crime data gathered by the police are subject to reporting biases (especially sexual crimes or hate crimes where victims might themselves be further at risk for even reporting the crime in certain jurisdictions).

Strengths and Limitations

As GIS data are often ubiquitous in many cities, it facilitates the examination of multiple neighborhood features. Indeed, with an address, one can obtain a variety of neighborhood-level information. This is an objective approach to measuring neighborhood characteristics, which might be more relevant to policymakers. Whereas GIS data can be useful for measuring neighborhood features, this method has caveats and limitations. Limitations include the fact that using GIS software often requires specialized expertise, and the creation of neighborhood-level variables from GIS information can be time intensive to obtain and compute. Another limitation is potential data availability issues—GIS data layers might not be available or readily accessible for all study areas or may not be readily up-to-date, which especially may be the case in rural neighborhoods and non-Western geographic locations. In addition, there are potential data quality issues (such as differential quality of measurement across geographies). In fact, GIS data quality can vary vastly from one municipality to another. Finally, GIS data can be quite costly to obtain when part of commercial data sets.

Web-Based Geospatial Data

A range of Web-based geospatial tools can be used to measure neighborhood characteristics, including Walk Score, Park Score, State of Place, and Google Places. We will discuss Walk Score® (a popular measure of neighborhood walkability) because it is arguably the most widely used Web-based geospatial tool (summarized in Duncan, 2013). Originally developed and launched in 2007 by Front Seat Management, Walk Score® allows a user to enter a location into the online interface on the Walk Score® website (www.walkscore.com). Users receive the numerical Walk Score® assigned to any address free of charge. Walk Score has become increasingly recognized in the study of walkability due to its accessibility, international scale, and use of dynamic (or up-to-date) data that are constantly being corrected.

The Walk Score® algorithm calculates walkability score based on distance to various categories of amenities (e.g., schools, stores, parks, and libraries). If the closest amenity in a specific category is within a quarter-mile radius, Walk Score® assigns the maximum number of points (100) for that type. If no facilities are within a 1-mile radius of the input location, that location will be assigned a score of zero. The algorithm uses a distance-decay function; the number of points declines as the distance approaches 1 mile and no points are awarded for amenities further than 1 mile. Each category is weighted equally and the points are summed to produce a score ranging from 0 to 100, with 0 being the lowest (lowest walkability/car dependent) and 100 being the highest (most walkable). The Walk Score® website has five categories designated by Walk Score®: "Very Car-Dependent" (score below 25, almost all errands require a car); "Car-Dependent" (25–49, a few amenities within walking distance); "Somewhat Walkable" (50–69, some amenities within walking distance); "Very Walkable" (70–89, most errands can be accomplished on foot); and "Walker's Paradise" (90–100, daily errands do not require a car).

The traditional Walk Score® measurement uses straight-line distances (also known as uses an "as the crow flies" distance). The "Street Smart" Walk Score® is a newer metric based on the traditional Walk Score®, and this new metric calculates "network distances." That is, this measurement takes walking distances, intersection density, and average block length into account. Comparison of the traditional and "Street Smart" Walk Scores® has shown that the "Street Smart" Walk Score® and the traditional Walk Score® were highly correlated (Hirsch, Moore, Evenson, Rodriguez, & Roux, 2013).

Front Seat Management also calculates Transit Score® and Bike Score®. Transit Score® measures how well a location is served by public transit and the new Bike Score® metric is a measure of whether a location is good for travel by biking. The Transit Score® algorithm locates the 16 closest transit stops and calculates the straight-line distances from the input location to each stop. A linear combination of these distances is calculated, using a distance decay function based on priority of the transit type served at that stop (e.g., subway, bus) and the frequency of service to the stop. The weighted sum is then normalized to the 0–100 scale. Like Walk Score®, Transit Score® has five categories: "Minimal Transit" (score below 25, it is possible to get on a bus); "Some Transit" (25–49, a few nearby public transportation options); "Good Transit" (50–69, many nearby public transportation options); "Excellent" (70–89, transit is convenient for most trips); and "Rider's Paradise" (90–100, world-class public transportation).

The Bike Score® metric assesses four qualities of a neighborhood—the presence of bike lanes, the presence of hills, road connectivity, and bike commuting mode share (the percentage of travelers in an area using bicycles)—in order to determine whether the neighborhood is suitable for biking. Each of these components is then weighted equally to calculate an overall Bike Score. Bike Scores can range from 0 to 100. Bike Scores has four categories: "Somewhat Bikeable" (0 to 49, minimal bike infrastructure); "Bikeable" (50–69, some bike infrastructure); "Very Bikeable" (70–89, biking is convenient for most trips); and "Biker's Paradise" (90–100, daily errands can be accomplished on a bike).

Reliability and Validity

Concerns come with use of Web-based geospatial data, including reliability and validity concerns. This is especially the case with newer Web-based geospatial tools and those less frequently used such as Walk Shed (available at www.walkshed.com). Although there is a need for more research on Walk Score® validation in rural and international contexts, the current scholarship establishes that Walk Score® is a valid measure of estimating neighborhood walkability, especially in multiple urban locations and at multiple spatial scales (Carr, Dunsiger, & Marcus, 2010, 2011; Duncan, Aldstadt, Whalen, & Melly, 2013; Duncan, Aldstadt, Whalen, Melly, & Gortmaker, 2011; Nykiforuk, McGetrick, Crick, & Johnson, 2016), bolstering the use of the website in neighborhood walkability assessment. This research shows that Walk Score® is a valid measure of estimating certain aspects of neighborhood walkability (such as density of retail destinations, density of recreational open space, intersection density, residential density, and density of subway stops), and Walk Score works best at larger spatial scales, especially a 1-mile buffer around an individual's residence. For example, using residential addresses of 733 children participating in an after-school obesity prevention intervention (2006–2007) in four U.S. metropolitan areas, one study found significant correlations between Walk Score® and several measures of walkability derived from GIS, especially at a 1,600-meter (approximately 1-mile) buffer (Duncan et al., 2011). In addition, Walk Score® has been associated with individuals' perception of their built environment (e.g., perceived access to facilities for physical activity) (Carr et al., 2010). Transit Score® has also been validated (Duncan et al., 2013). For example, a study conducted in Boston suggests that Transit Score® is a convenient tool to measure certain aspects of transit availability (such as density of subway stops) (Duncan et al., 2011).

Strengths and Limitations

Overall, strengths of using Web-based geospatial tools include consideration of up-to-date neighborhood conditions and use of data that is, in general, relatively easy to obtain. Regarding Walk Score (and its related Transit Score and Bike Score metrics), advantages include that it is quick, free, and easy to obtain; has an international scale (e.g., United States, Canada, France, United Kingdom, Ireland, Australia, and New Zealand); uses a dynamic data set (i.e., the data are updated regularly); and eliminates the necessity to gather data sets from different agencies. Using a network-based algorithm that counts amenities along street routes rather than simplistic straight-line distances, the "Street Smart" Walk Score® can provide insight into the depth of choice among amenities, and it penalizes locations with lower pedestrian friendliness. Although a benefit is that a single Walk Score® is rapid and inexpensive to acquire, one must pay for access to Walk Scores for a large number of addresses simultaneously. Furthermore, composite measures of neighborhood walkability such as Walk Score® might be more useful as predictors of health outcomes and health behaviors—as studies that use singe components of neighborhood walkability often generally document fewer relationships and are much more inconsistent regarding direction of effect (Duncan, 2013).

In terms of Walk Score® in particular, disadvantages include the fact that its traditional measure uses "as the crow flies" distance calculations, which are straight-line distances that do not account for routes individuals may actually take to get to specific destinations. Furthermore, Walk Score® weights all destinations equally and does not distinguish between the potential impact of these destinations on health (e.g., the benefits of products available at a health food store compared to the potential health consequences of products for sale at liquor stores), thereby limiting the specificity and precision of information provided by the site and the questions it can be used to answer. Moreover, Walk Score® does not consider the size or quality of these destinations (such as parks), nor does it consider how frequently these amenities are used. Walk Score® does not account for other features that may influence walkability, such as crime rates, neighborhood aesthetics, weather, traffic speed, and topography. Regarding this latter point, existing research shows moderate significant correlations between crime rates (especially property crime rates) and neighborhood walkability, including neighborhood walkability as measured by Walk Score® (Carr et al., 2010). Walk Score® and related Web-based GIS tools do not allow for much customization or "tweaking" by research staff. Because Walk Score® does not consider certain neighborhood-related characteristics that may decrease walkability (e.g., traffic) and weights all destinations equally, it may result in misclassification compared to a "true" walkability indicator. Therefore, Walk Score® should not be considered a complete measure of neighborhood walkability. Additionally, historical Walk Scores® are currently not available, which would be useful for integration into existing population health data sets to conduct longitudinal analyses. Furthermore, like traditional GIS data, there are potential errors of omission, features that no longer exist and positional errors with Web-based geospatial data. We discussed many strengths and limitations with current methods for measuring neighborhood characteristics. Some of the limitations of using these current methods can be overcome with emerging methods.

EMERGING METHODS FOR MEASURING NEIGHBORHOOD CHARACTERISTICS

Emerging methods to study neighborhood characteristics include use of wearable geospatial monitors, crowdsourcing geospatial data, and the use of social media platforms and other Internet-sourced data sources to create neighborhood-level indicators.

Reliability and Validity

The reliability and validity of emerging methods have rarely been examined. In fact, studies using these emerging methods are predominantly "proof-of-concept" studies; in the coming years, we suspect rigorous reliability and validity research will be conducted. However, we provide select examples of reliability and validity research when discussing the specific emerging method for measuring neighborhood characteristics.

Wearable Geospatial Technologies

Researchers can obtain "real-time" geospatial data using wearable devices and sensors, including wearable cameras, such as Microsoft's SenseCam (Kelly et al., 2011), to measure neighborhood characteristics. SenseCam is a life-logging camera that is usually worn around the neck. Its successors, Narrative Clip and Memoto, are small wearable life-logging cameras that can be clipped onto one's clothes. Other cameras in the form of glasses can be used as well, including Google Glasses and glasses often worn during extreme sports to provide point-of-view perspectives on performance. Although Google is perhaps best known for its namesake search engine, Google Glasses work with voice commands to display information in a smartphone-like, hands-free format. The product also comes with a camera attached to it and can be linked to other Google projects such as Google Goggles (an image recognition application), making it a potential tool for neighborhoods and health research. PivotHead, a wearable camera often used in extreme sports, represents another example of wearable computing that can also be used in neighborhoods and health research. These devices allow for the generation of photographs of neighborhood conditions as they are experienced by their wearers to create measures similar to those derived from systematic field observation; however, when using wearable cameras, we can ensure that the participant has indeed been exposed to the neighborhood features shown in the image because they provide a "first-person point-of-view."

Strengths and Limitations

Strengths of using wearable cameras for neighborhood health research include that the researcher sees what the individual participant sees (literally). As discussed, this is known as "first-person point-of-view" and, as such, provides very unique and nuanced data. Research has shown that SenseCam, for example, can be used to measure built environment features (Oliver et al., 2013). Although important, using wearable cameras also has limitations. The constraints include the coding of the generated images to create neighborhood-level variables, which can be difficult and time-consuming, especially when there is inconsistency in image quality. This may render certain photographs as unable to be coded. For example, Oliver et al. (2013) examined the utility of SenseCam to audit and quantify environment features along work-related walking and cycling routes among a sample of 15 employed adults in New Zealand over the span of three weekdays. In reference to the coding of the generated images, they stated that the "[manual] coding of the data was time consuming, taking approximately 25 researcher hours to process the 2,292 images (equivalent to approximately 6.4 hours of journey time)" (p. 6). Machine learning algorithms can be applied to code these images in future research to automate the process. Other limitations include high participant burden and participant reactivity (including the Harkness effect, where individuals may change their behavior because they know it is being monitored). This approach requires specialized training to code and interpret, and there are high costs associated with the equipment used, along with numerous privacy and ethical issues (e.g., data collection in sensitive situations, data collection from nonconsenting third parties). The ethics of using wearable cameras in research has unique considerations and has been discussed in detail (Kelly et al., 2013).

Crowdsourcing Geospatial Data

Crowdsourcing is the practice of obtaining needed services, ideas, or content by soliciting contributions from a large group of people, especially from online communities. In relation to neighborhoods, researchers can evaluate data on neighborhood features such as food stores, including whether a food store exists or on the quality of a food sold at a food store, as well as noise levels, among other nuanced features of neighborhoods and neighborhood amenities, using crowdsourced methods. Examples of pertinent websites that use crowdsourced data include Yelp and Foursquare. Yelp, for example, is a commercial website that provides user-contributed information and reviews of local businesses. The website was founded in 2004 to help people find local businesses and contribute different kinds of content, including reviews, rating scores, and photos of the businesses. A recent publication by Gomez-Lopez and colleagues (Gomez-Lopez et al., 2017) assessed the validity of Yelp in creating a data set of full-line grocery stores in Detroit compared to a business and consumer research database available from Reference USA and the Detroit Food Map, a community-based initiative aimed at creating accurate maps of healthy food retailers. Their results suggest that Yelp served as a more accurate data source than the Reference USA data set in identifying healthy food stores in urban areas when comparing both to the Detroit Food Map. In addition, another study investigated whether Yelp can be used to identify accurately the number of hookah bars in New York State, assess the distribution and characteristics of hookah bars, and monitor temporal trends in their presence (Cawkwell, Lee, Weitzman, & Sherman, 2015). This study found that Yelp data allowed for estimating the presence of such venues and demonstrated that new bars were not randomly distributed, but rather were clustered near colleges and in specific racial/ethnic neighborhoods. In addition, compared with the number that existed prior to 2009, New York has seen a substantial increase in hookah bars in 2012–2014.

Crowdsourcing can be used to process data collected via other approaches. For example, researchers (Ilakkuvan et al., 2014) have used Amazon Mechanical Turk (MTurk), a Web-based marketplace where "requestors" create open calls for "workers" to complete specified human intelligence tasks in return for a small payment (as low as a few cents per task), to annotate photographs of storefronts and point-of-sale terminals of tobacco retailers to enhance tobacco control surveillance. MTurk is often used for tasks, such as image annotation, that humans can achieve more effectively than computers. In this study, MTurk "workers" were used to identify advertisements for electronic cigarettes (e-cigarettes), to identify the lowest advertised price for a cigarette, and to identify the characteristics of individual advertisements on stores. This can decrease the burden of processing images collected from wearable cameras or systematic field observations at a relatively low cost.

Strengths and Limitations

The book *The Wisdom of Crowds* by James Surowiecki (2005) suggests that aggregated answers to questions involving quantity estimation, general world knowledge, and spatial reasoning from a large group of people can outperform the answer given by any of the individuals within the group. However, simultaneously, crowdsourcing introduces challenges such as reliability and validity concerns; differential quality across geographies; and quality control for coding. Crowdsourcing platforms such as MTurk, for example, include the "Work HIT" approval rate, which requestors can incorporate into task qualification requirements (e.g., requiring that over 95% of prior HITS completed by the worker must have been accepted as high quality by the requester) to ensure high-quality service is provided in completing a task.

Social Media and Other Internet-Sourced Data

Recently, researchers have started to apply computational epidemiological methods, such as those used to obtain social media and other Internet-sourced data, to measure neighborhood-level characteristics. This has included data from platforms such as Google, Instagram, and Twitter, to characterize community sentiments and perceptions on specific topics or constructs. We discuss specific applications of Internet-sourced data in the remaining part of this chapter.

Google Searches

Google is a company specializing in a variety of Internet-related services and products and is most well-known for its namesake search engine. Recent research has used Google searches to create an neighborhood-level measure of racism (Chae et al., 2015, 2017). Chae and colleagues (2015) used Google queries containing the "N-word" to predict anti-Black racism within 196 of 210 designated market areas (DMAs) in the United States. Neighborhood racism was defined as the proportion of Google searches containing the "N-word" in 196 DMAs. This study found that rural areas of the Northeast as well as Southern regions of the United States had greater proportions of Google search queries containing the "N-word" and that a one standard deviation increase in the proportion of racist Google searches was associated with an 8.2% increase in the all-cause mortality rate among Blacks in those areas. This measure was also linked to county-level birth data among Blacks collected by the National Center for Health Statistics. Each standard deviation increase in neighborhood-level racism was associated with relative increases of 5% in the prevalence of preterm birth (defined as birth at less than 37 weeks of gestation) and 5% in the prevalence of low birthweight (defined as a weight of less than 2,500 grams at birth) among all Black births.

Instagram

Instagram (acquired by Facebook in April 2012) is a highly popular mobile photosharing application and platform, which allows users to share pictures and videos either publicly or privately. An Instagram account can be also linked to other social networking platforms, such as Facebook, Twitter, Tumblr, and Flickr, to create larger platforms to share images. Users can apply digital filters to their images, and these images can be geotagged with the location of where the user took the image. With each image there is also an opportunity for users to add any comments. Instagram can be used to measure neighborhood-level characteristics, either through the examining of text captions or the images themselves. Studies based in locations in the United States have observed that Instagram posts geotagged in food deserts indicate consumption of food high in fat, cholesterol, and sugar at a rate higher by 5%–17% compared to non–food desert areas (De Choudhury, Sharma, & Kiciman, 2016; Sharma & De Choudhury, 2015). In addition, we have a study to assess the food environment using Instagram as the measurement instrument in the United Arab Emirates (UAE), where it is estimated that 56.37% of the population is considered to be active on social media and 1.72 million individuals in the UAE are active Instagram users (Blogger, 2015). The UAE is considered to be a unique environment in which to conduct such research because of cultural considerations. Religious and cultural norms in the UAE and the Arab world in general imply that photos of family members, specifically women of the family, are to be kept in private, and should not be shared publicly, including platforms such as Instagram. This has been previously recommended by the Islamic religion, as women should not be seen without a specific respectful dress code in front of people that are not family. These recommendations have been integrated with the culture and extended to the use of social media nowadays, as keeping photos of individuals is ultimately considered a way of worship and abiding to the religion's recommendations, as well as a method of maintaining respect to the privacy of individuals' personal life, the family's honor, and the women in the society. Consequently, these cultural aspects among UAE residents made the use of Instagram for neighborhoods and health research particularly useful, as it is more common to use Instagram as a tool to post images of environments, including the food environment, as opposed to posting images of people. In this study, we are using posts from the Instagram application programming interface (API) that are geolocated to UAE. To map Instagram post data of nutritional information, we are first developing a regular expression-matching framework in which each tag on a given post is compared to items in a list of canonical food names. A second matching step is being performed to map the canonical food names corresponding to a post's tags to United States Department of Agriculture food descriptors to associate a nutritional profile with each post to assess the nutritional quality of the overall food environment in the UAE, where GIS data sets on such a topic are unavailable to us.

Twitter

Twitter is a popular online news and social networking service wherein users post and interact with short messages (known as "Tweets"). Approximately 51 million people in the United States use Twitter, with use especially prevalent in urban areas. Tweets are restricted to 140 characteristics, and users can access Twitter via its website or a mobile device app (thus offering the potential to link geolocation to any Tweet where allowed by the user). We recently used geolocated Twitter data retrieved from the Twitter API from January 2014 to June 2014 in New York City as part of our research funded by the National Institute on Mental Health to measure aspects of the neighborhood social environment related to prejudice (Relia, Duncan, & Chunara, 2017). Tweets were classified as homophobic or racist using standard machine language approaches, including (1) labeling a set of Tweets (e.g., each Tweet is assigned a label regarding whether it is "racist" or "not racist"), (2) developing a machine learning algorithm to identify common words or phrases (hereby referred to as "features") that are most frequent in Tweets labeled as racist or homophobic, and (3) labeling the entire data set based on these features. After these Tweets have been classified, their linked geographic location can be used to map them to neighborhoods. Associations between these measures of the neighborhood environment derived from social media and selected health outcomes can then be assessed.

Nguyen and colleagues (2016) also recently utilized the Twitter API to assess neighborhood-level indicators. They also used publically available data from the Twitter API from April 2015 to March 2016, resulting in a collection of 80 million geotagged Tweets from 603,363 unique users across the United States. The authors used machine learning algorithms to construct indicators of happiness, food, and physical activity for census tracts and ZIP code areas and assessed the association of these indicators with neighborhood demographic, economic, business, and health characteristics. In these analyses, greater numbers of fast food restaurants predicted a higher frequency of fast food mentions in Tweets, but greater numbers of fitness centers and nature parks were only modestly associated with higher frequency of physical activity mentions in Tweets. When linked to state-level data collected as part of the United States Behavioral Risk Factor Surveillance System, a higher frequency of Tweets about happiness and physical activity at the state level were associated with lower state-level adult all-cause mortality rates, a lower percentage of adults who were obese, and a lower percentage of adults who rated their health as fair or poor.

Strengths and Limitations

Newly available methods for using Internet-based sources can help researchers to identify novel neighborhood-level risk factors infrequently examined. Earlier, we discussed research that used Google to measure neighborhood-level racism across the United States (Chae et al., 2015, 2017) and work that we conducted using Twitter to measure neighborhood-level racism and homophobia in New York City (Relia et al., 2017). Neighborhood indicators derived from Google and Twitter data, for example, can be used as novel neighborhood-level correlates of a wide variety of relevant health outcomes. Thus, the information derived from social media and other Internet sources provides valuable pieces of information, which have been shown to be linked to vital offline outcomes. Because the content of social media data is unlikely to suffer from censoring, it is easier to express taboo thoughts online rather than through face-to-face interactions or survey instruments (Kreuter, Presser, & Tourangeau, 2008). In addition, relative to many survey measures, online social media measures are also meaningfully available at a finer geographic level, use more recent data, and aggregate information from much larger samples, all relevant for assessing social determinants of health at the neighborhood level. Research using social media and other Internet-sourced data can inform how and what further research is necessary, for example, to use Twitter to construct indicators of neighborhood characteristics consistently and cost-effectively.

Using social media and other Internet-sourced data to measure neighborhood characteristics also has limitations. These include reliability and validity concerns, differential quality across geographies, and opaque reference populations (Chunara, Wisk, & Weitzman, 2017). Related to quality, people can be more likely to Tweet in certain geographies: Twitter data can be biased by the number of people who are regular Twitter users. Regarding the population posting on Twitter, among other social media platforms, it must be recognized that the data used to produce Internet-based measures are created by select populations of those who use these platforms. For example, younger populations might be more technologically literate and use technology more than older populations. One cannot avoid this factor but must be cognizant of it. Researchers should do their best to characterize sociodemographics of social media users, where possible, and report it.

Additionally, it is possible that the search terms and words contained in posts could be incorrect in characterizing certain neighborhood characteristics. For example, if a gay man uses a homophobic term as a term of endearment as a means of reappropriating a slur, this Tweet may incorrectly be classified as "homophobic." However, researchers can develop a protocol in the natural language processing pipeline to address potential issues such as this. More specifically, regarding measuring sentiment correctly, to alleviate capturing terminology incorrectly, natural language processing techniques can go beyond keyword-level filtering. A machine learning algorithm can be implemented to further classify the posts appropriately by using human-labeled examples of, for example, Twitter posts that represent actual instances of homophobic or racist Tweets and instances that represent other ways in which these vernacular terms may be used. We have successfully implemented this in other areas; for example, we implemented a text-based classifier for real-time surveillance of social and news media at a local scale to detect influenza-like illness (Nagar et al., 2014). This required encoding Internet vernacular indicative of "fever," drawing on labeled Tweets that had to rule in appropriate semantic inferences (i.e., body temperature) while ruling out inappropriate ones (i.e., excited).

SUMMARY

Good measures of neighborhoods are critical in studying neighborhoods, including studying how neighborhoods can influence health. As we discussed earlier in this chapter, research connecting neighborhoods and health has characterized neighborhood features in multiple ways. In this chapter, we discussed a range of methods used to assess neighborhood characteristics, including emerging methodological approaches (such as the use of social media and other Web-based data). We discussed the strengths and limitations of each neighborhood characteristic assessment method (e.g., ease of administration, reliability and validity, cost). Given that we presented a range of methods, this may lead to the question—*Is there a "right" way to study neighborhood characteristics?* We note that there is no one correct approach to measure a given neighborhood characteristic. Robert Sampson (2012), in *Great American City: Chicago and the Enduring Neighborhood Effect*, stated that "[the] choice of method depends on the question and the nature of the phenomena under study" (p. 384). In addition, among other issues, we note that the choice depends on the construct being studied and the financial resources available to the investigative team. For example, employing systematic field observation may not be feasible or may not be suited to the assessment of certain constructs (e.g., neighborhood social cohesion).

In addition, it is important to note that each method facilitates understanding the neighborhood environment and yields important insights through a different lens. The different methods may be measuring different dimensions of the same latent construct. However, it is important to underscore that the constructs that each method are tapping into are likely highly interconnected. For example, neighborhood residents might know how much crime happens in their neighborhood (i.e., have some idea of crime statistics of their neighborhood [which may be driven by the media coverage of neighborhood crime often informed by local crime incidents]); this knowledge may in turn impact one's perceptions of safety in that neighborhood. Therefore, moderate correlations between neighborhood crime measured via self-report and via crime statistics are reasonable to expect. Using data from the Detroit Area Study (Lee & Marans, 1980), a study indeed found that objective measures of crime correlated modestly with respondents' subjective feelings of safety in their neighborhoods. Triangulation of methods is important and may paint a truer understanding of the neighborhood environment; however, a few examples exist in the field. In one study, Quinn and colleagues (2016) conducted a study of neighborhood physical disorder (defined as the deterioration of urban environments) in New York City, given that this neighborhood characteristic has been associated with poor mental and physical health outcomes. In this study, 11 trained neighborhood raters used a Web-based system for conducting reliable virtual street audits to collect data on nine indicators of neighborhood physical disorder using Google Street View imagery of 532 block faces in New York City. These researchers estimated neighborhood physical disorder at the center point of each sampled block. Subsequently, they used ordinary kriging to interpolate estimates of disorder levels throughout New York City (Quinn et al., 2016). Taking a triangulation approach to measuring neighborhood characteristics explicitly recognizes that each method has strengths and weaknesses, and the weaknesses of one approach could be compensated by the strengths of another approach.

ACKNOWLEDGMENTS

Dr. Dustin Duncan was funded in part by National Institutes of Health grants R01MH112406, R21MH110190, and R03DA039748 and the Centers for Disease Control and Prevention grant U01PS005122. Dr. Rumi Chunara was funded in part by National Institutes of Health grant R21MH110190. We thank Mr. Seann Regan and Dr. Jessica Athens for commenting on an earlier iteration of this chapter. In addition, we thank the following research assistants in NYU's Spatial Epidemiology

Lab for providing comments and for conducting background research: Aisha Khan and Yazan Al-Ajlouni. We are also grateful for the comments on an earlier, spoken version of this chapter from participants at the Neighborhoods and Health Authors Workshop in Boston in April 2017. We thank the Harvard Center for Population and Development Studies for their support in hosting the Neighborhoods and Health Authors Workshop.

REFERENCES

Auchincloss, A. H., Roux, A. V. D., Brown, D. G., Raghunathan, T. E., & Erdmann, C. A. (2007). Filling the gaps: Spatial interpolation of residential survey data in the estimation of neighborhood characteristics. *Epidemiology (Cambridge, Mass.)*, *18*(4), 469.

Block, J. P., Christakis, N. A., O'Malley, A. J., & Subramanian, S. (2011). Proximity to food establishments and body mass index in the Framingham Heart Study offspring cohort over 30 years. *American Journal of Epidemiology*, *174*(10), 1108–1114.

Blogger, G. (2015). *UAE social media statistics 2015. Global Media Insight: Infographics, Social Media Marketing*. Dubai: Global Media Insight. Retrived from http://www.globalmediainsight.com/blog/uae-social-media-statistics-2015/

Boone, J. E., Gordon-Larsen, P., Stewart, J. D., & Popkin, B. M. (2008). Validation of a GIS facilities database: Quantification and implications of error. *Annals of Epidemiology*, *18*(5), 371–377.

Carr, L. J., Dunsiger, S. I., & Marcus, B. H. (2010). Walk Score™ as a global estimate of neighborhood walkability. *American Journal of Preventive Medicine*, *39*(5), 460–463.

Carr, L. J., Dunsiger, S. I., & Marcus, B. H. (2011). Validation of Walk Score for estimating access to walkable amenities. *British Journal of Sports Medicine*, *45*(14), 1144–1148.

Caspi, C. E., Kawachi, I., Subramanian, S., Adamkiewicz, G., & Sorensen, G. (2012). The relationship between diet and perceived and objective access to supermarkets among low-income housing residents. *Social Science & Medicine*, *75*(7), 1254–1262.

Cawkwell, P. B., Lee, L., Weitzman, M., & Sherman, S. E. (2015). Tracking hookah bars in New York: Utilizing Yelp as a powerful public health tool. *JMIR Public Health Surveillance*, *1*(2), e19. doi:10.2196/publichealth.4809

Cerin, E., Saelens, B. E., Sallis, J. F., & Frank, L. D. (2006). Neighborhood Environment Walkability Scale: Validity and development of a short form. *Medicine & Science in Sports & Exercise*, *38*(9), 1682–1691.

Chae, D. H., Clouston, S., Hatzenbuehler, M. L., Kramer, M. R., Cooper, H. L., Wilson, S. M., Stephens-Davidowitz, S. I., & Gold, R. S., Link, B. G. (2015). Association between an internet-based measure of area racism and black mortality. *PloS One*, *10*(4), e0122963. Reference link is here: https://www.ncbi.nlm.nih.gov/pubmed/25909964

Chae, D. H., Clouston, S., Martz, C. D., Hatzenbuehler, M. L., Cooper, H. L., Turpin, R., Stephens-Davidowitz, S., & Kramer, M. R. (in press). Area racism and birth outcomes among Blacks in the United States. *Social Science & Medicine*.

Chunara, R., Wisk, L. E., & Weitzman, E. R. (2017). Denominator issues for personally generated data in population health monitoring. *American Journal of Preventive Medicine*, *52*(4), 549–553.

De Choudhury, M., Sharma, S., & Kiciman, E. (2016). *Characterizing dietary choices, nutrition, and language in food deserts via social media*. Paper presented at the Proceedings of the 19th ACM Conference on Computer-Supported Cooperative Work & Social Computing.

Duncan, D. T. (2013). What's Your Walk Score®? *American Journal of Preventive Medicine, 45*(2), 244–245.

Duncan, D. T., Aldstadt, J., Whalen, J., & Melly, S. J. (2013). Validation of Walk Scores and Transit Scores for estimating neighborhood walkability and transit availability: A small-area analysis. *GeoJournal, 78*(2), 407–416.

Duncan, D. T., Aldstadt, J., Whalen, J., Melly, S. J., & Gortmaker, S. L. (2011). Validation of Walk Score® for estimating neighborhood walkability: An analysis of four US metropolitan areas. *International Journal of Environmental Research and Public Health, 8*(11), 4160–4179.

Duncan, D. T., Goedel, W. C., Stults, C. B., Brady, W. J., Brooks, F. A., Blakely, J. S., & Hagen, D. (2016). A study of intimate partner violence, substance abuse, and sexual risk behaviors among gay, bisexual, and other men who have sex with men in a sample of geosocial-networking smartphone application users. *American Journal of Men's Health*, pii, 1557988316631964.

Duncan, D. T., & Hatzenbuehler, M. L. (2014). Lesbian, gay, bisexual, and transgender hate crimes and suicidality among a population-based sample of sexual-minority adolescents in Boston. *American Journal of Public Health, 104*(2), 272–278.

Duncan, D. T., Hatzenbuehler, M. L., & Johnson, R. M. (2014). Neighborhood-level LGBT hate crimes and current illicit drug use among sexual minority youth. *Drug and Alcohol Dependence, 135*, 65–70.

Duncan, D. T., Kawachi, I., Kum, S., Aldstadt, J., Piras, G., Matthews, S. A., Arbia, G., Castro, M.C., White, K., & Williams, D. R. (2014). A spatially explicit approach to the study of socio-demographic inequality in the spatial distribution of trees across boston neighborhoods. *Spatial Demography, 2*(1), 1–29.

Duncan, D. T., Park, S. H., Goedel, W. C., Kreski, N. T., Morganstein, J. G., Hambrick, H. R., Jean-Louis, G., & Chaix, B. (2017). Perceived neighborhood safety is associated with poor sleep health among gay, bisexual, and other men who have sex with men in Paris, France. *Journal of Urban Health, 94*(3), 399–407.

Duncan, D. T., Ruff, R. R., Chaix, B., Regan, S. D., Williams, J. H., Ravenell, J., Bragg, M. A., Ogedegbe, G., & Elbel, B. (2016). Perceived spatial stigma, body mass index and blood pressure: A global positioning system study among low-income housing residents in New York City. *Geospatial Health, 11*(2), 399.

Duncan, D. T., Sharifi, M., Melly, S. J., Marshall, R., Sequist, T. D., Rifas-Shiman, S. L., & Taveras, E. M. (2014). Characteristics of walkable built environments and BMI z-scores in children: Evidence from a large electronic health record database. *Environmental Health Perspectives, 122*(12), 1359.

Dunton, G. F., Kawabata, K., Intille, S., Wolch, J., & Pentz, M. A. (2012). Assessing the social and physical contexts of children's leisure-time physical activity: An ecological momentary assessment study. *American Journal of Health Promotion, 26*(3), 135–142.

Echeverria, S. E., Diez-Roux, A. V., & Link, B. G. (2004). Reliability of self-reported neighborhood characteristics. *Journal of Urban Health, 81*(4), 682–701.

Epstein, D. H., Tyburski, M., Craig, I. M., Phillips, K. A., Jobes, M. L., Vahabzadeh, M., Mezghanni, M., Lin, J. L., Furr-Holden, C. D. M., & Preston, K. L. (2014). Real-time tracking of neighborhood surroundings and mood in urban drug misusers: Application of a new method to study behavior in its geographical context. *Drug and Alcohol Dependence, 134*, 22–29.

Frey, N. (2016). Equity in the distribution of urban environmental amenities: The case of Washington, DC. *Urban Geography*, 1–16. Retrived from http://www.tandfonline.com/doi/abs/10.1080/02723638.2016.1238686?journalCode=rurb20

Gibbs, J. J., & Rice, E. (2016). The social context of depression symptomology in sexual minority male youth: Determinants of depression in a sample of Grindr users. *Journal of Homosexuality*, *63*(2), 278–299.

Goedel, W. C., & Duncan, D. T. (2015). Geosocial-networking app usage patterns of gay, bisexual, and other men who have sex with men: Survey among users of Grindr, a mobile dating app. *JMIR Public Health and Surveillance*, *1*(1), e4.

Goedel, W. C., Hagen, D., Halkitis, P. N., Greene, R. E., Griffin-Tomas, M., Brooks, F. A., Hickson, D., & Duncan, D. T. (2017). Post-exposure prophylaxis awareness and use among men who have sex with men in London who use geosocial-networking smartphone applications. *AIDS Care*, *29*(5), 579–586.

Goedel, W. C., Halkitis, P. N., Greene, R. E., & Duncan, D. T. (2016). Correlates of awareness of and willingness to use pre-exposure prophylaxis (PrEP) in gay, bisexual, and other men who have sex with men who use geosocial-networking smartphone applications in New York City. *AIDS and Behavior*, *20*(7), 1435–1442.

Goedel, W. C., Safren, S. A., Mayer, K. H., & Duncan, D. T. (2017). Community-level norms and condomless anal intercourse among gay, bisexual, and other men who have sex with men who use geosocial-networking smartphone applications in the Deep South. *Journal of HIV/AIDS & Social Services*, 1–8. Retrived from http://www.tandfonline.com/doi/abs/10.1080/15381501.2017.1344599

Goedel, W. C., Schneider, J. A., Hagen, D., & Duncan, D. T. (2017). Serodiscussion, perceived seroconcordance, and sexual risk behaviors among dyads of men who have sex with men who use geosocial-networking smartphone applications in London. *Journal of the International Association of Providers of AIDS Care (JIAPAC)*, *16*(3), 233–238.

Gomez-Lopez, I. N., Clarke, P., Hill, A. B., Romero, D. M., Goodspeed, R., Berrocal, V. J., Vinod Vydiswaran, V. G., & Veinot, T. C. (2017). Using social media to identify sources of healthy food in urban neighborhoods. *Journal of Urban Health*, *94*(3), 429–436.

Heynen, N., Perkins, H. A., & Roy, P. (2006). The political ecology of uneven urban green space: The impact of political economy on race and ethnicity in producing environmental inequality in Milwaukee. *Urban Affairs Review*, *42*(1), 3–25.

Hirsch, J. A., Moore, K. A., Evenson, K. R., Rodriguez, D. A., & Roux, A. V. D. (2013). Walk Score® and Transit Score® and walking in the multi-ethnic study of atherosclerosis. *American Journal of Preventive Medicine*, *45*(2), 158–166.

Huang, E., Marlin, R. W., Young, S. D., Medline, A., & Klausner, J. D. (2016). Using Grindr, a smartphone social-networking application, to increase HIV self-testing among Black and Latino men who have sex with men in Los Angeles, 2014. *AIDS Education and Prevention*, *28*(4), 341–350.

Ilakkuvan, V., Tacelosky, M., Ivey, K. C., Pearson, J. L., Cantrell, J., Vallone, D. M., Abrams, D. M., & Kirchner, T. R. (2014). Cameras for public health surveillance: A methods protocol for crowdsourced annotation of point-of-sale photographs. *JMIR Research Protocols*, *3*(2), e22.

Kelly, P., Doherty, A., Berry, E., Hodges, S., Batterham, A. M., & Foster, C. (2011). Can we use digital life-log images to investigate active and sedentary travel behaviour? Results from a pilot study. *International Journal of Behavioral Nutrition and Physical Activity*, *8*(1), 44.

Kelly, P., Marshall, S. J., Badland, H., Kerr, J., Oliver, M., Doherty, A. R., & Foster, C. (2013). An ethical framework for automated, wearable cameras in health behavior research. *American Journal of Preventive Medicine*, *44*(3), 314–319.

Kirchner, T. R., & Shiffman, S. (2016). Spatio-temporal determinants of mental health and well-being: Advances in geographically-explicit ecological momentary assessment (GEMA). *Social Psychiatry and Psychiatric Epidemiology*, *51*(9), 1211–1223.

Kreuter, F., Presser, S., & Tourangeau, R. (2008). Social desirability bias in CATI, IVR, and web surveys: The effects of mode and question sensitivity. *Public Opinion Quarterly*, *72*(5), 847–865.

Landry, S. M., & Chakraborty, J. (2009). Street trees and equity: Evaluating the spatial distribution of an urban amenity. *Environment and Planning A*, *41*(11), 2651–2670.

Lebel, A., Daepp, M. I., Block, J. P., Walker, R., Lalonde, B., Kestens, Y., & Subramanian, S. (2017). Quantifying the foodscape: A systematic review and meta-analysis of the validity of commercially available business data. *PloS One*, *12*(3), e0174417.

Lee, T., & Marans, R. W. (1980). Objective and subjective indicators: Effects of scale discordance on interrelationships. *Social Indicators Research*, *8*(1), 47–64.

Liao, Y., Intille, S. S., & Dunton, G. F. (2015). Using Ecological Momentary Assessment to understand where and with whom adults' physical and sedentary activity occur. *International Journal of Behavioral Medicine*, *22*(1), 51–61.

Marco, M., Gracia, E., Martín-Fernández, M., & López-Quílez, A. (2017). Validation of a Google street view-based neighborhood disorder observational scale. *Journal of Urban Health*, *94*(2), 190–198.

Messer, L. C., Laraia, B. A., Kaufman, J. S., Eyster, J., Holzman, C., Culhane, J., Elo I, Burke J. G., & O'campo, P. (2006). The development of a standardized neighborhood deprivation index. *Journal of Urban Health*, *83*(6), 1041–1062.

Mitchell, J. T., Schick, R. S., Hallyburton, M., Dennis, M. F., Kollins, S. H., Beckham, J. C., & McClernon, F. J. (2014). Combined ecological momentary assessment and global positioning system tracking to assess smoking behavior: A proof of concept study. *Journal of Dual Diagnosis*, *10*(1), 19–29.

Molnar, B. E., Gortmaker, S. L., Bull, F. C., & Buka, S. L. (2004). Unsafe to play? Neighborhood disorder and lack of safety predict reduced physical activity among urban children and adolescents. *American Journal of Health Promotion*, *18*(5), 378–386.

Mujahid, M. S., Diez Roux, A. V., Morenoff, J. D., & Raghunathan, T. (2007). Assessing the measurement properties of neighborhood scales: From psychometrics to ecometrics. *American journal of epidemiology*, *165*(8), 858–867.

Mujahid, M. S., Roux, A. V. D., Morenoff, J. D., Raghunathan, T. E., Cooper, R. S., Ni, H., & Shea, S. (2008). Neighborhood characteristics and hypertension. *Epidemiology*, *19*(4), 590–598.

Nagar, R., Yuan, Q., Freifeld, C. C., Santillana, M., Nojima, A., Chunara, R., & Brownstein, J. S. (2014). A case study of the New York City 2012–2013 influenza season with daily geocoded Twitter data from temporal and spatiotemporal perspectives. *Journal of Medical Internet Research*, *16*(10), e236.

Nguyen, Q. C., Li, D., Meng, H.-W., Kath, S., Nsoesie, E., Li, F., & Wen, M. (2016). Building a national neighborhood dataset from geotagged Twitter data for indicators of happiness, diet, and physical activity. *JMIR Public Health and Surveillance*, *2*(2), e158.

Nykiforuk, C. I., McGetrick, J. A., Crick, K., & Johnson, J. A. (2016). Check the score: Field validation of Street Smart Walk Score in Alberta, Canada. *Preventive Medicine Reports*, *4*, 532–539.

Odgers, C. L., Caspi, A., Bates, C. J., Sampson, R. J., & Moffitt, T. E. (2012). Systematic social observation of children's neighborhoods using Google Street View: A reliable and cost-effective method. *Journal of Child Psychology and Psychiatry, 53*(10), 1009–1017.

Oliver, M., Doherty, A. R., Kelly, P., Badland, H. M., Mavoa, S., Shepherd, J., Kerr, J., Marshall, S., Hamilton, A., & Foster, C. (2013). Utility of passive photography to objectively audit built environment features of active transport journeys: An observational study. *International Journal of Health Geographics, 12*(1), 20.

Oyeyemi, A. L., Sallis, J. F., Deforche, B., Oyeyemi, A. Y., De Bourdeaudhuij, I., & Van Dyck, D. (2013). Evaluation of the neighborhood environment walkability scale in Nigeria. *International Journal of Health Geographics, 12*(1), 16.

Quinn, J. W., Mooney, S. J., Sheehan, D. M., Teitler, J. O., Neckerman, K. M., Kaufman, T. K., Lovasi, G. S., Bader, M. D., & Rundle, A. G. (2016). Neighborhood physical disorder in New York City. *Journal of Maps, 12*(1), 53–60.

Raudenbush, S. W., & Sampson, R. J. (1999). Ecometrics: toward a science of assessing ecological settings, with application to the systematic social observation of neighborhoods. *Sociological Methodology, 29*(1), 1–41.

Relia, K., Duncan, D. T., & Chunara, R. (2017). *What is a neighborhood? Using social media to assess relevant geographies for social processes.*

Rosenberg, D., Ding, D., Sallis, J. F., Kerr, J., Norman, G. J., Durant, N., Harris, S. K., & Saelens, B. E. (2009). Neighborhood Environment Walkability Scale for Youth (NEWS-Y): Reliability and relationship with physical activity. *Preventive Medicine, 49*(2), 213–218.

Rothman, E. F., Johnson, R. M., Young, R., Weinberg, J., Azrael, D., & Molnar, B. E. (2011). Neighborhood-level factors associated with physical dating violence perpetration: Results of a representative survey conducted in Boston, MA. *Journal of Urban Health, 88*(2), 201–213.

Roux, A.-V. D. (2007). Neighborhoods and health: Where are we and were do we go from here? *Revue d'epidemiologie et de sante publique, 55*(1), 13–21.

Ruff, R. R., Ng, J., Jean-Louis, G., Elbel, B., Chaix, B., & Duncan, D. T. (2016). Neighborhood stigma and sleep: Findings from a pilot study of low-income housing residents in New York City. *Behavioral Medicine, 5*, 1–6.

Rundle, A. G., Bader, M. D., Richards, C. A., Neckerman, K. M., & Teitler, J. O. (2011). Using Google Street View to audit neighborhood environments. *American Journal of Preventive Medicine, 40*(1), 94–100.

Saelens, B. E., Frank, L. D., Auffrey, C., Whitaker, R. C., Burdette, H. L., & Colabianchi, N. (2006). Measuring physical environments of parks and playgrounds: EAPRS instrument development and inter-rater reliability. *Journal of Physical Activity and Health, 3*(s1), S190–S207.

Saelens, B. E., Sallis, J. F., Black, J. B., & Chen, D. (2003). Neighborhood-based differences in physical activity: An environment scale evaluation. *American Journal of Public Health, 93*(9), 1552–1558.

Safren, S. A., Hughes, J. P., Mimiaga, M. J., Moore, A. T., Friedman, R. K., Srithanaviboonchai, K., Limbada, M., Williamson, B. D., Elharrar, V., Cummings, V., Magidson, J. F., Gaydos, C. A., Celentano, D. D., Mayer, K. H., & HPTN063 Study Team. (2016). Frequency and predictors of estimated HIV transmissions and bacterial STI acquisition among HIV-positive patients in HIV care across three continents. *Journal of the International AIDS Society, 19*(1), 21096.

Sampson, R. J. (2012). *Great American city: Chicago and the enduring neighborhood effect.* Chicago, IL: University of Chicago Press.

Sampson, R. J., & Raudenbush, S. W. (1999). Systematic social observation of public spaces: A new look at disorder in urban neighborhoods. *American Journal of Sociology, 105*(3), 603–651.

Sampson, R. J., Raudenbush, S. W., & Earls, F. (1997). Neighborhoods and violent crime: A multilevel study of collective efficacy. *Science, 277*(5328), 918–924.

Schwarz, K., Fragkias, M., Boone, C. G., Zhou, W., McHale, M., Grove, J. M., O'Neil-Dunne, J., McFadden, J. P., Buckley, G. L., Childers, D., Ogden, L., Pincetl, S., Pataki, D., Whitmer, A., & Cadenasso, M, L. (2015). Trees grow on money: Urban tree canopy cover and environmental justice. *PloS One, 10*(4), e0122051.

Sharma, S. S., & De Choudhury, M. (2015). *Measuring and characterizing nutritional information of food and ingestion content in instagram.* Paper presented at the Proceedings of the 24th International Conference on World Wide Web.

Shiffman, S. (2013). Conceptualizing analyses of ecological momentary assessment data. *Nicotine & Tobacco Research, 16*(Suppl 2), S76–S87.

Shiffman, S., Stone, A. A., & Hufford, M. R. (2008). Ecological momentary assessment. *Annual Review of Clinical Psychology, 4*, 1–32.

Stone, A. A., & Shiffman, S. (1994). Ecological momentary assessment (EMA) in behavorial medicine. *Annals of Behavioral Medicine, 16*(3), 199–202.

Stone, A. A., & Shiffman, S. (2002). Capturing momentary, self-report data: A proposal for reporting guidelines. *Annals of Behavioral Medicine, 24*(3), 236–243.

Surowiecki, J. (2005). *The wisdom of crowds.* New York, NY: Anchor.

Van Dyck, D., Sallis, J. F., Cardon, G., Deforche, B., Adams, M. A., Geremia, C., & De Bourdeaudhuij, I. (2013). Associations of neighborhood characteristics with active park use: An observational study in two cities in the USA and Belgium. *International Journal of Health Geographics, 12*(1), 26.

Zenk, S. N., Horoi, I., Jones, K. K., Finnegan, L., Corte, C., Riley, B., & Wilbur, J. (2017). Environmental and personal correlates of physical activity and sedentary behavior in African American women: An ecological momentary assessment study. *Women & Health, 57*(4), 446–462.

Zenk, S. N., Horoi, I., McDonald, A., Corte, C., Riley, B., & Odoms-Young, A. M. (2014). Ecological momentary assessment of environmental and personal factors and snack food intake in African American women. *Appetite, 83*, 333–341.

4

STATISTICAL METHODS IN SPATIAL EPIDEMIOLOGY

Samson Y. Gebreab

Historically, analysis of spatial distribution of disease has long played a major role in epidemiology and often underscored the effect of "place" on health—for example, in John Snow's classic 1854 study of cholera distribution in Soho, London. Snow mapped public wells and all the known cholera deaths using dots on a map background, which subsequently formed a pattern of clustering around the fecal-contaminated Broad Street pump as source of the cholera outbreak (Snow, 1855). Ultimately, this study led to better sanitation measures and healthier neighborhoods. Since then, advances in geographic information systems (GIS), global positioning systems (GPS), and availability of geo-referenced health data combined with improved computing power and statistical methods have equipped researchers to perform more sophisticated and, above all, more accurate spatial analyses of disease occurrence. So much so that a new subfield of spatial epidemiology, a hybrid of epidemiology, statistics and geography, has emerged and is increasingly being used to describe the spatial distributions of health outcomes and their relationships with broad placed-based factors at small-area level, with much emphasis on disease mapping, spatial cluster analysis, and ecological analysis (Elliott et al., 2000; Elliott & Wartenberg, 2004).

As with spatial epidemiology, studies of neighborhood health effects share the common goal of investigating how "place" or neighborhood contexts may influence individual behaviors and health outcomes alike (Diez Roux, 2001; Diez Roux & Mair, 2010; Kawachi & Berkman, 2003; Macintyre et al., 2002). Over the last few decades, such studies have indeed contributed significantly to our understanding of how health outcomes are affected by neighborhood contexts (Diez Roux, 2007; Oakes, 2004; O'Campo, 2003). However, many studies of neighborhood effects have traditionally focused on the "internal" characteristics of immediate neighborhood but neglected the effects of the broader spatial environment concerned (Chaix et al.,

2005a, 2005b; Downey, 2006; Morenoff & Sampson, 1997). Analytically, these studies often employ traditional regression, generalized estimating equation (GEE), and/or multilevel models (discussed in the first edition of the textbook; see Subramanian, Jones, & Duncan, 2003), all of these in ways which tend to treat neighborhoods as spatially independent and disconnected units. Often, moreover, for convenience's sake, the neighborhood being investigated is defined on the basis of census or administrative boundaries (Caughy et al., 2007; Coulton et al., 2001; Diez Roux, 2000). (See Chapter 2 for a discussion of how "neighborhood" is defined in relation to health research.) The problem with this assumption is that neighborhoods are rarely spatially independent of each other, as they are most often embedded in, and shaped by, a wider geographical space (Caughy et al., 2007; Chaix et al., 2005a, 2005b; Mennis et al., 2011; Morenoff & Sampson, 1997; Sampson et al., 1999; Sampson & Wilson, 2012; Vogel & South, 2016).

Indeed, previous studies have shown that individuals' behaviors and health outcomes are affected not only by the contexts of their immediate neighborhoods but also by the contexts of those surrounding neighborhoods (Auchincloss et al., 2007a; Chaix et al., 2005a, 2005b; Chen & Wen, 2010; Graif et al., 2014; Morenoff, 2003; Sampson et al., 1999; Sampson & Wilson, 2012), commonly referred to as "spatially proximate" or "extralocal" or "egocentric" or "extended" neighborhoods (Crowder & South, 2011; Graif, 2015; Vogel & South, 2016). For instance, birthweight in Chicago has been found to be affected not only by the contexts of the immediate neighborhood but also by the social environment of the surrounding neighborhoods (Morenoff, 2003). This evidence suggests that neighborhood processes are inherently spatial in nature and that they may display varying degrees of spatial dependence, depending on the scale on which the data are collected and investigated (here, "spatial dependence" describes a geographical phenomenon that observations taken near each other in space are likely to be more similar than those observations taken farther apart). Taking spatial dependence into account is therefore fundamentally important for drawing appropriate inferences from, and making meaningful interpretations of, neighborhood health effects (Legendre, 1993).

Various spatial statistics tools, which spatial epidemiology has developed for dealing with spatial dependence, are pertinent to the study of neighborhood health effects (Anselin, 2013; Auchincloss et al., 2012; Elliott, 2000; Lawson et al., 2003; Waller & Gotway, 2004). However, those methods have been slow to permeate this field, owing to the widespread lack of quality spatial data, of training in spatial thinking, and of access to spatial-statistics software tools (Auchincloss et al., 2012). Today, however, cutting-edge technologies (e.g., GPS and accelerometers) relevant to such study have become more readily available and are capable of generating large amounts of spatially referenced data at multiple levels. Likewise, GIS and spatial statistics tools are growing more accessible. Large-scale integration of spatial epidemiology into the study of neighborhood health effects is therefore the next logical step for addressing a multitude of this discipline's conceptual and methodological challenges (Auchincloss et al., 2012; Dietz, 2002; Matthews & Parker, 2013).

By offering new insights into the direct influence of spatially proximate neighborhoods, as well as their moderating role on the association of immediate neighborhoods contexts with behaviors and health outcomes, spatial epidemiology approaches can greatly enrich our understanding of neighborhood health effects (Chaix et al., 2005a, 2005b; Diez Roux & Mair, 2010; Morenoff, 2003). Spatial epidemiology methods can also allow us to assess directly the spatial scale on which neighborhood processes influence health outcomes beyond the commonly used fixed neighborhood boundaries (Chaix et al., 2005a, 2005b). Additionally, identifying the spatial scale appropriate for addressing given areas of real concern can be a serious contribution to the development of effective health interventions and to the efficient allocation of health resources (Brännström et al., 2015). Finally, spatial epidemiology methods can be valuable tools for generating more reliable and more valid measures of neighborhood context, particularly when the data are missing or sparse (Auchincloss et al., 2007b; Savitz & Raudenbush, 2009).

Although an exhaustive or even comprehensive review of the relevant spatial methods would be beyond this chapter, the present author's objective is to provide readers with a coherent review of the most popular spatial statistics methods useful for the study of neighborhood health effects. Thus, we discuss the strengths and weakness of these methods and examine several examples of their application to neighborhood health research. The discussion is rounded out both by a summary of certain software tools/packages available for implementing the spatial methods and by references pointing the reader to more thorough and comprehensive information about each method described here.

The chapter is organized as follows. In the second section, we provide an overview of the concept of spatial autocorrelation and illustrate its implications for the study of neighborhood health effects. In the third section, we present the specific statistical methods that have been developed for assessing spatial autocorrelation and for detection of clusters. In the fourth section, we review spatial regression models that account explicitly for spatial autocorrelation in the modeling of the relationships between neighborhood contexts and health outcomes. This review includes spatial econometrics and geographical weighted regression; on a more sophisticated level, Bayesian spatial models; and multilevel spatial models.

SPATIAL AUTOCORRELATION

The fundamental concept underlying spatial autocorrelation is Tobler's First Law of Geography: "Everything is related to everything else, but near things are more related than distant things" (Tobler, 1970, p. 236). Although this law was first applied to urban growth systems, its relevance is widely felt in various other applications and in particular in the study of neighborhood health effects. Indeed, several studies have shown that health outcomes and the neighborhood contexts behind them are not randomly distributed in space. On the contrary, they tend to show some degree of clustering across space, depending on the scale at which they are collected and investigated (Elliott, 2000; Elliott & Wartenberg, 2004; Jerrett et al., 2010). This spatial clustering (called "spatial autocorrelation" or "spatial dependence") denotes the pattern in which observations (e.g., cardiovascular disease mortality rates or rates of obesity) that are distributed closely to each other tend to have more similar values than would be expected from mere random chance (Anselin, 1988).

The sources of spatial autocorrelation are manifold (Jerrett et al., 2010; Morenoff, 2003; Waller & Gotway, 2004). (1) It can be generated by diffusion process/"spillover" effect; that is, the reality that spatial autocorrelation is an inherent property of the health outcome. For instance, a health outcome in a given neighborhood may be affected by the health outcomes of the surrounding neighborhoods. This is usually the result of social interactions and movements among individuals located in a close spatial proximity which extends beyond the arbitrarily defined neighborhood boundaries (e.g., census tract or ZIP code) (Browning & Soller, 2014; Sampson et al., 2002). (2) Spatial autocorrelation can be induced by spatial externalities resulting from spatially structured neighborhood contexts (e.g., socioeconomic status or availability of healthy foods), which in turn cause health outcomes to be spatially dependent. (3) Also, a nuisance spatial autocorrelation can be caused by measurement error or by a contextual mismatch due to discrepancies between researchers' respective definitions of neighborhood and the spatial scale on which neighborhood processes actually operate (Coulton et al., 2001; Waller & Gotway, 2004).

Regardless of the sources, the presence of spatial autocorrelation poses serious methodological and substantive challenges, because it violates any assumption of independence and identically distributes errors required by many of the standard nonspatial statistical models used in the study of neighborhood health effects (Legendre, 1993; LeSage & Pace, 2009). Thus, ignoring spatial autocorrelation can lead to inaccurate estimates of, and mistaken inferences about, neighborhood health effects. For instance, an appearance of large and highly inflated neighborhood effect could be generated by spatial autocorrelation rather than reflect a "true" causal relationship, thereby considerably affecting our ability to draw meaningful conclusions about that presumed neighborhood effect. Yet, far from being merely a statistical nuisance that should be corrected, spatial autocorrelation can provide substantive insights into the spatial determinants of health outcomes and into their relevant spatial scales (Brännström et al., 2015; Chaix et al., 2005a, 2005b). For example, a spatial dependence over some given large spatial scale may suggest the influence of large-scale contextual factors, such as health care infrastructure, air or water pollution, state- or federal-level polices, or other massive interventions. Alternatively, spatial dependence between proximate neighborhoods might suggest the influence of local contextual factors, such as local access to healthy foods or local facilities for physical activity, as well as local social environments in which individuals live. Furthermore, identifying the scale at which spatial dependence occurs can also facilitate measurements, and predictions, of neighborhood processes and of health outcomes. It is therefore imperative that quantification and accommodation of spatial autocorrelation should be a routine procedure in the modeling of neighborhood health effects. The following section reviews methods that allow us to assess the presence of spatial autocorrelation and local clusters.

SPATIAL CLUSTER ANALYSES

Investigation of spatial clusters of disease occurrence has been an integral component of spatial epidemiology since at least John Snow's famous mapping of cholera in London (Snow, 1855). A disease cluster is defined as a "geographically and/or temporally bounded group of occurrences of sufficient size and concentration to be unlikely to have occurred by chance" (Knox, 1964). Such investigations of disease clusters in space or in time or both can be useful for addressing public health concerns about environmental hazards and can likewise generate possible etiological clues (Olson et al., 2006). Over the past few decades, several statistical methods have been developed for assessing spatial clustering, and local clusters in spatial epidemiology (a more detailed review of these methods is available in Wakefield et al. (2000a) and in Waller and Gotway (2004).

These methods differ from each other in their objectives and with regard to the types of data they use. The methods can be distinguished from each other as being respectively tests for either "global" or "local" clustering. Tests for global clustering are designed to determine the existence of spatial autocorrelation/clustering across the study area without pinpointing the specific locations of clusters, whereas tests for local cluster detection are used to identify the location of local clusters characterized by elevated (or reduced) disease rates and to determine their level of significance (Anselin, 1995; Waller & Gotway, 2004). There are several methods used to test for global clustering or for local clusters (see Table 4-1). Some of these methods use point data (e.g., case-control data) and others aggregated data (e.g., census tracts or county-level). Point data involve actual locations of cases and of controls, with the controls providing background information on the spatial distribution of the population at risk. However, confidentiality and privacy issues will more often than not restrict point-data use. In such instances, aggregated data, where the cases are aggregated up to some geographical unit level (e.g., census tract, or ZIP code), are more commonly made available for purposes of research, with any privacy concerns being safeguarded in a suitable manner (Olson et al., 2006). Next we provide an overview of the Moran's *I* and of the spatial scan statistic, because these two methods are popular and widely used in various applications, including the study of neighborhood health effects.

Table 4-1 Summary of the Most Commonly Used Tests for Spatial Clustering and for Detection of Clusters

Statistical Methods	*Test of Cluster Type*	*Data Type*	*Author*
Moran's *I* statistic	Global	Area	(Moran, 1950)
Geary's *C* statistic	Global	Area	(Geary, 1954)
Tango's *MEET*	Global	Area	(Tango, 1995)
Oden's *I*pop*	Global	Area	(Oden, 1995)
Cuzick-Edwards' *k*-NN	Global	Point	(Cuzick & Edwards, 1990)
Diggle and Chetwynd's *D* function	Global	point	(Diggle & Chetwynd, 1991)
Besag-Newell's *R*	Global/local	Point	(Besag & Newell, 1991)
Turnbull's CEPP	Local	Point	(Turnbull et al., 1990)
Whitmore's Test	Global	point	(Whittemore et al., 1987)
Geographical Analysis Machine (GAM)	Local	Point	(Openshaw et al., 1987)
Spatial Scan Statistic	Global/local/ space-time	Point/area	(Kulldorff & Nagarwalla, 1995)
Getis-Ord *G* statistic	Local	Area	(Getis & Ord, 1992)
Local Indicators of Spatial Association (LISA)	Local	Area	(Anselin, 1995)

Moran's *I* Statistic

Moran's *I* statistic is one of the oldest and best known for evaluating spatial autocorrelation of continuous outcome data, such as physical activity score and body mass index (BMI) as well as regression residuals (Cliff & Ord, 1981; Moran, 1950). It measures whether observations for neighboring areas are more similar (i.e., spatial autocorrelation) than would be expected under a null hypothesis of no spatial autocorrelation (or no global clustering). A Moran's *I* value ranges between −1.0 and 1.0. A significant positive value of *I* indicates positive spatial autocorrelation, suggesting the clustering of areas with similar high or low values. A significant negative value of *I* indicates a negative spatial autocorrelation, showing neighboring areas have dissimilar values like a chessboard pattern. When Moran's *I* value is close to zero, it indicates "no spatial autocorrelation" or "complete spatial randomness." Statistical significance (*p* value) for Moran's *I* is usually determined by using an asymptotic normality or Monte Carlo tests. Moran's *I* statistic is calculated as

$$I = \frac{n \sum_{i=1}^{n} \sum_{j=1}^{n} w_{ij} \left(Y_i - \overline{Y}\right)\left(Y_j - \overline{Y}\right)}{\sum_{i=1}^{n} \sum_{j=1}^{n} w_{ij} \sum_{i=1}^{n} \left(Y_i - \overline{Y}\right)^2}$$

where Y_i is the value of interest (e.g., mortality rates) in area *i*, $\overline{Y}$ is the mean of the variable of interest, and w_{ij} is an $n \times n$ spatial weight matrix that measures the "closeness" between area *i* and its neighbor *j*. Oftentimes, the spatial weight matrix is symmetric and row standardized so that the sum of neighbors' weights for any particular observation equals 1. There are various ways of defining spatial weights matrix, as defined next.

The adjacency-based spatial weight matrix is defined as

$$w_{ij} = \begin{cases} 1 & \text{if areas } i \text{ and } j \text{ are adjacent} \\ 0 & \text{otherwise} \end{cases}$$

The *k*-nearest neighbors spatial weight matrix is defined as

$$w_{ij} = \begin{cases} 1 & \text{if area } j \text{ is a } k \text{ order neighbor of area } i \\ 0 & \text{otherwise} \end{cases}$$

The distance-based spatial weight matrix is defined as

$$w_{ij} = \begin{cases} 1 & \text{if } d_{ij} < d \text{ for some fixed distance } d \\ 0 & \text{otherwise} \end{cases}$$

where d_{ij} is the Euclidean distance in kilometers between the centroids of neighborhoods i and j, and d is a user-specified spatial autocorrelation scale. In practice, we have no a priori knowledge of the scale of spatial autocorrelation for the variable of interest. Thus, one can calculate Moran's I at successive values of d to plot spatial correlogram and visualize the extent of spatial autocorrelation, as well as select the most appropriate distance beyond which the data are not spatially autocorrelated.

The Moran's I statistic is extensively used in epidemiologic studies for checking the presence of spatial autocorrelation in outcomes and regression residuals (Auchincloss et al., 2012a; Duncan et al., 2013a; Morenoff, 2003). For instance, Duncan et al. used Moran's I when examining the spatial relationship between various built environment features and BMI among a sample of adolescents from a range of racial/ethnic minority groups. The authors found significant spatial autocorrelation after adjusting in the residuals of ordinary least square (OLS) regression, which warranted fitting spatial regression models (Duncan et al., 2013a). A substantive application of the Moran's I statistic is demonstrated by Laraia et al. (see Box 4-1, Case Study 1), who examined the extent of spatial clustering of extreme BMI among diabetic adults from Northern California (Laraia et al., 2014). However, it is important to note that the Moran's I statistic does not account for population heterogeneity. Therefore, a significant-looking positive spatial autocorrelation may be entirely

Box 4-1 Case Study 1: Spatial Clustering of Extreme Body Mass Index Values in Northern California

Using the Moran's I statistic and local clusters using LISA, Laraia et al. evaluated the extent to which spatial clustering of extreme body mass index (BMI) values was explained by either individual-level characteristics or contextual-level factors, in a large sample of diabetic adults in a diabetes survey of Northern California (Laraia et al., 2014). The study found significant global clustering and local clustering of extremely high/low BMI values. However, individual characteristics accounted for more of the clustering of the extreme BMI values than did neighborhood characteristics. The study concluded that the choices, conditions, and preferences of individuals might play a more important role than do neighborhood contexts with regard to how individuals self-select into neighborhoods.

due to clustering in areas with similar high/low population. As alternatives, a modified version of Moran's *I*, Oden I^*_{pop} (Oden, 1995), or Tango's maximized excess events (Tango, 2000) that adjust for a heterogeneous background population are to be recommended. For example, Kulldorff and colleagues reported that Moran's *I* had only a limited ability to detect global clustering of Nasopharynx mortality in the United States, as compared to five other global clustering tests where there was true spatial clustering in the data and suggested that the Moran's *I* should be used for continuous attribute data, for which it was originally designed, and recommended Tango's MEET for global clustering tests for count, or incidence data (Kulldorff et al., 2006b).

Spatial Scan Statistic

The spatial scan statistic is one of the most highly preferred and popular tools for detecting local clusters in various applications, because it offers several advantages over the other methods (Kulldorff, 1997; Kulldorff et al., 2006b). The spatial scan statistic detects clusters, and identifies their location, without prior specification of the suspected location or size, thereby overcoming preselection bias while correcting for multiple comparisons. In addition, it allows adjusting for heterogeneous background population densities. Furthermore, it also allows adjustment for confounding covariates (e.g., demographic variables or socioeconomic status). Finally, the method is applicable to either point or aggregated data and allows detection of spatial, temporal, and space-time clusters as well.

The general statistical theory behind the spatial scan statistic is described in detail by Kulldorff and Nagarwalla (1995). Briefly, the method imposes a circular window on the map and allows the circle centroid to move across the map. For any given position of the centroid, the circle radius varies continuously in size, taking value between zero and some predefined upper limit, common choices being 20% or 50% of the total population. In this way, the method creates an infinite number of distinct circles, each with a different location and size, and each being a possible candidate for a cluster. The method considers both the Poisson and the binomial distribution for modeling disease counts and cases and controls, respectively.

Under the alternative hypothesis, there exists at least one circle with a higher relative risk compared to what lies outside. For every circle, it calculates a likelihood that takes into account the observed number of cases inside and outside the circle. Under the Poisson assumption, the likelihood ratio statistic *LR(z)* given *z* is expressed as

$$LR(z) = \left(\frac{C_z}{E_z}\right)^{C_z} \left(\frac{C-C_z}{C-E_z}\right)^{C-C_z} I\left(\frac{C_z}{E_z} > \frac{C-C_z}{C-E_z}\right)$$

where *LR* is the maximum likelihood ratio within a circular window *z*, C_z is the observed number of cases within window *z*, E_z is the expected number of cases in circle *z*, *C* is the total number of cases in the whole study region, and *I(.)* is the indicator function, which is equal to "1" when the window has more cases than expected under the null hypothesis (otherwise, it is equal to "0"). The circle with the maximum likelihood ratio among all radius sizes at all possible locations is considered as the most likely cluster, also known as the *primary cluster*. In addition to the most likely cluster, the method also identifies other, nonoverlapping, secondary clusters and orders them according to their likelihood ratios. The significance of the most likely cluster is estimated through a Monte Carlo simulation.

Circular spatial scan statistic has been used in numerous epidemiological studies (see details in Auchincloss et al., 2012), including detection of local clusters of prostate cancer grade and stage diagnosis in Maryland (Klassen et al., 2005), brain cancer mortality in the United States (Fang et al., 2004), mental disorder in Sweden (Chaix et al., 2006), and youth substance use in Boston (see Box 4-2, Case Study 2). A limitation of the circular spatial scan statistic is that it is unsuitable for detection of noncircular clusters which tend to follow either rivers or overhead power lines. To address this limitation, the method has been expanded to detect irregularly shaped clusters, including elliptical-shaped spatial scan statistic (Kulldorff et al., 2006a), flexible spatial scan statistic (Tango & Takahashi, 2005), and the maxima-likelihood-first algorithm and the non–greedy growth algorithm (Yao et al., 2011). For example, Doi et al. (2008) adopted a flexible spatial scan statistic over the circular spatial scan statistic to detect clusters Creutzfeldt-Jakob disease (CJD) mortality

Box 4-2 Case Study 2: Spatial Clustering of Youth Substance Use in Boston, Massachusetts

Duncan et al. examined the spatial clustering of youth use of tobacco, alcohol, and marijuana, all this in a sample of 1,292 high-school students aged 13–19 years, from the 2008 Boston Youth Survey Geospatial Dataset (Duncan et al., 2016). In their analysis, the authors used Bernoulli spatial scan models to identify local clusters before and after adjusting for covariates, including age, gender, and race/ethnicity. The study identified one cluster of elevated past tobacco use among Boston youths, which was in the South Boston neighborhood and exhibited a relative risk of 5.37 ($p < 0.001$) after adjustment for the covariates. However, the authors found no significant local cluster in youthful past alcohol or marijuana use before or after adjusting covariates. The study suggested that evaluating spatial clusters of youth substance use can help identify local drug abuse so as to generate etiological clues and devise prevention interventions.

in Japan between 1995 and 2004. This was because the circular scan fails to detect noncircular clusters along the coast of Japan where there is clearly no elevated risk. The study revealed one primary cluster of CJD mortality in Northwest region of Mt. Fuji with a relative risk of 2.28. The study concluded that such spatial cluster analysis can inform potential avenues for future epidemiological studies of CJD etiology and for planning of prevention and health care services. In addition, the spatial scan statistic has likewise been extended for cluster detection of survival data using an exponential probability model (Gregorio et al., 2002; Huang et al., 2007).

Statistical Software Packages

Several software packages are available for spatial cluster analysis. For example, Bivand developed an R "*spdep*" package that allows testing for global and local clustering, including Moran's *I*, LISA, and spatial scan statistic (Bivand et al., 2013). The open-source SaTScan software can also be used to implement spatial scan statistic for detecting purely spatial, purely temporal, or space-time clusters for point- or area-level data (Kulldorff, 2015). GeoDA is another such (free and user-friendly) software, which provides a quick and easy way to calculate, and visualize, Moran's *I* and LISA statistic (Anselin et al., 2006).

SPATIAL REGRESSION MODELS

It is now widely recognized that spatial dependence and spatial heterogeneity are common occurrences in the study of neighborhood health effects. As mentioned in the introduction to this chapter, however, previous studies of neighborhood health effects tend to treat neighborhoods as isolated islands and neglect to examine the effects that spatially proximate neighborhoods may have on health outcomes. Furthermore, many of these studies have analyzed neighborhood health effects using standard nonspatial regression models, such as OLS, GEE, or multilevel models. These models do not take into account the underlying spatial dependence and/or spatial heterogeneity inherent in the data. Although it is very difficult to distinguish these two spatial effects from each other (Anselin, 2001), their presence in neighborhood health data is a serious problem for hypothesis testing and prediction, because they violate the assumptions of independently and identically distributed errors and/or stationarity that many standard nonspatial regression models require (Anselin, 2002). As a result, nonspatial models have been criticized for providing biased estimates and often inflated statistical significance, leading to erroneous conclusions about neighborhood health effects (Anselin, 2002; Chaix et al., 2005a; Havard et al., 2009; Legendre & Fortin, 1989; Legendre, 1993; Xu, 2014).

Spatial regression deals with the estimation and prediction of the association between neighborhood contexts and health outcomes while explicitly incorporating spatial dependence. In recent decades, a variety of spatial regression models have been developed and are increasingly being employed in the study of neighborhood health effects (Auchincloss et al., 2012). It is common practice, however, to first check the presence of spatial autocorrelation in the residuals from standard regression models using Moran's *I* prior to using any of the spatial regression models. If Moran's *I* value shows a significant spatial autocorrelation in the residuals, theoretically one can add all the relevant neighborhood contexts until the spatial autocorrelation is eliminated from the residuals (Wagner & Fortin, 2005). However, this is rarely possible, because of unmeasured or unmeasurable neighborhood contexts, measurement errors, and other model misspecifications. In such instances, it is appropriate to employ spatial regression models that account for the spatial autocorrelation in the model, so as to avoid both bias and inflated significance levels. The following section reviews various spatial regression modeling approaches, starting with simultaneous autoregressive models.

Simultaneous Autoregressive Models

Simultaneous autoregressive (SAR) models are among the most commonly used regression models that account for spatial autocorrelation and examine "spillover" effects (Anselin, 1988, 2002, 2003, 2009; Getis et al., 2004; Morenoff, 2003). SAR models are derived from spatial econometrics and augment the standard linear regression model with an additional term that incorporates spatial autocorrelation. This spatial autocorrelation term is implemented by using a "spatial weights matrix," which specifies the spatial relationships between neighboring data points (either defined by adjacency or distance based), in order to account for the influence that neighboring data points exercise on the variable of interest. In this situation, neighboring data points receive a higher spatial weight. The spatial weights can be applied to dependent variable, independent variable, or error terms, depending on where the spatial autocorrelation is believed to occur. Accordingly, there are three different formulations of SAR models.

The SAR lag model assumes that spatial autocorrelation is an inherent property of the dependent variable itself and accounts for spatial autocorrelation by including a spatially lagged dependent variable (Wy), as an additional predictor, in the model. The SAR lag model is appropriate when the spatial autocorrelation is caused by spatial "spillover effects," reflecting social interactions that extend beyond neighborhood boundaries. Thus, this model has a "substantive" interpretation when used in examining neighborhood "spillover" effects. The spatial lag model builds on the OLS model and can be expressed as:

$$y = \rho Wy + X\beta + \varepsilon$$

where y is a vector of dependent variable of interest, Wy is the spatial lagged dependent variable for y, representing the weighted average of the dependent variable of neighboring areas, W is the spatial weights matrix as defined in the third section of this chapter, X is a matrix of observations of the independent variables, β is a vector coefficient for the independent variables, and ε is the vector of independent and identically distributed random error terms. The term ρ is the spatial autoregressive coefficient for the lagged variable Wy. The ρ value ranges between -1 and 1, while a value >1 indicates that neighborhoods surrounding each other have similar values relative to outcome (e.g., high or low mortality rates), whereas $\rho < 0$ indicates that high-values neighborhoods are typically surrounded by low-values neighborhoods, and vice versa. If $\rho = 0$, then there is no spatial dependence, and the first part on the right-hand side cancels out, leaving us with OLS as an appropriate model.

In contrast, the spatial error model assumes that the spatial autocorrelation is found only in the error term and treats spatial autocorrelation as a "nuisance" parameter by putting a spatially lagged error term (Wu) into the model. This model is appropriate when the spatial autocorrelation is caused by omitted, or unmeasured, spatially correlated variables or by model misspecifications or by contextual mismatch (e.g., mismatch between neighborhood boundaries and the actual phenomenon being examined). The spatial error model can be expressed as:

$$y = X\beta + \lambda Wu + \varepsilon$$

where λ is the spatial autoregressive coefficient for the error terms, Wu is the spatially lagged error term, and the remaining parameters are as described earlier.

Finally, the SAR lagged-mixed model assumes that spatial autocorrelation affects both dependent and explanatory variables, and thus spatially lagged dependent variables and spatially lagged explanatory variables are added to the model. The SAR lagged-mixed is particularly useful in a more complex situation in which the spatial autocorrelation is not fully accounted for by either SAR-lag or SAR-error model.

$$y = \rho Wy + X\beta + WX\gamma + \varepsilon$$

Here, γ denotes the regression coefficients of the spatially lagged independent variables WX.

There are several freely available software packages suitable for implementing the different SAR models. The "*spdep*" package in *R* software has various functions applicable to the SAR models and to the relevant model-selection procedures (Bivand et al., 2013). GeoDa software also provides fast and user-friendly tools for implementing OLS, spatial lag, and error models. In addition, the software provides various diagnostic and model-selection tools that help decide whether any of the SAR models is preferable to the standard regression models and which SAR model specification is appropriate (Anselin et al., 2006).

A first step in determining whether a spatial regression model is preferable to an OLS model is to assess the presence of spatial autocorrelation in the model residuals, by using Moran's *I* or by comparing standard OLS and SAR models through use of the Akaike Information Criterion (AIC). Here, a model with a lower AIC value is a better fit (Akaike, 1974). The second step is to conduct Lagrange Multiplier (LM) testing to determine whether an SAR error or SAR lag model would be most appropriate for modeling the spatial process underlying the relationships between neighborhood contexts and health outcomes (Anselin, 2009). The rule of thumb is that, if only one of the LM-Lag or LM-error tests proves significant, that model should be chosen; if both LM tests are robust and prove significant, the model with the larger test statistic value is to be favored.

SAR models are widely used in social studies but have only just begun to appear in epidemiologic studies (Auchincloss et al., 2012; Duncan et al., 2012, 2013b; Havard et al., 2009). For example, Havard et al. (2009) used the SAR lag model to take into account spatial autocorrelation and obtain more accurate parameter estimates and clarify the association between exposure to air pollution and deprivation index (see Box 4-3, Case Study 3). Other researchers, however, have coupled SAR models with multilevel or standard regression models in two-step procedures to examine "spillover" effects from nearby neighborhoods, also known as spatial externalities (Mennis et al., 2011; Morenoff & Sampson, 1997; Morenoff et al., 2001; Morenoff, 2003) (see Box 4-4, Case Study 4).

Although potentially useful in taking account of spatial dependence in respect of neighborhood health effects, SAR models suffer from several methodological limitations. First, these models are limited to aggregated data; thus, they do not make use of the multilevel structure data in which individuals are nested within neighborhoods. Consequently, findings from these models can be subject to the *ecological fallacy*, a bias that consists of drawing unwarranted individual-level inferences from aggregated-level data when the models are not coupled with traditional multilevel modeling. Second, these models are also prone to the "modifiable areal unit problem (MAUP)," a phenomenon whereby different results are obtained in analyses of the same data by changing the scale and definition of neighborhood units (Openshaw,

Box 4-3 Case Study 3: Simultaneous Autoregressive Lag Model for Accurate Parameter Estimates

Havard et al. investigated the association between traffic-related air pollution and deprivation index over a small area of Strasbourg (France) and assessed the impact of spatial autocorrelation on the association (Havard et al., 2009). The authors first assessed the association between exposure to NO_2 and the deprivation index by using an ordinary least square (OLS) model. However, the Moran's *I* value showed significant autocorrelation in the residuals, which warranted a spatial regression model to avoid violating the assumptions of OLS. The authors then used the simultaneous autoregressive (SAR) lag model to control for the spatial autocorrelation in the data. The results from this study showed significant nonlinear association between the deprivation index and NO_2 levels in both regression models. However, controlling for spatial autocorrelation strongly reduced the strength of the association while highly improving the model's goodness-of-fit. This study suggests a need to take spatial autocorrelation into account in studying the role of air pollution in social inequalities of health, so as to avoid biased and unreliable estimates and therefore erroneous conclusions.

Box 4-4 Case Study 4: Spatial Dynamics of Birthweight in Chicago Using the Simultaneous Autoregressive Lag Model

Morenoff, in his famously seminal work and using data from the Project on Human Development in Chicago Neighborhoods (PHDCN) study, examined the spatial dynamics of birthweight in a large sample of birthweight (n = 101,662) within 342 Chicago neighborhoods (Morenoff, 2003). For this, he followed a two-stage procedure in order to examine the influence of neighborhood contexts, and of spatial externalities (neighborhood "spillover" effects), on birthweight. In the first stage, the author adjusted for individual-level covariates by using a multilevel model. Thereafter, the adjusted birthweight was regressed in respect of neighborhood-level covariates and a spatial lag term using a simultaneous autoregressive (SAR) lag model. The study results showed that violent crime and exchange/voluntarism were significant neighborhood predictors of birthweight. Moreover, the findings also demonstrated significant spatial clustering of birthweight, a result which then warranted the introduction of a spatially lagged exchange/voluntarism component into the multilevel model. The results further indicated that spatial lag in exchange/voluntarism had a positive and significant effect on birthweight. The study concluded that contextual effects on birthweight extend to the social environment beyond the immediate neighborhood.

1984). Furthermore, these models do not allow direct assessment of the spatial scale on which variations in health outcomes operate, unless different neighborhood definitions are specified and tested separately, which can lead to multiple testing problems. Finally, SAR models do not account for the possible nonlinear relationship between health outcomes and neighborhood contexts.

Geographical Weighted Regression

As has already been discussed, most previous neighborhood health effects studies using either standard regression or multilevel models assumed that the relationships between neighborhood contexts and health outcomes are homogenous (characterized by stationarity) over a large study area, an assumption also commonly true of those studies that use spatial econometrics models. These studies typically provide "global" parameter estimates, which implies that the influences of neighborhood effects and contextual policies on health outcomes operate more or less homogeneously over a large study area. In the real world, this is often an unreasonable expectation, given the significantly heterogeneous ways in which actual individual people interact with their respective neighborhoods on different spatial scales. Consequently, one can frequently expect the relationships between neighborhood contexts and health outcomes to vary notably across space—a phenomenon called "spatial heterogeneity" (or "spatial nonstationarity").

In recent years, geographically weighted regression (GWR) has been developed to explore the spatial heterogeneity frequently encountered in the relationships between dependent and explanatory variables across space. The GWR model provides a set of local regression coefficients, which can be mapped and visualized, in order to explore the varying spatial relationships between health outcomes and explanatory variables (Fotheringham et al., 2002, 2003). Moreover, the GWR model also provides other useful local regression results, including the values of t-testing with respect to local parameter estimates, the local R^2 values, and the local residuals for each regression point. The GWR can be expressed as:

$$y_i = \beta_{0i} + \sum_{k=1}^{p} \beta_{ik} X_{ik} + \varepsilon_i, \quad k = 1,\ldots,p, \quad i = 1,\ldots,n,$$

where y_i is the value outcome variable for location i, β_{i0} is the intercept coefficient specific to location i, x_{ik} is the value of the kth explanatory variable specific to location i, β_{ik} denotes the local regression coefficients for the kth explanatory variable specific to location i, and ε_i is the random error terms at location i, which is assumed to follow an independent normal distribution with zero mean and homogeneous variance.

In contrast to the OLS model, which provides a fixed β_k for the whole study area, the β_{ik} local regression coefficients from the GWR model are allowed to vary in magnitude and direction for each location i. The local regression coefficients are calculated by applying a weighting scheme using a distance-decay function, which gives more weight to nearby observations than to those farther away. Typically, the kernel bandwidth can be a fixed or adaptive kernel function (Fotheringham et al., 2002). Fixed kernel uses a fixed bandwidth throughout the study area and is appropriate in situations where data are regularly spaced. On the other hand, adaptive kernels allow varying bandwidth such that small bandwidths are used in areas where the data are dense over space and relatively large bandwidths where the data are sparse over space. Hence, the size of the kernel bandwidth has a large impact on the outcome of the GWR analysis and should be selected carefully. Increasingly smaller bandwidths result in parameter estimates that are highly localized and have a great degree of variance, whereas increasingly larger bandwidths tend toward the normal global regression estimate.

$$w_{ij} = \exp\left[-\frac{\left(d_{ij}/h\right)^2}{2}\right]$$

where d_{ij} is the Euclidean between observations i and j, and h, the bandwidth beyond which the weights are zero and no longer influence the local estimates. The kernel bandwidth is usually determined by using cross-validation calibration methodology (Fotheringham et al., 2002) or by minimizing the Akaike's Information Criterion (AIC) value for the fitted regression model (Akaike, 1974). The AIC is a relative goodness-of-fit statistic for comparing competing models, where the model with the smallest AIC provides the closest approximation to reality.

The GWR model is increasingly being used to explore spatial heterogeneity in epidemiologic studies (Chen et al., 2010, 2012; Gebreab & Diez Roux, 2012; Graif & Sampson, 2009). For instance, Graif and Sampson used GWR to examine the spatial heterogeneity in the association of neighborhood immigrant concentration and language diversity with homicide rates at census-tract level in Chicago using data from the Neighborhood database (Graif & Sampson, 2009). Their results showed language diversity was consistently linked to lower homicide, whereas the level of immigrant concentrations was found to be either unrelated or inversely associated with homicide rates, suggesting substantial evidence that neighborhood characteristics vary in their relationships with homicide across space. Gebreab and Diez Roux also demonstrated the importance of spatial heterogeneity for understanding and

Box 4-5 Case Study 5: Spatial Heterogeneity in Understanding Racial Disparities of Coronary Heart Disease in the United States

Gebreab and Diez Roux examined the spatial heterogeneity involved in Black-White differences with regard to coronary heart disease (CHD) mortality across the United States and assessed the contributions of poverty and segregation to the spatial heterogeneity (Gebreab & Diez Roux, 2012). Age-adjusted county-level CHD mortality rates data for Blacks and Whites in the continental United States between 1996 and 2006 were obtained from the Center for Disease Control and Prevention WONDER online database. The authors used both ordinary least square (OLS) and geographically weighted regression (GWR) models in their analysis. The results from the OLS model showed that, on average for the whole United States, CHD mortality was significantly higher in Blacks than in Whites (mean difference = 27.8 per 100,000). Using a GWR model, however, the result showed significant spatial heterogeneity in Black-White differences in CHD mortality (a median Black-White difference of 17.7 per 100,000, with interquartile range [IQR]: 4.0, 34.0). Moreover, GWR results also showed that segregation was positively associated with CHD mortality in some counties while negatively associated in other counties. However, the study found that the heterogeneity was no longer present after accounting for county differences in race-specific poverty and segregation and for interactions of these variables with race. The study demonstrated the importance of spatial heterogeneity in understanding, and eliminating, racial disparities in CHD mortality, and it suggested that this heterogeneity might not be "natural" or "biologically" determined but, on the contrary, malleable and context dependent.

eliminating racial disparities in coronary heart disease (CHD) mortality between Blacks and Whites across the United States (Gebreab & Diez Roux, 2012) (see Box 4-5, Case Study 5).

Despite its utility as a descriptive and exploratory tool for the study of spatial heterogeneity, GWR has some limitations. The GWR model does not provide exact statistical inference on regression relationships and so should be regarded as a supplement to the standard regression models. Additionally, the GWR model can be unstable, and its local coefficients may suffer from multicollinearity, particularly when variables are correlated or the sample sizes are small (Páez et al., 2011; Wheeler, 2007). GWR modeling is also very sensitive to the choice of kernel bandwidth, and the selection of optimal bandwidth using cross-validation can be computationally demanding, especially when the data are extensive (Wheeler & Tiefelsdorf, 2005). Given these limitations, it is recommended that researchers do model selection and diagnosis as part of their analyses when using GWR (Wheeler & Tiefelsdorf, 2005).

Other researchers have also suggested alternative approaches, such as Bayesian spatially varying coefficient (BSVC) models for modeling spatial heterogeneity in the relationships between explanatory variables and outcomes (Finley, 2011; Waller et al., 2007). For example, Waller et al. compared GWR to BSVC modeling and suggested that BSVC models not only perform better but offer several advantages over GWR (Waller et al., 2007).

The GWR analysis can be implemented by using GWR 3.0 software (Fotheringham et al., 2002), and Wheeler has developed an R package called "*gwrr*" that includes diagnostic tests for collinearity in GWR models (Wheeler, 2007).

Bayesian Spatial Models

The SAR and GWR models outlined in previous sections are based on frequentist approaches where model estimation is largely dependent on the maximum likelihood. However, these models are very limited in their ability both to handle complex modeling characterized by a large number of parameters and to fully account for uncertainties resulting from missing or sparse data or from measurement errors, all of these being problems that can have considerable implications for risk estimations (Carlin & Louis, 2008; Gelman & Price, 1999). Alternatively, Bayesian spatial models offer more flexible approaches than do SAR models with regard to estimating relative risks (disease mapping) and evaluating the effects of neighborhood contexts on health outcomes at a small-area level (ecological analysis). In contrast to frequentist approaches, Bayesian spatial models assume all unknown parameters (e.g., relative risk) as random variables with probability distributions. These Bayesian models combine prior distributions and likelihood data to obtain posterior distributions for the parameters of interest (Carlin & Louis, 2008). Although the implementation of such models requires computer-intensive Markov Chain Monte Carlo (MCMC) simulations, such as Gibbs sampler (Gilks et al., 1995), the availability of the WinBUGS software package (Spiegelhalter et al., 2002a) for implementing MCMC has facilitated the adoption of Bayesian spatial models for disease mapping and for ecological modeling of health outcomes (Best et al., 2005).

One of the main advantages of Bayesian spatial models is that they allow incorporating one or more random effects into the modeling of neighborhood contexts, and health outcomes, at the small-area level (Lawson, 2013; MacNab, 2004). These random effects capture unobserved spatial heterogeneity and/or spatial autocorrelation that cannot be explained by available covariates (Besag et al., 1991). In essence, the random effects can be thought of as latent variables that capture the effects of unmeasured and/or unobserved covariates that are either randomly distributed or spatially structured (Clayton et al., 1993; Richardson, 1992). Additionally, Bayesian spatial models account for different sources of uncertainty related to sparse data, to missing data, and to measurement errors occurring in the modeling process (Bernardinelli et al., 1997; Xia & Carlin, 1998). For example, incorporating spatially correlated random effects permits spatial smoothing by "borrowing strength" from neighboring areas to generate more stable and more reliable risk estimates when the diseases concerned are rare or the data sparse (Besag et al., 1991; MacNab, 2004). Finally, these models can be naturally extended to handle more complicated data structures, such as multilevel data, survival data, and space-temporal data.

There are different formulations of Bayesian spatial models (for more details on those specific formulations, see Best et al., 2005; Lee, 2011). Here, I focus on the Besag York and Mollie (BYM) model, also known as the "convolution model" (Besag et al., 1991), because it is the most popular and benchmark model for disease mapping and for ecological analysis at the small-area level (Best et al., 2005).

The BYM Model

Suppose one wants to study the spatial distribution of cardiovascular disease (CVD) mortality in a study region partitioned into n nonoverlapping neighborhoods (e.g., census tract-level, or county-level), and y_i is the number of CVD cases in the ith neighborhood. The BYM model aims to model the spatial distribution of CVD via a three-stage hierarchical model (Lawson et al., 2003; Wakefield et al., 2000b).

First-Stage Model

The observed number of CVD mortality cases in each neighborhood is assumed to follow a Poisson distribution with mean $R_i E_i$.

$$y_i | R_i \sim Poisson(R_i E_i), \quad i = 1, \ldots, n,$$

where R_i represents the relative risk of CVD mortality in the ith neighborhood, which is our parameter of interest, and E_i is the expected number of CVD cases in the ith neighborhood, typically adjusted for age and sex.

The BYM model assumes that the log relative risk of CVD mortality can be broken down into two random effects: a spatially uncorrelated random effect and a spatially correlated random effect.

$$\log(R_i) = \log(E_i) + \beta_0 + X_i\beta + V_i + U_i$$

where $\log(E_i)$ is an offset term, β_0 is the intercept, X_i represents the matrix of covariates for the ith neighborhood, with coefficients β, V_i is the spatial uncorrelated random effect, and U_i is the spatial correlated random effect.

Second-Stage Model

Within the Bayesian framework, a prior distribution for the random effects, an intercept term, and coefficients are specified. The spatially uncorrelated random effect V_i is assumed to be independent and identically distributed with normal distribution of zero mean and common variance σ_v^2.

$$V_i \sim N(0, \sigma_v^2),$$

The spatially correlated random effect U_i is assumed to follow an intrinsic conditional autoregressive (ICAR) model (Besag et al., 1991), which accounts for spatial correlation for area i through a weighted average of the random effects for areas that are neighbors of i. The ICAR model is expressed as:

$$U_i | U_{j, j \neq i} \sim N\left(\frac{\sum_j w_{ij} u_j}{\sum_j w_{ij}}, \frac{\sigma_u^2}{\sum_j w_{ij}}\right), \quad i = 1, \ldots, n,$$

where w_{ij} is the spatial weight matrix defining the spatial adjacency of neighborhood i and its neighbor j. If two neighborhoods, i and j, are adjacent (i.e., share a common border), $w_{ij} = 1$; otherwise, $w_{ij} = 0$. Thus, the estimated risk for CVD mortality in each neighborhood i is conditional on the risks of the surrounding neighborhoods. The precision parameters σ_v^2 and σ_u^2 control the amount of variability in V_i and U_i, respectively. The BYM can therefore be useful in determining the extent, and the amount of spatial clustering in the data. For example, one can compute the relative importance of spatially correlated random effects compared to uncorrelated heterogeneity random effects from the posterior distribution of ψ as shown here (Best et al., 1999; Eberly & Carlin, 2000):

$$\psi = \frac{sd(u)}{sd(v) + sd(u)}$$

where *sd(v)* and *sd(u)* are the empirical marginal standard deviations of V_i and U_i, respectively. The parameter ψ ranges between 0 and 1. If the estimate of ψ is close to

1, then the total variation is dominated by the spatial clustering, while a value close to 0 indicates that the spatial clustering is negligible.

Third-Stage Model

Under the fully Bayesian settings, hyperprior distributions are specified for the hyperparameters of intercept β_0, the regression coefficients β, and precision parameters σ_ν^2 and σ_ν^2. For the parameters of β_0 and β, improper uniform or normal priors with large variance are often specified as representative of vague beliefs. Gamma prior distributions are typically specified for the inverse of the two precisions parameters σ_ν^2 and σ_ν^2 (Wakefield et al., 2000a). For more detailed information on issues related to the selection and interpretation of the various hyper-prior distributions, readers can refer to Bernardinelli et al. (1995) and Kelsall and Wakefield (1999). The BYM model can be fitted by using MCMC simulation, which is implemented by using WinBUGS software (Spiegelhalter et al., 2002c). The software also provides a deviance information criterion (DIC) for checking both goodness-of-fit and model comparison (Spiegelhalter et al., 2002b).

A number of studies have used the BYM CAR model for disease mapping and for ecological analysis (Auchincloss et al., 2012; Dominguez-Berjon et al., 2010; Goovaerts & Gebreab, 2008; MacNab, 2004; Wakefield, 2007). For example, Dominguez Berjoni et al. examined the geographic variation of CVD mortality in relation to deprivation index and environments variables using the BYM Poisson model at the census tract level within Madrid, Spain (see Box 4-6, Case Study 6, for details) (Dominguez-Berjon et al., 2010). Although most studies use BYM model for single disease outcome, other studies expanded the BYM CAR model into shared component models (SCM) or multivariate CAR (MCAR) models for joint spatial modeling of bivariate or multiple disease outcomes. For example, Liese et al. examined similarities of the spatial patterns between type 1 diabetes mellitus (T1DM) and type 2 diabetes mellitus (T2DM) using the sparse Poisson MCAR (SPMCAR) model among youth aged 10–19 years in four US states using data from the *SEARCH* for diabetes in Youth study (Liese et al., 2010). The SPMCAR is an extension of MCAR model, which accounts for sparseness of data by adding an indicator term for areas with zero and nonzero count. The authors found evidence of geographical variation in T1DM and T2DM incidence and evidence for joint spatial correlation between the two types of diabetes. In addition, the BYM CAR model has been expanded for spatial-temporal and survival analysis (Casper et al., 2016; Kleinschmidt et al., 2001). Recently, for example, Casper et al. used the Bayesian spatial-temporal model to investigate changes in geographic patterns of heart disease mortality in the United States during 40 years (Casper et al., 2016; see Box 4-7, Case Study 7). Finally, few

Box 4-6 Case Study 6: Geographic Variation of Cardiovascular Disease Mortality in Spain Using the Bayesian Spatial Model

Dominguez Berjoni et al. used a Bayesian spatial model to examine the geographic variation of cardiovascular disease (CVD) mortality at census-tract levels in Madrid, using data from the Madrid Regional Statistics Institute and from Spain's national Census. First, the authors calculated raw standardized mortality ratios (SMRs) of CVD mortality (Dominguez-Berjon et al., 2010). Second, the authors used the Besag York and Mollie (BYM) model, where the spatial correlation in one census tract and its neighbors was accounted for by a conditional autoregressive (CAR) model, to estimate smoothed relative risks (RRs) of CVD mortality and to evaluate the association with deprivation-index and environmental variables. The study results showed that the BYM model produced more precise estimates of CVD mortality RRs compared to the SMRs and identified census tracts with excess risk of CVD mortality. Furthermore, the CVD mortality was strongly associated with deprivation, but that finding was slightly attenuated after adjusting for perceived lack of green spaces and for delinquency. The study demonstrated BYM modeling's usefulness for accurate estimation of RRs of CVD mortality and for identifying areas of real excess mortality as well as for accurate targeting of public health interventions.

Box 4-7 Case Study 7: Spatial-Temporal Bayesian Modeling of Heart Disease Mortality in the United States

Casper et al. used a spatial-temporal Bayesian model to examine changes in geographic patterns of heart disease mortality in the United States from 1973 to 2010 (during 40 years) using data from the National Vital Statistics System of the National Center for Health Statistics (Casper et al., 2016). In their approach, a fully Bayesian spatial temporal model that accounts for temporal correlation of rates within a given county and spatial correlation of rates across adjacent counties was used to borrow strength across both space and time. In this way, the model produced precise rate estimates, especially in areas with sparse populations. Results from this study showed significant geographic changes in heart disease mortality observed over a relatively short period of time, with a shift of high-rate counties from the Northeast to the Deep South. Furthermore, the rates in the Northeast were found to have declined much faster than those in the Deep South. The study suggested that these dramatic changes in geographic patterns of heart disease mortality may be due to variability in biomedical, behavioral, and socioenvironmental factors.

studies have also used Bayesian geostatistical models for examining the spatial variation of health outcomes across continuous spaces using either point-referenced data or multilevel data (Chaix et al., 2005a, 2005b; Gemperli et al., 2004).

Multilevel Spatial Models

In studies of neighborhood health effects, we are interested in investigating the individual's health outcome as a phenomenon embedded in neighborhood contexts. To that end, we often collect data at multiple levels where individuals are nested within neighborhoods, other communities, cities, or states. In such situations, standard regression models are not appropriate for the hierarchal-level data concerned, because individual-level observations are not independent. Researchers traditionally use multilevel models that allow simultaneous examination of the effects that individual- and neighborhood-level factors alike have on health outcomes. These models account for nonindependence of observations within neighborhoods (i.e., clustering of individuals within those neighborhoods) and thus provide correct standard errors, and thereby robust estimates, for the association between neighborhood-level factors and health outcomes (Bryk & Raudenbush, 1992). Furthermore, these models also allow researchers to quantify both within- and between-neighborhood variations in health outcomes, such as the intraclass correlation coefficient (ICC) (Snijders & Bosker, 2011) as well as the contribution of individual- and neighborhood-level factors to the variations at either level (Diez Roux, 2000). For example, multilevel models can be used to estimate the ICC, which represents the percentage of variance between neighborhoods.

However, one of the major limitations of multilevel modeling is that it treats neighborhoods as spatially independent from each other. This is often an imprudent expectation, because neighborhoods that are close to each other tend to have similar health outcomes as the result of "spillover" effects, spatial externalities, or omitted, unmeasured, and/or contextual mismatch. Failure to take such spatial dependence into account can lead to overestimation of the statistical significance and distort understanding of neighborhood health effects (Chaix et al., 2005b; Dietz, 2002; Xu, 2014). Furthermore, traditional multilevel models are notorious for relying on arbitrary definition of census-based or administrative neighborhood boundaries, which do not always reflect the actual residents' neighborhood activities (Coulton et al., 2001). Often, that kind of misperception results in MAUP (Openshaw, 1984) and more generally in inaccurate conclusions about neighborhood health effects. Finally, traditional multilevel models may not provide enough detail on the geographic scale at which variations in health outcomes operate, unless one tests different neighborhood definitions, a course which itself can result in multiple testing problems (Xu, 2014).

Although many of the spatial regression models outlined in the previous sections are useful for incorporating spatial dependence between neighborhoods, they are limited to aggregate-level data, and thus they do not take advantage of the multilevel data structures encountered in neighborhood health studies (admittedly, though, BYM modeling has been extended to handle multilevel data structures). To address the limitations of purely spatial models and of traditional multilevel models, some researchers have offered solutions by adding spatial dependence to the residuals of the traditional multilevel models via two-stage procedures (Morenoff et al., 2001; Sampson et al., 1999). In the first stage, the outcome variables are fitted to multilevel models adjusting for potentially confounding effects of individual-level covariates. In the second stage, the adjusted outcomes (residuals) from the multilevel models were regressed on neighborhood-level covariates using spatial lag models (see Case Study 4). This way the spatial lag models explicitly account for the spatial dependence in the residuals between neighborhoods. However, the two-stage procedures are statistically inefficient and may produce insufficiently precise estimates, especially when the sample size is small. Furthermore, the two-stage approaches are also subject to some of the limitations of the SAR models discussed previously.

Recently, a very few researchers have developed multilevel spatial models that integrate both spatial models and traditional multilevel models. These models explicitly consider both the spatial autocorrelation between neighborhoods and within-neighborhood correlation (Chaix et al., 2005a, 2005b; Savitz & Raudenbush, 2009; Xu, 2014). Chaix and colleagues are the first to have introduced multilevel-spatial models, which they termed "hierarchical geostatistical logistic models" (Chaix et al., 2005a, 2005b). In one study modeling healthcare utilization in France (Chaix et al., 2005a) and in another modeling mental disorder in Malmo in Sweden (Chaix et al., 2005b), these authors compared traditional multilevel models with hierarchical geostatistical logistic ones, which incorporate spatial correlation in a continuous space rather than rely on administrative boundaries. The conclusion was that, in both those two studies, hierarchical geostatistical logistic models provided more accurate standard errors for risk factors than did traditional multilevel modeling, which did not account for spatial autocorrelation. Furthermore, the authors indicated that the hierarchical geostatistical logistic models provided detailed information on the scale of spatial variations, and that this latter information facilitated a better understanding of the spatial variations in health outcomes and of those variations' relationships with neighborhood contexts. Similarly, Xu has conducted simulation-based comparison between traditional multilevel, pure spatial, and multilevel spatial models and found that multilevel spatial modeling provides better estimates of random effects variance with regard to both within-neighborhood correlation and between-neighborhoods spatial autocorrelation (Xu, 2014).

Other researchers too have developed innovative formulations of multilevel spatial models. For example, Arcaya et al. used a conditional autoregressive (CAR) model to incorporate spatial dependence into traditional multilevel modeling to capture place and spatial variations simultaneously in US county-level life expectancy study in which states are treated as a higher level of hierarchy (Arcaya et al., 2012). Dong and Harris developed hierarchical spatial autoregressive models for geographically hierarchical data in which spatial dependence is simultaneously modeled at higher and lower level units (Dong & Harris, 2015). Browne and colleagues also developed a more complex spatial multiple membership model that incorporates spatial dependence while individuals are allowed to be influenced by both their immediate and neighboring contexts. Savitz and Raudenbush adopted an empirical Bayes approach to extend the traditional multilevel model by adding spatial dependence, using spatial contiguity at the neighborhood level, which is referred to as empirical Bayes spatial (EBS) estimator (Savitz & Raudenbush, 2009). The authors demonstrated that the EBS model provided more precise, more stable estimation of neighborhood social processes than did the OLS estimator and the empirical Bayes estimator (EBE) based on the traditional multilevel (Savitz & Raudenbush, 2009).

We refer to Xu (2014) for a detailed description of the multilevel spatial model. A general formulation of the multilevel spatial model takes the form of a generalized linear mixed model and consists of within-neighborhood correlation and between-neighborhood spatial correlation random effects as shown:

$$y_{ij} = \beta_{0j} + X_{ij}\beta + Z_j\gamma + V_j + U_j$$

where y_{ij} is the health outcome of the ith individual in neighborhood j, β_{0j} and β_j are the individual-level intercept and coefficients, respectively, X_{ij} represents the individual-level covariates in neighborhood j, and Z_j signifies the neighborhood-level variables in neighborhood j and γ represents the coefficients associated with neighborhood-level variables Z_j, while V_j represents within-neighborhood correlation, which is assumed to be a normally distributed random intercept with mean 0 and variance σ_v^2, and U_j represents the spatial random effects term, which captures spatial dependence between neighborhoods.

There are different ways of modeling the spatial random effects, U_i. One approach is to use an ICAR model (Besag et al., 1991). However, the ICAR model relies on a spatial lattice based on predefined neighborhood boundaries, which may be regular or irregular in shape and thus may not be optimal for modeling spatial variations across a continuous space. A second approach to modeling spatial random effects is to adopt an isotropic geostatistical model. This model assumes that the correlation between observations is a function of distance and one or more function parameters; thus, it allows us to model spatial variations across continuous space (Chaix et al., 2005b). In this approach, the spatial random effects, U_i, is commonly modeled using stationary, isotropic Gaussian process with mean zero.

$$U_j \sim N\left(0, \sigma_u^2 \Phi(\theta)\right)$$

where σ_u^2 is the spatial variance also known as sill, Φ is the correlation matrix that specifies the rate at which the spatial correlation declines as the distance between the two locations *i* and *j* increases. One can use the individual-level locations, although these data are often unavailable due to confidentiality considerations. Instead, the centroid of the neighborhoods can be used as a proxy for the individual location when the individual-level locations are unavailable (Chaix et al., 2005a, 2005b) or when a large number of different locations are computationally too expensive to be fully incorporated (Clark & Gelfand, 2006). The most popular choice of correlation matrix is the exponential decay model and takes the following form:

$$\Phi_{ij} = \exp\left(-\theta d_{ij}\right)$$

where d_{ij} is the Euclidean distance between locations *i* and *j*, θ is the range parameter that models the decay of spatial correlation with distance, with a large value of θ indicates a rapid decline in the spatial correlation while a small value indicates a slow decline in spatial autocorrelation. In practice, the effective range (θ) is often estimated as the distance where the spatial correlation drops below 5% (Banerjee et al., 2004). Analytically, most of the multilevel-spatial models described earlier are implemented under a fully Bayesian setting, using MCMC simulations performed with either WinBUGS (Spiegelhalter et al., 2002c) or MLwiN software (Browne, 2017). However, a simpler form of multilevel spatial modeling based on an empirical Bayes approach can be implemented via HLM 7 software (Raudenbush, 2013).

SUMMARY

This chapter responds to a pressing need for spatial statistical methods in neighborhood health studies. It has been widely recognized that neighborhoods are not independent from each other and that spatial dependence is a common occurrence in the study of neighborhood health effects. Yet, thus far, epidemiologists have too often tended not to incorporate spatial dependence between neighborhoods into their research. Spatial epidemiology has nonetheless developed a wide variety of readily accessible spatial statistical methods that potentially allow researchers to take spatial dependence into account so as to attain a better understanding of neighborhood health effects than has previously been known. It is regrettable that researchers have proven very slow to integrate these methods into their work in that field. The chapter facilitates this integration by describing the concepts of spatial dependence and/or spatial heterogeneity and providing an overview of the most popular and widely used spatial methods applicable to spatial epidemiology.

These methods range from tools for assessing spatial autocorrelation to more sophisticated Bayesian approaches and multilevel spatial models that take into consideration not only within-neighborhood correlations but also spatial correlations between neighborhoods. The author highlights the strengths and weaknesses of the methods and provides guidance for the appropriate choice of such tools in the study of neighborhood health effects. As researchers become more comfortable with including spatial methods in their analyses, one can anticipate that these methodologies will prove to be routine components in the study of neighborhood health effects and ultimately provide opportunities for researchers to look anew at the contributions of both space- and place-based factors to individual behaviors and health outcomes alike.

REFERENCES

Akaike, H. (1974). A new look at the statistical model identification. *IEEE Transactions on Automatic Control, 19*(6), 716–723.

Anselin, L. (1988). *Spatial econometrics: Methods and models*. Dordrecht: Kluwer Academic.

Anselin, L. (1995). Local Indicators of Spatial Association—LISA. *Geographical Analysis, 27*(2), 93–115.

Anselin, L. (2001). Spatial econometrics. In B. H. Baltagi (Eds.), *A companion to theoretical econometrics* (pp. 310–330). Malden, MA: Blackwell.

Anselin, L. (2002). Under the hood: Issues in the specification and interpretation of spatial regression models. *Agricultural Economics, 27*, 247–267

Anselin, L. (2003). Spatial externalities, spatial multipliers, and spatial econometrics. *International Regional Science Review, 26*(2), 153–166.

Anselin L (2009). Spatial Regression. In A. S. Fotheringham & P. A. Rogerson (Eds.), *The SAGE Handbook of Spatial Analysis* (pp. 254–270). London: SAGE Publications.

Anselin, L., Syabri, I., & Kho, Y. (2006). GeoDa: An introduction to spatial data analysis. *Geographical Analysis, 38*(1), 5–22.

Arcaya, M., Brewster, M., Zigler, C. M., & Subramanian, S. V. (2012). Area variations in health: A spatial multilevel modeling approach. *Health Place, 18*(4), 824–831.

Auchincloss, A. H., Diez Roux, A. V., Brown, D. G., O'Meara, E. S., & Raghunathan, T. E. (2007a). Association of insulin resistance with distance to wealthy areas: the multi-ethnic study of atherosclerosis. *American Journal of Epidemiology, 165*(4), 389–397.

Auchincloss, A. H., Diez Roux, A. V., Brown, D. G., Raghunathan, T. E., & Erdmann, C. A. (2007b). Filling the gaps: Spatial interpolation of residential survey data in the estimation of neighborhood characteristics. *Epidemiology, 18*(4), 469–478.

Auchincloss, A. H., Gebreab, S. Y., Mair, C., & Diez Roux, A. V. (2012). A review of spatial methods in epidemiology, 2000–2010. *Annual Review of Public Health, 33*, 107–122.

Banerjee, S., Carlin, B. P., & Gelfand, A. E. (2004). *Hierarchical modeling and analysis for spatial data.* Boca Raton, FL: CRC Press.

Bernardinelli, L., Clayton, D., & Montomoli, C. (1995). Bayesian estimates of disease maps: How important are priors? *Statistics in Medicine, 14*(21–22), 2411–2431.

Bernardinelli, L., Pascutto, C., Best, N. G., & Gilks, W. R. (1997). Disease mapping with errors in covariates. *Statistics in Medicine, 16*(7), 741–752.

Besag, J., & Newell, J. (1991). The detection of clusters in rare diseases. *Journal of the Royal Statistical Society. Series A (Statistics in Society), 154*(1), 143–155.

Besag, J., York, J., & Mollie, A. (1991). Bayesian image restoration with two applications in spatial statistics. *Annals of the Institute of Statistical Mathematics 43*, 1–20.

Best, N., Richardson, S., & Thomson, A. (2005). A comparison of Bayesian spatial models for disease mapping. *Statistical Methods in Medical Research, 14*(1), 35–59.

Best, N. G., Arnold, R. A., Thomas, A., Waller, L. A., & Conlon, E. M. (1999). Bayesian models for spatially correlated disease and exposure data. In J. M. Bernardo, J. O. Berger, A. P. Dawid, & A. F. M. Smith (Eds.), *Bayesian Statistics 6* (pp. 131–156). Oxford, UK: Oxford University Press.

Bivand, R. S., Pebesma, E., & Gómez-Rubio, V. (2013). *Applied spatial data analysis with R.* New York, NY: Springer.

Brännström, L., Trolldal, B., & Menke, M. (2015). Spatial spillover effects of a community action programme targeting on-licensed premises on violent assaults: evidence from a natural experiment. *Journal of Epidemiology and Community Health.* doi:10.1136/jech-2015-206124

Browne, W. J. (2017). MCMC estimation in MLwiN v3.00. Centre for Multilevel Modelling, University of Bristol.

Browning, C. R., & Soller, B. (2014). Moving beyond neighborhood: Activity spaces and ecological networks as contexts for youth development. *Journal of Policy Development Research, 16*(1), 165–196.

Bryk, A. S., & Raudenbush, S. W. (1992). *Hierarchical linear models: Applications and data analysis methods.* Thousand Oaks, CA: Sage.

Carlin, B. P., & Louis, T. A. (2008). *Bayesian methods for data analysis* (3rd ed.). Boca Raton, FL: CRC Press.

Casper, M., Kramer, M. R., Quick, H., Schieb, L. J., Vaughan, A. S., & Greer, S. (2016). Changes in the geographic patterns of heart disease mortality in the United States: 1973 to 2010. *Circulation, 133*(12), 1171–1180.

Caughy, M. O. B., Hayslett-McCall, K. L., & O'Campo, P. J. (2007). No neighborhood is an island: Incorporating distal neighborhood effects into multilevel studies of child developmental competence. *Health & Place, 13*(4), 788–798.

Chaix, B., Leyland, A. H., Sabel, C. E., Chauvin, P., Råstam, L., Kristersson, H., & Merlo, J. (2006). Spatial clustering of mental disorders and associated characteristics of the neighbourhood context in Malmö, Sweden, in 2001. *Journal of Epidemiology and Community Health, 60*(5), 427–435.

Chaix, B., Merlo, J., & Chauvin, P. (2005a). Comparison of a spatial approach with the multilevel approach for investigating place effects on health: the example of healthcare utilisation in France. *Journal of Epidemiology and Community Health, 59*(6), 517–526.

Chaix, B., Merlo, J., Subramanian, S. V., Lynch, J., & Chauvin, P. (2005b). Comparison of a spatial perspective with the multilevel analytical approach in neighborhood studies: The case of mental and behavioral disorders due to psychoactive substance use in Malmo, Sweden, 2001. *American Journal of Epidemiology, 162*(2), 171–182.

Chen, D.-R., & Wen, T.-H. (2010). Elucidating the changing socio-spatial dynamics of neighborhood effects on adult obesity risk in Taiwan from 2001 to 2005. *Health & Place, 16*(6), 1248–1258.

Chen, V. Y., Deng, W. S., Yang, T. C., & Matthews, S. A. (2012). Geographically weighted quantile regression (GWQR): An application to U.S. mortality data. *Geographical Analysis, 44*(2), 134–150.

Chen, V. Y., Wu, P. C., Yang, T. C., & Su, H. J. (2010). Examining non-stationary effects of social determinants on cardiovascular mortality after cold surges in Taiwan. *Science of the Total Environment, 408*(9), 2042–2049.

Clark, J. S., & Gelfand, A. E. (2006). *Hierarchical modelling for the environmental sciences: Statistical methods and applications.* Oxford, UK: Oxford University Press.

Clayton, D. G., Bernardinelli, L., & Montomoli, C. (1993). Spatial correlation in ecological analysis. *International Journal of Epidemiology, 22*(6), 1193–1202.

Cliff, A. D., & Ord, J. K. (1981). *Spatial processes: Models & applications.* London: Pion.

Coulton, C.J., Korin, Chan, T., & Su, M. (2001). Mapping residents' perceptions of neighborhood boundaries: A methodological note. *American Journal of Community Psychology, 29*(2), 371–382.

Crowder, K., & South, S. J. (2011). Spatial and temporal dimensions of neighborhood effects on high school graduation. *Social Science Research, 40*(1), 87–106.

Cuzick, J., & Edwards, R. (1990). Spatial clustering for inhomogeneous populations. *Journal of the Royal Statistical Society. Series B (Methodological), 52*(1), 73–104.

Dietz, R. D. (2002). The estimation of neighborhood effects in the social sciences: An interdisciplinary approach. *Social Science Research, 31*(4), 539–575.

Diez Roux, A. V. (2000). Multilevel analysis in public health research. *Annual Review of Public Health, 21*, 171–192.

Diez Roux, A. V. (2001). Investigating neighborhood and area effects on health. *American Journal of Public Health, 91*(11), 1783–1789.

Diez Roux, A. V. (2007). Neighborhoods and health: Where are we and were do we go from here? *Review of Epidemiology Sante Publique, 55*(1), 13–21.

Diez Roux, A. V., & Mair, C. (2010). Neighborhoods and health. *Annals of the New York Academy of Sciences, 1186*(1), 125–145.

Diggle, P. J., & Chetwynd, A. G. (1991). Second-order analysis of spatial clustering for inhomogeneous populations. *Biometrics, 47*(3), 1155–1163.

Doi, Y., Yokoyama, T., Sakai, M., Nakamura, Y., Tango, T., & Takahashi, K. (2008). Spatial clusters of Creutzfeldt-Jakob disease mortality in Japan between 1995 and 2004. *Neuroepidemiology, 30*(4), 222–228.

Dominguez-Berjon, M. F., Gandarillas, A., Segura del Pozo, J., Zorrilla, B., Soto, M. J., Lopez, L., . . . Abad, I. (2010). Census tract socioeconomic and physical environment and cardiovascular mortality in the region of Madrid (Spain). *Journal of Epidemiology and Community Health, 64*(12), 1086–1093.

Dong, G., & Harris, R. (2015). Spatial autoregressive models for geographically hierarchical data structures. *Geographical Analysis, 47*(2), 173–191.

Downey, L. (2006). Using geographic information systems to reconceptualize spatial relationships and ecological context. *American Journal of Sociology, 112*(2), 567–612.

Duncan, D. T., Castro, M. C., Gortmaker, S. L., Aldstadt, J., Melly, S. J., & Bennett, G. G. (2012). Racial differences in the built environment—body mass index relationship? A geospatial analysis of adolescents in urban neighborhoods. *International Journal of Health Geographics, 11*(1), 11.

Duncan, D. T., Kawachi, I., White, K., & Williams, D. R. (2013a). The geography of recreational open space: Influence of neighborhood racial composition and neighborhood poverty. *Journal of Urban Health: Bulletin of the New York Academy of Medicine, 90*(4), 618–631.

Duncan, D. T., Piras, G., Dunn, E. C., Johnson, R. M., Melly, S. J., & Molnar, B. E. (2013b). The built environment and depressive symptoms among urban youth: A spatial regression study. *Spatial and Spatio-temporal Epidemiology, 5*, 11–25.

Duncan, D. T., Rienti, M., Jr., Kulldorff, M., Aldstadt, J., Castro, M. C., Frounfelker, R., . . . Williams, D. R. (2016). Local spatial clustering in youths' use of tobacco, alcohol, and marijuana in Boston. *American Journal of Drug and Alcohol Abuse, 42*(4), 412–421.

Eberly, L. E., & Carlin, B. P. (2000). Identifiability and convergence issues for Markov chain Monte Carlo fitting of spatial models. *Statistics in Medicine, 19*(17–18), 2279–2294.

Elliot, P., Wakefield, J. C., Best, N. G, & Briggs, D. J. (2000). *Spatial epidemiology: Methods and applications*. Oxford, UK: Oxford University Press.

Elliott, P., & Wartenberg, D. (2004). Spatial epidemiology: Current approaches and future challenges. *Environmental Health Perspectives, 112*(9), 998–1006.

Fang, Z., Kulldorff, M., & Gregorio, D. I. (2004). Brain cancer mortality in the United States, 1986 to 1995: A geographic analysis. *Neuro-Oncology, 6*(3), 179–187.

Finley, A. O. (2011). Comparing spatially-varying coefficients models for analysis of ecological data with non-stationary and anisotropic residual dependence. *Methods in Ecology and Evolution, 2*(2), 143–154.

Fotheringham, S., Brunsdon, C., & Charlton, M. (2002). Geographically weighted summary statistics- a framework for localized exploratory data analysis. *Computers, Environment and Urban Systems, 26*(6), 501–524.

Fotheringham, A. S., Brunsdon, C., & Charlton, M. (2003). *Geographically weighted regression: The analysis of spatially varying relationships*. Hoboken, NJ: Wiley.

Geary, R. C. (1954). The contiguity ratio and statistical mapping. *The Incorporated Statistician, 5*(3), 115–146.

Gebreab, S. Y., & Diez Roux, A. V. (2012). Exploring racial disparities in CHD mortality between blacks and whites across the United States: A geographically weighted regression approach. *Health & Place, 18*(5), 1006–1014.

Gelman, A., & Price, P. N. (1999). All maps of parameter estimates are misleading. *Statistics in Medicine, 18*(23), 3221–3234.

Gemperli, A., Vounatsou, P., Kleinschmidt, I., Bagayoko, M., Lengeler, C., & Smith, T. (2004). Spatial patterns of infant mortality in Mali: The effect of malaria endemicity. *American Journal of Epidemiology, 159*(1), 64–72.

Getis, A., Mur, J., Zoller, H. G. (2004). *Spatial econometrics and spatial statistics*. London: Palgrave Macmillan.

Getis, A., & Ord, J. K. (1992). The analysis of spatial association by use of distance statistics. *Geographical Analysis, 24*(3), 189–206.

Gilks, W. R., Richardson, S., & Spiegelhalter, D. (1995). *Markov chain Monte Carlo in practice.* Boca Raton, FL: CRC Press.

Goovaerts, P., & Gebreab, S. (2008). How does Poisson kriging compare to the popular BYM model for mapping disease risks? *International Journal of Health Geographics, 7*(1), 6.

Graif, C. (2015). Delinquency and gender moderation in the moving to opportunity interventions: The role of extended neighborhoods. *Criminology, 53*(3), 366–398.

Graif, C., Gladfelter, A. S., & Matthews, S. A. (2014). Urban poverty and neighborhood effects on crime: Incorporating spatial and network perspectives. *Sociology Compass, 8*(9), 1140–1155.

Graif, C., & Sampson, R. J. (2009). Spatial heterogeneity in the effects of immigration and diversity on neighborhood homicide rates. *Homicide Studies, 13*(3), 242–260.

Gregorio, D. I., Kulldorff, M., Barry, L., & Samociuk, H. (2002). Geographic differences in invasive and in-situ breast cancer incidence according to precise geographic coordinates, Connecticut, 1991–1995. *International Journal of Cancer, 100*, 194–198

Havard, S., Deguen, S., Zmirou-Navier, D., Schillinger, C., & Bard, D. (2009). Traffic-related air pollution and socioeconomic status: A spatial autocorrelation study to assess environmental equity on a small-area scale. *Epidemiology, 20*(2), 223–230.

Huang, L., Kulldorff, M., & Gregorio, D. (2007). A spatial scan statistic for survival data. *Biometrics, 63*(1), 109–118.

Jerrett, M., Gale, S., & Kontgis, C. (2010). Spatial modeling in environmental and public health research. *International Journal of Environmental Research and Public Health, 7*(4), 1302–1329.

Kawachi, I., & Berkman, L. F. (2003). *Neighborhoods and health.* New York, NY: Oxford University Press.

Kelsall, J. E., & Wakefield, J. C. (1999). Discussion on Bayesian models for spatially correlated disease and exposure data. In J. M. Bernardo, J. O. Berger, A. P. Dawid, & A. F. M. Smith (Eds.), *Bayesian statistics 6* (p. 151). Oxford, UK: Oxford University Press.

Klassen, A. C., Kulldorff, M., & Curriero, F. (2005). Geographical clustering of prostate cancer grade and stage at diagnosis, before and after adjustment for risk factors. *International Journal of Health Geographics, 4*(1), 1.

Kleinschmidt, I., Sharp, B. L., Clarke, G. P., Curtis, B., & Fraser, C. (2001). Use of generalized linear mixed models in the spatial analysis of small-area malaria incidence rates in Kwazulu Natal, South Africa. *American Journal of Epidemiology, 153*(12), 1213–1221.

Knox, E. G. (1964). The detections of space-time interactions. *The Royal Statistical Society Series C-Applied Statistics, 13*(1), 25–29.

Kulldorff, M. (1997). A spatial scan statistic. *Communications in Statistics: Theory and Methods, 26.*

Kulldorff, M. (2015). SaTScanTM v9.4: Software for the spatial and space-time scan statistics. Information Management Services, Inc.

Kulldorff, M., Huang, L., Pickle, L., & Duczmal, L. (2006a). An elliptic spatial scan statistic. *Statistics in Medicine, 25*(22), 3929–3943.

Kulldorff, M., & Nagarwalla, N. (1995). Spatial disease clusters: Detection and inference. *Statistics in Medicine, 14*(8), 799–810.

Kulldorff, M., Song, C., Gregorio, D., Samociuk, H., & DeChello, L. (2006b). Cancer map patterns: Are they random or not? *American Journal of Preventive Medicine, 30*(2 Suppl), S37–S49.

Laraia, B. A., Blanchard, S. D., Karter, A. J., Jones-Smith, J. C., Warton, M., Kersten, E., . . . Kelly, M. (2014). Spatial pattern of body mass index among adults in the diabetes study of Northern California (Distance). *International Journal of Health Geographics, 13*(1), 48.

Lawson, A. B. (2013). *Bayesian disease mapping: Hierarchical modeling in spatial epidemiology* (2nd ed.). Boca Raton, FL: CRC Press.

Lawson, A. B., Browne, W., & Rodeiro, C. V. (2003). *Disease mapping in WinBUGS and MLwiN*. New York, NY: Wiley.

Lee, D. (2011). A comparison of conditional autoregressive models used in Bayesian disease mapping. *Spatial and Spatio-temporal Epidemiology, 2*(2), 79–89.

Legendre, P. (1993). Spatial autocorrelation: Trouble or new paradigm? *Ecology, 74*(6), 1659–1673.

Legendre, P., & Fortin, M. J. (1989). Spatial pattern and ecological analysis. *Vegetatio, 80*(2), 107–138.

LeSage, J., & Pace, R. K. (2009). *Introduction to spatial econometrics*. Boca Raton, FL CRC Press.

Liese, A. D., Lawson, A., Song, H.-R., Hibbert, J. D., Porter, D. E., Nichols, M., . . . D'Agostino, R. B. (2010). Evaluating geographic variation in Type 1 and Type 2 diabetes mellitus incidence in youth in four U.S. regions. *Health & Place, 16*(3), 547–556.

Macintyre, S., Ellaway, A., & Cummins, S. (2002). Place effects on health: how can we conceptualise, operationalise and measure them? *Social Science and Medicine, 55*(1), 125–139.

MacNab, Y. C. (2004). Bayesian spatial and ecological models for small-area accident and injury analysis. *Accident Analysis & Prevention, 36*(6), 1019–1028.

Matthews, S., & Parker, D. M. (2013). Progress in spatial demography. *Demographic Research, S13*(10), 271–312.

Mennis, J., Harris, P. W., Obradovic, Z., Izenman, A. J., Grunwald, H. E., & Lockwood, B. (2011). The effect of neighborhood characteristics and spatial spillover on urban juvenile delinquency and recidivism. *The Professional Geographer, 63*(2), 174–192.

Moran, P. A. (1950). Notes on continuous stochastic phenomena. *Biometrika, 37*(1–2), 17–23.

Morenoff, J. D. (2003). Neighborhood mechanisms and the spatial dynamics of birth weight. *Ajs, 108*(5), 976–1017.

Morenoff, J. D., & Sampson, R. J. (1997). Violent crime and the spatial dynamics of neighborhood transition: Chicago, 1970–1990. *Social Forces, 76*(1), 31–64.

Morenoff, J. D., Sampson, R. J., & Raudenbush, S. W. (2001). Neighborhood inequality, collective efficacy, and the spatial dynamics of urban violence. *Criminology, 39*(3), 517–558.

Oakes, J. M. (2004). The (mis)estimation of neighborhood effects: causal inference for a practicable social epidemiology. *Social Science and Medicine, 58*(10), 1929–1952.

O'Campo, P. (2003). Invited commentary: Advancing theory and methods for multilevel models of residential neighborhoods and health. *American Journal of Epidemiology, 157*(1), 9–13.

Oden, N. (1995). Adjusting Moran's I for population density. *Statistics in Medicine, 14*(1), 17–26.

Olson, K. L., Grannis, S. J., & Mandl, K. D. (2006). Privacy protection versus cluster detection in spatial epidemiology. *American Journal of Public Health, 96*(11), 2002–2008.

Openshaw, S. (1984). *The modifiable areal unit problem*. Norwich, UK: Geobooks.

Openshaw, S., Charlton, M., Wymer, C., & Craft, A. (1987). A Mark 1 Geographical Analysis Machine for the automated analysis of point data sets. *International Journal of Geographical Information Systems, 1*(4), 335–358.

Páez, A., Farber, S., & Wheeler, D. (2011). A simulation-based study of geographically weighted regression as a method for investigating spatially varying relationships. *Environment and Planning A, 43*(12), 2992–3010.

Raudenbush, S. W., Bryk, A.S, Congdon, R. (2013). HLM 7.01 for Windows [Computer software]. Skokie, IL: Scientific Software International, Inc.

Richardson, S., (1992). Statistical methods for geographical correlation studies. In P. Elliott, J. Cuzick, D. English, & R. Stern (Eds.), *Geographical and environmental epidemiology, Methods for small-area studies* (pp. 181–204). Oxford, UK: Oxford University Press.

Sampson, R. J., Morenoff, J. D., & Gannon-Rowley, T. (2002). Assessing "neighborhood effects": Social processes and new directions in research. *Annual Review of Sociology, 28*(1), 443–478.

Sampson, R. J., Morenoff, J. D., & Earls, F. (1999). Beyond social capital: Spatial dynamics of collective efficacy for children. *American Sociological Review, 64*(5), 633–660. doi:10.2307/2657367

Sampson, R. J., & Wilson, W. J. (2012). *Great American City: Chicago and the enduring neighborhood effect.* Chicago, IL: University of Chicago Press.

Savitz, N. V., & Raudenbush, S. W. (2009). Exploiting spatial dependence to improve measurement of neighborhood social processes. *Sociological Methodology, 39*(1), 151–183.

Snijders, T. A. B., & Bosker, R. J. (2011). *Multilevel analysis: An introduction to basic and advanced multilevel modeling.* Thousand Oaks, CA: Sage.

Snow, J. (1855). *On the mode of communication of cholera.* London, UK: John Churchill.

Spiegelhalter, D., Thomas, A., Best, N., & Lunn, D. (2002a). *WinBUGS: Bayesian inference using Gibbs Sampling Manual,* Version 1.4. London: Imperial College: MRC Biostatistics Unit.

Spiegelhalter, D. J., Best, N. G., Carlin, B. P., & Van Der Linde, A. (2002b). Bayesian measures of model complexity and fit. *Journal of the Royal Statistical Society: Series B (Statistical Methodology), 64*(4), 583–639.

Spiegelhalter, D. J., Thomas, A., Best, N. G., & Lunn, D. J. (2002c). *WinBUGS: Bayesian inference using Gibbs Sampling Manual, Version 1.4.* London: Imperial College: MRC Biostatistics Unit.

Subramanim, S.V., Jones, K., & Duncan, C. (2003). Multilevel methods for public health research. In L. F. Berkman & I. Kawachi (Eds.), *Neighborhoods and health* (pp. 65–111). New York, NY: Oxford University Press.

Tango, T. (1995). A class of tests for detecting "general" and "focused" clustering of rare diseases. *Statistics in Medicine, 14* (21–22), 2323–2334.

Tango, T. (2000). A test for spatial disease clustering adjusted for multiple testing. *Statistics in Medicine, 19*(2), 191–204.

Tango, T., & Takahashi, K. (2005). A flexibly shaped spatial scan statistic for detecting clusters. *International Journal of Health Geographics, 4*(1), 11.

Tobler, W. R. (1970). Computer movie simulating urban growth in Detroit region. *Economic Geography, 46*(2), 234–240.

Turnbull, B. W., Iwano, E. J., Burnett, W. S., Howe, H. L., & Clark, L. C. (1990). Monitoring for clusters of disease: Application to leukemia incidence in upstate New York. *American Journal of Epidemiology, 132*(1 Suppl), S136–S143.

Vogel, M., & South, S. J. (2016). Spatial dimensions of the effect of neighborhood disadvantage on delinquency. *Criminology, 54*(3), 434–458.

Wagner, H. H., & Fortin, M.-J. (2005). Spatial analysis of landscapes: Concepts and statistics. *Ecology, 86*(8), 1975–1987.

Wakefield, J. (2007). Disease mapping and spatial regression with count data. *Biostatistics, 8*(2), 158–183. doi:10.1093/biostatistics/kxl008

Wakefield, J., Kelsall, J. E., & Morris, S. E. (2000a). Clustering, cluster detection and spatial variation in risk. In P. Elliott, J. C. Wakefield, N. G. Best, & D. Briggs (Eds.),

Spatial Epidemiology: Methods and Applications (pp. 128–152). New York, NY: Oxford University Press.

Wakefield, J. C., Best, N. G., & Waller, L. A. (2000b). Bayesian approaches to disease mapping. In P. Elliott, J. C. Wakefield, N. G. Best, & D. Briggs (Eds.), *Spatial epidemiology: Methods and applications* (pp. 104–127). New York, NY: Oxford University Press.

Waller, L. A., & Gotway, C. A. (2004). *Applied spatial statistics for public health data.* Hoboken, NJ: Wiley.

Waller, L. A., Zhu, L., Gotway, C. A., Gorman, D. M., & Gruenewald, P. J. (2007). Quantifying geographic variations in associations between alcohol distribution and violence: A comparison of geographically weighted regression and spatially varying coefficient models. *Stochastic Environmental Research and Risk Assessment, 21*(5), 573–588.

Wheeler, D., & Tiefelsdorf, M. (2005). Multicollinearity and correlation among local regression coefficients in geographically weighted regression. *Journal of Geographical Systems, 7*(2), 161–187.

Wheeler, D. C. (2007). Diagnostic tools and a remedial method for collinearity in geographically weighted regression. *Environment and Planning A, 39*(10), 2464–2481.

Whittemore, A. S., Friend, N., Brown, B. W., & Holly, E. A. (1987). A test to detect clusters of disease. *Biometrika, 74*(3), 631–635.

Xia, H., & Carlin, B.P. (1998). Spatio-temporal models with errors in covariates: mapping Ohio lung cancer mortality. *Statistics in Medicine, 17*, 2025–2043.

Xu, H. (2014). Comparing spatial and multilevel regression models for binary outcomes in neighborhood studies. *Sociological Methodology, 44*(1), 229–272.

Yao, Z., Tang, J., & Zhan, F. B. (2011). Detection of arbitrarily-shaped clusters using a neighbor-expanding approach: A case study on murine typhus in south Texas. *International Journal of Health Geographics, 10*, 23.

5

AGENT-BASED MODELS

Brenda Heaton, Abdulrahman El-Sayed, and Sandro Galea

There is a growing recognition in the health and social sciences research literature that population health is produced through a complex set of pathways and mechanisms that cut across multiple levels of influence (Diez Roux, 2007; Mabry, Milstein, Abraido-Lanza, Livingood, & Allegrante, 2013). These levels of influence constitute a complex system, and the health of a population emerges from the functioning of a system in which the levels of influence interact to produce patterns of health and disease that are not adequately described by the sum of the individual component parts. This perspective on health has introduced "systems thinking" (Luke & Stamatakis, 2012; Trochim, Cabrera, Milstein, Gallagher, & Leischow, 2006) to population health, echoing the embrace of this approach by disciplines ranging from the social sciences to the natural sciences. Systems thinking encourages a focus on the interactions between components of the system that dynamically adapt over time, rather than the characteristics of the individual components themselves (Diez Roux & Auchincloss, 2009).

Agent-based models (ABMs) are computer representations of complex adaptive systems and have gained currency as one flexible approach to the modeling of complex systems. Computational models, such as ABM, use simulation methods to evaluate the collective effects that the behaviors of autonomous individuals or entities, that is, agents, have on a system. ABM specifically employs computer simulation to allow the user to explore feedback among its individual constituents and between the individual constituents and emergent properties of the system as a whole. In this way, ABMs allow for the study of processes we know to be important but that may be too complex to study in more simple, traditional models. For these reasons, the application of ABM has experienced a sharp uptick in the population health research literature since the turn of the century (El-Sayed, Scarborough, Seemann, & Galea, 2012; Hammond, 2009; Li, Lawley, Siscovick, Zhang, & Pagan, 2016; Maglio & Mabry, 2011; Marshall & Galea, 2015; Nianogo & Arah, 2015), with more recent applications to the neighborhoods and health literature (Auchincloss & Diez Roux, 2008).

In this chapter, we introduce ABMs as a tool for modeling the interactive and adaptive processes that occur within a system, such as a neighborhood. The chapter is meant to provide a basic introduction to the concepts of complexity and the implementation of complex models, specifically ABM, in order to ground the reader in their potential utility for the study of neighborhoods and health. There are ample reviews, commentaries, and technical overviews of ABMs in the public health literature that are available for additional reference (Auchincloss & Diez Roux, 2008; Auchincloss & Garcia, 2015; Bonabeau, 2002; Borshchev & Filippov, 2004; Diez Roux & Auchincloss, 2009; El-Sayed et al., 2012; Galea, Riddle, & Kaplan, 2010; Giabbanelli & Crutzen, 2017; Hammond, 2009; Li et al., 2016; Luke & Stamatakis, 2012; Mabry et al., 2013; Marshall & Galea, 2015; Nianogo & Arah, 2015). There are several terms used throughout the chapter that are defined for the reader in Table 5-1.

Table 5-1 Common Terminology Used in the Agent-Based Research Literature

adaptation	the ability to change in response to the environment
agent	simulated individuals or components of a model
autonomous	refers to the capacity for making independent decisions
collective	refers to the combined effect or to the whole of something
complex system	the behavior or attributes of the system cannot be explained by the sum of its parts
dynamic	continuous or occurring over time
emergence	the production of higher level outcomes resulting from synergies on lower levels
entities	a broader term used to refer to multiple components of a system or computer model
feedback loop	the outcome of an action informs future actions
heterogeneity	differing in some quality or characteristic
individual agents	simulated agents that represent people
interaction	communication or experience with another entity
interdependence	the actions or behaviors of two or more entities are dependent on one another
simulation	a computer model used to artificially recreate system entities and their behaviors for analysis
spatial agents	simulated agents that represent the environment
system	a collection of related or connected parts; a neighborhood system could refer to the collection of facilities, properties, homes, and people

CONCEPTS OF COMPLEXITY

A complex system can be defined as one in which the collective behaviors of the system are a result of dynamic interactions between the autonomous entities, or agents, that make up that system. Specifically, agents of a complex system interact in multiple ways, and these interactions occur "locally," meaning that the agents of the system interact with their neighbors or those who are close to them in space and time. Further, the result of these interactions and interdependencies is the emergence of system-level properties that cannot be explained by the independent behaviors of the systems' agents. Complex systems are also adaptive in that agent- and system-level properties can change over time as a product of feedback loops.

These basic concepts of complexity and complex systems can be readily explained and understood by considering examples from nature—the flocking behaviors of birds, the swarming behaviors of bees, or the schooling of fish, to name a few, are all examples of emergent properties of complex systems, patterned behavior that cannot be observed by studying the individual agent alone but which are clear when one looks at the whole system. In each of these examples, the individual entities, that is, birds, bees, or fish, operate autonomously according to a set of simple rules that are implemented locally: (1) move in the same direction as your neighbors (alignment), (2) remain close to your neighbors (cohesion), and (3) avoid collisions with your neighbors (separation). The emergent behavior of the group (e.g., flocking, swarming, or schooling) is a product of the local interactions that the individual entities have with those around them. In the implementation of these simple rules, the entities of the system can learn from their experiences and adapt accordingly. In this way, the entities, or agents, of the system can be thought of as both autonomous and heterogeneous, possessing the ability to act on their own and according to their own experiences, traits, or characteristics. Further, the autonomous and heterogeneous nature of the agents allows for adaptive processes that can be reflected locally and at the level of the system. The adaptive processes of a system can easily be observed when watching the early formations of a flock, or as a flock of birds shifts direction or speed. In nature, these emergent and adaptive properties also provide an evolutionary advantage over individual entities operating independently, such as protection from predators or greater access to food in neighborhoods, the benefits of which encourage the organization of individual entities into such groups. Importantly, the collective behavior of the group requires no central coordination, reflecting the nature of health as an emergent property from complex population systems.

Neighborhoods as Complex Adaptive Systems

Neighborhoods reflect the physical and social environment within which people live and interact. Their features can dictate how individuals interact with others, what resources are available to them, and the physical and social barriers they may experience in attempting to access those resources. These individual-social-geographic interactions have been shown to influence neighborhood-specific levels of physical activity, diet, social capital, drug use, utilization of healthcare, and more (Diez Roux, 2016; Diez Roux & Mair, 2010). Most important to our discussion of complex systems is that neighborhood characteristics and resources evolve and adapt as the individuals living within them change and vice versa. In this way, neighborhoods represent a complex adaptive system and represent a clear illustration of individuals and their environment forming an interactive system. Changes in individuals or features of the environment make this an adaptive system. Next we provide three examples of adaptive features of a neighborhood.

Built Environment

The physical environment, referred to in this textbook as the built environment (see Chapter 8), can refer to the physical location of recreational spaces, green space, community spaces, sidewalks, and foot paths. Studies have observed associations between the built environment and the health of individuals residing in that environment (Lovasi, Grady, & Rundle, 2012). Specifically, the amount of green space or walking trails can predict how physically active individuals living in that area are, and the presence of community spaces can facilitate social interaction and access to resources. The physical environment and changes to the physical environment may also influence the movement of individuals in and out of a neighborhood (Handy, Cao, & Mokhtarian, 2006). For example, individuals with preferences for green space and good schools may be more or less inclined to move into a neighborhood with access to such features. Additionally, neighborhoods that undergo gentrification which results in higher rental prices, for example, may drive individuals with lower incomes out of the neighborhood. As such, the neighborhood system will adapt over time as a result of the dynamic interactions between individuals and the built environment.

Food Environment

The food environment, a subset of the physical environment, refers to the presence of foods available for purchase by residents of a neighborhood (see Chapter 9). The food environment is typically characterized by the quality and quantity of the foods available. For example, neighborhoods that lack access to a supermarket, large grocery store, or supercenter, where affordable fresh fruit, vegetables, and other whole foods may be found, are termed as "food deserts." The occurrence of food deserts is location specific and often associated with higher concentrations of low-income individuals. Chapter 9 includes added discussion of food deserts and their definitions. It has been hypothesized that the food environment can adapt based on the demand of residents for certain types of foods based either on preference or price. Anecdotally, the most common reason offered by storekeepers for why they do not stock specific products (e.g., reduced-fat dairy products) is because "my customers don't want it." Similarly, characteristics of the individuals residing in a neighborhood may adapt over time based on the availability of certain foods. In this way, the evolution of food deserts may be a result of dynamic interactions between individuals and their environment over time.

Social Environment

The social demographics of residents in a neighborhood such as income, education, race or ethnicity, gender, sexual orientation, and criminal records contribute to the social environment when the selection forces dictating entries and exits in and out of a neighborhood result in geospatial patterning by these characteristics. Specifically, in the presence of interaction between individuals and with their environment, patterns of residential crime, poverty, and social service resources available in a neighborhood system, for example, can emerge. In other words, the observed characteristics of the social environment are potential outcomes of feedback loops from interactions occurring within the social context of a neighborhood. Social networks of individuals are another feature of the social environment that dynamically changes and adapts over time (El-Sayed et al., 2012).

These features of the neighborhood system have displayed adaptive processes of their own. However, these features of the system cannot be viewed in isolation when we seek to understand the collective behavior of the neighborhood system. Rather, these features may also adapt as a function of another. Therefore, the adaptive nature of a neighborhood system incorporates feedback loops at multiple levels. For example, if the social environment of a neighborhood includes pockets of high crime, the physical environment may adapt to address this issue by relocating a local police station or redeveloping a dilapidated area previously known for facilitating criminal activities. In contrast, the added presence or removal of public transit options may result in changes to the social demography of a neighborhood's residents. We should also note that our discussion of neighborhood features is in no way exhaustive and that there are other features, such as the political environment, that interact with components of the neighborhood system and contribute to the adaptive processes discussed.

Modeling Complexity: An Illustration

Complex system behaviors, such as residential segregation, can be simulated in a computer environment by applying simple rules to the agents of the system. Briefly, a computational model is a purposeful simplification of a system and contains the algorithms and equations used to capture the behaviors of particular interest. Computer simulation refers to the running of the program that contains the algorithms and equations used to capture the behavior. In other words, computer simulation creates a prototype of processes and conditions that can be observed in a population in order to study a particular problem or process. Once the prototype is created, simulation methods then analyze that prototype to assess population outcomes over time under varying conditions. A simulation model can refer to the set of rules that determine *how* the system being modeled will change in the future given its present state (Borshchev & Filippov, 2004). In this way, simulation affords the opportunity to observe population-level outcomes that emerge over time as a result of making changes to one or more parameters in the model.

Similar to how fish organize into schools to avoid predators, groups of people self-organize into neighborhoods frequently influenced by characteristics such as race or ethnicity. The resultant spatial patterning at the macro level is referred to as residential segregation (discussed in Chapter 12) and provides an illustration of one of the earliest adoptions of complex systems approaches to understand neighborhood behavior. In 1969, Thomas Schelling developed an early computer model that was able to simulate patterns of residential segregation that were observable in the real world (Schelling, 1969, 1971). Desiring to understand how people's preferences to reside near those who shared their same trait(s) contributed to collective segregation, he developed a set of simple behavioral rules that dictated individual movements through space and time, according to their satisfaction with the diversity of traits around them. The basic model took the following form. First, agents (i.e., individuals) were assigned one of two colors. Second, agents were placed in space at random. Third, each agent was assigned rules of behavior as follows:

1. Agents were satisfied with their location in space if, between them and their four nearest neighbors, there was a minimum majority. For example, if the agent of interest was blue, two out of the four nearest neighbors would also have to be blue for there to be a local majority of blue agents.
2. Agents were dissatisfied when they were in the local minority.

3. Dissatisfied agents relocated to the nearest space where they could find at least half of the neighbors to be of the same color. If agents, though dissatisfied, preferred to reside in mixed neighborhoods, bounds were placed on the distance with which they would move to find a local majority.

Starting with an initial random distribution, individuals moved in the model until equilibrium was reached. This simple model demonstrated that with a limited number of runs of the model, complete segregation by agent color could be observed, even when varying the population ratio of the two colors, the preferences for neighbors of the same color, and the size of the local neighborhood within which individual preferences operated.

The Schelling model is simple, in that it ignores other processes that contribute to or are responsible for collective segregation, such as economic segregation or organized or externally imposed segregation (such as the practice of "redlining" of mortgage loans offered by commercial banks). That is not to say that these processes are less important or superseded by preferential segregation by individuals, but simply that they are different processes that operate according to a different set of rules. Therefore, though a simplistic reduction of a much more complex problem, the Schelling model affords exploration into a macro-level phenomenon by allowing for variations in the micro-level components of the model. For example, the model contained five components that could be varied—neighborhood size, preference percentage for one's own color, the ratio of colors in the total population, rules governing movement, and the initial configuration. The Schelling model was one of the earliest ABMs and has continued to be exploited for further understanding of mechanisms and processes underlying spatial patterns, such as residential segregation.

ABMs can provide certain advantages over traditional approaches. The emergence of macro-level spatial patterns, such as segregation, according to micro-level interactions cannot be easily explored with traditional analytic approaches. Traditional statistical methods have advanced in recent years to account for data collected at multiple levels of influence, as well as interactions between multilevel constructs. The most commonly known among them are hierarchical or multilevel models that can account for variability at multiple levels of influence (Subramanian, Jones, & Duncan, 2003). However, the main limitation of these models with respect to complex processes is that they cannot readily account for multidirectional feedback among variables, that is, complex adaptive processes. Specifically, these models rely on assumptions of linearity (X causes Y), whereas a hallmark of complex systems is nonlinear processes. Although the multilevel model does provide data that explain what happened, it does not provide a basis to explore *how* it happened. In other words, multilevel statistical models cannot handle the emergent processes that result from adaptation.

Computational models, like the agent-based Schelling model, offer greater flexibility with regard to adaptive processes. Specifically, they simulate the interactions and relationships between autonomous, decision-making entities (e.g., agents) in a system and the consequential adaptive processes that occur over time. By observing the explicitly programmed health behaviors, social interactions, and movements of simulated individuals over simulated time, we are able to gain unique insights into *how* the distribution of health and disease emerges on a population level (Bonabeau, 2002). Several papers highlight the differences, similarities, and relationships between simulation models, such as ABM, versus static analytical models, such as multilevel models (Rice, 2012). To be clear, we are not advocating the replacement of traditional models by ABMs, but rather aim to highlight the utility of these models as an adjunct approach to studying neighborhoods and health when complex processes are the focus of investigation. For example, ABMs are ideally suited for situations in which the agents of a system have real individual behaviors, meaning agents can adapt, change, or learn in response to other agents in the system; are capable of forming dynamic relationships; and interact spatially.

MODEL IMPLEMENTATION

The specific implementation of ABMs varies across fields of study and research questions of interest. However, ABMs generally contain a minimum set of components that are common across all applications. In this section, we focus on providing a technical overview of the modeling components, review common applications of the method, and discuss a general approach to model implementation, including resources available to facilitate model construction and implementation. The primary aim of this section is to enhance the reader's ability to become an informed consumer of applications of ABM in the research literature.

Technical Overview of Agent-Based Models

ABMs are "decentralized" models in that no one component controls how the system operates or adapts over time. If we think back to our earlier examples of birds, bees, and fish, the emergent behaviors of the flock, swarm, or school arise from the set of simple rules followed by each individual entity and do not require any central coordination. As such, an agent-based model is built from the "bottom up" by first determining model components and, second, assigning the agents' attributes, characteristics, interactions, and rules of behavior. Depending on the approach to modeling, initial characteristics, behavior states, and decision rules (i.e., model parameters) of individual agents may be assigned based on empirical data distributions. In this way, agents of the model are programmed to learn and adapt over time according to a set of rules which can be observed to be operational in the real-world setting.

The focus of the model is on interdependent processes, as compared to independent associations, which are the typical focus of empirical research. Like the earlier example of the Schelling model, the lower level processes under study are thought to only provide a sufficient explanation of the higher level phenomenon of interest, as opposed to a necessary one. This property of ABMs allows for the comparative evaluation of multiple structures and mechanisms that may similarly result in the outcome of interest (Marshall & Galea, 2015). For this reason, a common approach to modeling takes a minimalist approach in that models are to contain the minimal set of rules sufficient to observe the macro-level outcome (Conte & Paolucci, 2014).

Model Components

We have already referenced many of the basic components (e.g., "entities") that make up an ABM. For ease, we explicitly review them here.

Agents and Characteristics

We have already introduced the concept of agents. To review, the term "agents" is reserved for those independent individuals or components of the model that can learn and adapt. More specifically, the agents of a model refer to the micro-entities whose behaviors are collectively responsible for the emergent behaviors of the system. Simulated agents should be heterogeneous in their attributes and behaviors; able to form dynamic relationships with other agents; interact spatially with their local environment; and adapt, change, or learn based on those relationships or interactions. The term "agents" can refer to individual people as well as components of the environment, such as stores or schools, depending on the outcomes of interest. Simulated agents should reflect characteristics and behaviors that are grounded in reality. Agents exist within the simulated environment and follow programmed rules that use each agent's characteristics and information available to it to decide what it does at each time step in the model (see next section).

Environment

The model environment, often referring to the spatial context or simulation space, provides the backdrop for the spatial interactions that are observed in a system.

A simulated neighborhood environment may include the geographic patterns of households, schools, community health centers, and stores near where agents are placed. The environmental landscape of the model should constrain or dictate agent behaviors in meaningful ways and, therefore, should reflect only those features that relate to the question of interest. Attributes of the simulated environment should reflect those observed in the real world. The model environment is typically static in that it doesn't change or adapt over time.

With a basic understanding of the model environment and agents, we can now explain some disparate terminology that can be found in the research literature to refer to ABMs. The computer representation of the environment as a backdrop to agent interactions is different from what is referred to when ABMs are termed "spatial agent-based models" (Filatova, Verburg, Parker, & Stannard, 2013). If features of the spatial environment, such as the location of stores, for example, are instead heterogeneous and intended to dynamically interact with other components of the model, these environmental features are more appropriately characterized as "agents." When features of the environment are included in the model in this way, the model may qualify as a spatial ABM. Similarly, if the agents of the model are restricted to individuals, the model can be described as an individual-based model.

Rules of Behavior

Agent behaviors refer to the initial behavioral states as well as adaptation behavior as a result of interaction. Specifically, agents can adapt their behavior in response to their current state, other agents, and their environment. In a simulation model, the specific adaptive processes occur according to a set of behavioral rules that are explicitly programmed. Rules of behavior typically follow a stochastic probability model and are broken down into discrete steps. In the Schelling model, the rules of behavior included the predictive models for whether agents were satisfied with their local environment, as well as the models specifying their relocation based on their current state of satisfaction.

Time Steps

With each run of the simulation model, also referred to as a time step, the programmed processes are executed and the behavioral states of the agents are updated. To illustrate, one run of the Schelling model would assess the current state of satisfaction based on an agent's location and, secondly, relocate the agent in space accordingly. At the start of the next time step, the agent would reside in a new location and the state of satisfaction would again be determined and the agent's location updated at the end of the time step. The amount of time that passes with each run of the model can also be specified. Therefore, the time-relevant variables characterizing an agent's state or behavior, such as age, will be updated based on the time allocated to each run. If the amount of time specified is 1 year, for example, an agent's age will be advanced by 1 year at the end of each time step. This aspect of the model is what allows for adaptive and emergent processes to occur and their effects to be observed in real time. With each run of the model, one can observe or visualize the micro- and macro-level processes as they occur.

Model Development and Implementation

In addition to commonly agreed-upon model components, the general approach to model implementation and the modeling process is similar across applications of the method. In this section, a simple description of the modeling process is provided, including reference to the available software packages designed to facilitate implementation.

The steps to model implementation can generically be categorized into three procedures: development of a conceptual model, implementation of the computational or simulation model, and model validation and verification. For illustration purposes, we draw upon the model developed by Orr, Kaplan, and Galea (2016), which evaluates the role of the neighborhood environment in racial disparities in obesity.

Conceptual Model

Conceptual models are constructed as a first step to model development and specify the system, system entities, interactions and relations, and the collective behaviors of interest. They are often depicted graphically, with directed edges indicating relations between entities of the model. Composition of a conceptual model will give an initial sense for whether the planned model is too simple or too complex, and it can help to identify when the question posed is inappropriate or ill-focused. Specifically, it aids in the assembly of hypotheses for what processes and entities are essential to the question or problem to be addressed by the simulation model. To illustrate, Figure 5-1 depicts the variables hypothesized by Orr and colleagues that lead from potential policy intervention targets to agent-level body mass index (BMI). These policy targets were conceptualized as neighborhood-level variables and are lightly shaded in the model (Orr, Kaplan, & Galea, 2016).

In addition to graphical depictions of the planned model, some aspects of the ABM literature include the development of "conceptual frameworks" or "conceptual design checklists." Similar to a conceptual model, conceptual frameworks detail the list of design concepts to be addressed in the implementation of the model. In addition to the simplistic visual representation of the system processes depicted in

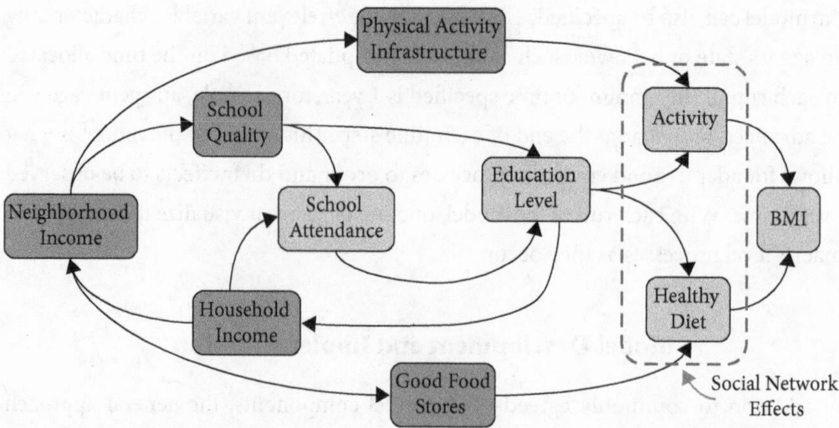

FIGURE 5-1 **A conceptual model of the hypothesized variables and relationships impacting obesity outcomes.**

the conceptual model, the conceptual framework describes the model from start to finish, including the model purpose, entities and process, design concepts such as prediction, interaction, adaptation, stochasticity, and emergence, and the initial conditions. Protocols have been developed to standardize the development of conceptual frameworks and to facilitate communication of assumed relations, interactions, interdependencies, and system feedback (Grimm et al., 2006).

Computational Model

The computational model refers to the collection of probability models that determine the initial states of the model entities and that implement the time steps and behavioral updates. The computational model also specifies the processes by which parameter estimation occurs. Implementation of the computational model follows a linear process in which the initial parameters are set, the model environment is initialized, and the prediction rules for each time step are implemented. Submodels refer to the models created for all of the major processes in the model. The models are typically independent of each other and can be designed and tested independently, hence the term. Typically, ABMs include several submodels with multiple parameters. Detailed descriptions of the computational model are typically included as supplementary files or appendices to published papers. To illustrate, we provide a brief description of some of the submodels used by Orr and colleagues to determine the agent health behaviors of activity and diet (see Figure 5-1). Descriptions of the model are simplified for the purposes of this textbook. (Full descriptions of the models implemented by Orr and colleagues can be found in the Model Documentation file included in the supplementary materials that were published along with their paper.)

Activity Level

The estimation of activity level for a given agent was informed by data from the National Health Interview Survey (NHIS). It was hypothesized that a person's activity level is predicted by two independent influences—personal propensity for physical activity (termed "self-activity" in the model) and pressure from friends to be active. Self-activity (SA) levels for each agent in the model were considered to be a function of the following:

Education influence (EI): Parameter value chosen to reflect the relationship between years of schooling and self-activity observed in the NHIS data.
Education level (EL): Refers to the agent's education level.
Exercise infrastructure (ExlL): Parameter value derived from published work that depicted the relationship between the neighborhood infrastructure and physical activity levels.
Agent predisposition (AP): Parameter value was drawn from a normal distribution to capture to idiosyncratic variation among agents.
Agent predisposition influence (API): A set measure based on NHIS data to reflect the amount of influence an agent's predisposition has on activity level.
Constant (C): A numerical constant that places bounds on the variation in activity level in order to reflect NHIS data.

The model determining the level of self-activity took the following form:

$$SA = EI * EL + ExlL * ExI + API * AP + C$$

Friend effects were determined separately in a model that considered all of the agent's friends at a given time step, their self-activity levels, and the proportion of the agent's friends above a certain threshold of activity. If the majority of friends exceeded the threshold, a positive influence was exerted; below it, a negative influence.

Diet

The modeling of an agent's diet followed a similar approach, hypothesizing the presence of two independent influences: personal preferences and the influence of friends. The model for self-diet took the following form:

$$SD = EI * EL + GFSI * GFS + API * AP + C$$

In this model, self-diet is similarly predicted by education influence on dietary choices, the agent's education level, the influence of an agent's predisposition for healthy eating based on empirical research, an agent's predisposition for dietary habits, and a numerical constant used to reflect age-appropriate intakes. In addition, the model included a measure of the availability of good-food stores (GFS) in the agent's neighborhood, as well as a measure of their influence on dietary choices (GFSI).

Model Calibration, Verification, and Validation

Several approaches to ensuring the appropriateness of the model can be found in the literature (Sargent, 2013). Commonly implemented methods include calibration and sensitivity analysis (Thiele, Kurth, & Grimm, 2014). Parameterization of the submodels can be difficult due to the lack of empirical data or the uncertainty of it. Parameter fitting or calibration methods can be used to find values that will reasonably reproduce observable patterns of the outcome of interest. Sensitivity analysis can help to identify the importance of uncertainty in the model parameters. For example, by varying the parameter values, changes to the model output can be observed. If the output is robust against variations in an uncertain parameter, the uncertainty is of low importance. Model calibration refers to comparisons of model output with the patterns of outcomes observed in the real world. Submodels and model parameters can be varied to calibrate the emergent properties of the model to those empirically observed. Throughout the computational model implemented by Orr and colleagues, calibration techniques were implemented to ensure that outcomes, such as activity level and diet (see earlier), were consistent with distributions observed in the empirical research literature. Model verification procedures ensure that the model is behaving as expected. Model verification can be compared to concepts of internal validity, while model validation and calibration can be compared to concepts of external validity.

Modeling Software

The implementation of ABMs is greatly aided by the well-developed software platforms that support execution of the modeling process. Common programming languages, such as Java, Python, and C ++, typically support these platforms. Commonly used packages or toolkits include open-source applications such as NetLogo and RePast (Nikolai & Madey, 2009; North et al., 2013; Railsback, Lytinen, & Jackson, 2006) and proprietary packages, such as AnyLogic (Macal & North, 2007). Among the benefits of these toolkits is that naïve users can explore model libraries which contain a collection of the types of models that have been made using the software, with accompanying documentation. They are also "user-friendly" in that parameters of the model are easily varied, in the case of NetLogo, with "sliders." Additionally, the toolkits contain some procedures that facilitate model calibration or verification, such as the BehaviorSearch tool in NetLogo, which explores combinations of parameters that will result in the target behavior.

Model Applications

Although the basic model components and approach to implementation in ABM are essentially the same, the purpose of the model may vary. Specific applications of the approach can range from simple models, like the Schelling model, sometimes referred to as a "toy" model, to more sophisticated models that make use of empirical data and where the predicted processes are grounded in reality. More specifically, the applications can range from early models which demonstrate *how* mechanisms or processes interact to produce observed outcomes, to later models which demonstrate *what* happens to outcomes when new model entities are introduced or parameters are modified, to reflect hypothetical interventions.

The focus of early models is typically on demonstrating general mechanisms capable of reproducing system behaviors, and they can provide generic insights or explanations for observed phenomena. They allow for exploration of processes through variation and visualization of the hypothesized mechanisms driving the outcomes of interest. Once a simplistic, exploratory model of sufficient processes that produces the collective system behavior of interest is constructed, the model can then be extended to include additional parameters of interest or purposeful modifications to reflect planned intervention. Alternatively, when key processes are sufficiently understood, the more complex model can be built independent of an exploratory model (Chalabi & Lorenc, 2013). To do this, these models increasingly use quantitative data and analyses to facilitate a better understanding of mechanisms and their linkages to real-world phenomena. Importantly, they incorporate ad hoc procedures like sensitivity analysis and calibration to empirical data sets and observed patterns to verify and validate those linkages to reality.

Each application along the spectrum highlights the potential benefits of simulation models and the modeling process. In addition to providing a deeper understanding of important mechanisms and processes, exploratory models also serve to highlight the dearth of empirical data available upon which model inputs can be based. For example, the original Schelling model was based on simplified assumptions about one's satisfaction with the heterogeneity of their environment and the thresholds of satisfaction that would predict movement. Explicating the assumptions of a model can highlight the amount of uncertainty present in the model and guide priorities for future data collection. More developed or quantitatively informed models can provide robust estimates for predicted impacts of hypothesized interventions. They also can serve to provide insight into the predictors of effect magnitude.

Next, we review the range of applications of ABMs using examples from the neighborhoods and health literature.

APPLICATIONS OF AGENT-BASED MODELS FOR THE STUDY OF NEIGHBORHOODS AND HEALTH

The contributions of ABMs to the neighborhoods and health literature to date reflect the unique insights into causal process that are afforded by simulation methods. Specifically, they have highlighted the ability to observe patterns of micro-level interactions that produce macro-level outcomes, the ability to measure differences and magnitudes of effect, the utility in comparing interventions, and the role of interdependent processes that result in unintended or previously unobserved impacts. Next, we provide an overview of the specific contributions of ABM to the study of neighborhood effects on health within three areas: the built environment, food environment, and the social environment.

Built Environment

There is a long-standing debate about the role that the built environment plays in the production of health and disease on a population level (see Chapter 8). Underlying this debate are the shortcomings of traditional statistical models, which cannot accommodate the myriad feedback loops and dynamic interactions that exist between individuals and their environment, thereby limiting the understanding of the responsible mechanisms and processes. Neighborhood walkability, for example, has been linked to health behaviors (especially physical activity) as well as obesity and cardiovascular outcomes (Lovasi et al., 2012). However, the uncertainty around the causal nature of the dynamic interactions that extend over space and time contributes to reluctance or skepticism for intervening on the built environment, which may be costly. ABMs have been employed to investigate how aspects of the built environment interact with personal characteristics and preferences to produce patterns of walking behaviors observed on a population level. Additionally, they have been used to evaluate the viability of intervention targets, predicted intervention impacts, and compared intervention effects.

To illustrate, Yang and colleagues developed a series of iterative ABMs simulating people's walking behaviors within a hypothetical city. The first in the series was a self-described exploratory spatial ABM designed to investigate *how* the spatial patterning of the built (and social) environment(s) contributed to social inequalities in walking behaviors (Yang, Roux, Auchincloss, Rodriguez, & Brown, 2011). The model components included an environment which incorporated geographically distributed grocery and nonfood stores, social places, workplaces, neighborhoods, and households. Neighborhood characteristics included the environmental properties of safety and aesthetics (i.e., land use). Individuals were heterogeneous with respect to gender, age, socioeconomic status, family size, friends, dog ownership, household, work, and workplace. Individuals were assigned a walking ability as a function of their age, and an attitude toward walking as a function of feedback from attitudes of family and friends, the environmental experience of walking, observations of others walking, and the distance walked. Walking decisions made by individuals followed a set of rules based on the purpose of travel, that is, to work, for leisure, or for things they need, such as food. Each individual was assigned a maximum walking distance in any direction. If the destination, that is, work, leisure, or food, was within that person-specific distance, the decision to walk was based on a random draw from a probability distribution. The time step for the model was equal to 1 day. Therefore, with each run of the model, the individuals advanced in age by 1 day, and attitudes toward walking were updated—influencing how much the person would walk the following day. The model was calibrated by comparing model output to data from the National Household Travel Survey and other observational data. To investigate the influence of interactions with the built and social (attitudes of friends and family) environments on socioeconomic differences in walking, two dimensions of the model were varied—the spatial distribution of nonhousehold locations and the spatial distribution of safe neighborhoods, thereby creating four scenarios for analysis. The location of households in the environment was held constant to maintain residential segregation by socioeconomic status. The outcomes of this simple model revealed several things. First, that the minimal set of entities and related mechanisms was able to generate empirically observed patterns of walking behaviors. Second, the scenario analysis facilitated an understanding of the *processes* that were largely responsible for differences by socioeconomic status that cannot be visualized or are difficult to understand with traditional statistical models. Lastly, aspects of the model, such as the influence of dog ownership, were informed by evidence, but the model highlighted the limitations of existing data with respect to the magnitude of differences in walking behaviors.

Using this exploratory model and the newfound understanding of processes, Yang and colleagues further examined the impact of interventions targeting people's attitudes toward walking (Yang, Roux, Auchincloss, Rodriguez, & Brown, 2012) in a further iteration of the model. Two hypothetical interventions, one individual based and one environment based, were examined and produced twelve scenarios for analysis. Among the key findings, the model revealed that increases in walking due to increases in positive attitude toward walking diminish over time if other features of the environment (such as safety) are not conducive to walking. Additionally, the model allowed for evaluation of determinants of the magnitude of intervention effects.

In a second series of models, Yang and colleagues developed an ABM simulating children's school travel within a hypothetical city. The initial model was developed specifically to address yet unanswered questions about children's active travel to school (Yang & Diez-Roux, 2013). As stated by the authors, the impact of school location, catchment area definition, school size, and population density, and the impact of changing traffic safety levels were still largely unknown. Outcomes of the model revealed the ideal geographic locations of schools within the city and child's distance to the assigned school in order to maximize the proportion of children who walk to school. Additionally, ideal combinations of intervention intensity and areas targeted for traffic safety were provided. In a second iteration of the model, Yang and colleagues evaluated the impact of the walking school bus, a community-based program in which groups of children walk to school together, accompanied by adults, picking up additional children at "bus stops" along the way (Yang, Diez-Roux, Evenson, & Colabianchi, 2014). When the walking school bus was combined with interventions like those evaluated in the initial model, synergistic effects on children's active travel were identified.

These applications, as well as others (Badland et al., 2013; Zhu et al., 2013), highlight the dynamic and complex interactions between individuals and the built environment and call for the development of complex interventions. However, built environment interventions using traditional designs are not always possible and previous evaluations have highlighted the shortcomings (McCormack & Shiell, 2011; Northridge, Sclar, & Biswas, 2003). For these reasons, ABMs have been highlighted as helpful alternatives to traditional approaches (Chalabi & Lorenc, 2013).

Food Environment

Applications of ABM to the food environment are driven by similar pitfalls of traditional approaches, given that the food environment can often be considered as a subenvironment of the built environment. In addition to the weak and inconsistent associations observed in studies of the built environment and health, studies of the food environment are additionally fraught with issues of measurement error and available data that capture the multiple systems of influence that drive the specifics of the food environment, such as distribution and price (see Chapter 9) (Hammond & Dube, 2012). Furthermore, food behaviors (i.e., food-related decisions) are influenced through many sources, again highlighting the need for complex interventions.

To date, applications of the method to the study of the food environment and health fall into two general areas: (1) models that explore key processes influencing inequalities in diet and (2) models that evaluate policy-based interventions to modify food behaviors.

Auchincloss and colleagues developed the initial model of income inequalities in diet in the contexts of residential segregation (Auchincloss, Riolo, Brown, Cook, & Diez Roux, 2011). Similar to the Schelling model, this model was built on little to no empirical data on the complex processes at play and was self-ascribed as a simple model, built to stimulate further questions about processes involved. In this way, the model provided a conceptual framework for thinking about income inequalities in food consumption. Importantly, the intent of the model was not to present a full representation of the processes that create differences in diet but to explore key processes that had been hypothesized in the literature. The model interactions included where people live, healthy food resources, income constraints, and personal food preferences. The model was not able to verify common assumptions in the field about the relationship between food preferences and market demands; specifically, that if low-income individuals shift their preferences toward healthier foods, the market will respond accordingly and income differentials in diet will be reduced. Rather, both favorable preferences and favorable prices had to be present in order to observe reductions in the diet differentials.

The conceptual framework and modeling approach undertaken in the Auchincloss model has served to inspire additional models exploring income inequalities. Widener et al. developed a spatially explicit model to explore food purchasing behaviors of low-income residents in Buffalo, New York, using empirical resident data (Widener, Metcalf, & Bar-Yam, 2013). It expanded the work done in the Auchincloss model by integrating empirical spatial data and further included spatiotemporal patterns of food availability, such as increases in stock during the summer months as a result of farmers' markets. Blok et al. similarly applied the Auchincloss framework to the modeling of interventions addressing residential segregation, food prices, and health education. This model was able to estimate the length of time to observed intervention impacts (5–10 years), as well as to evaluate unintended effects of single interventions to other components of the model.

These and other examples from the literature (Orr, Galea, Riddle, & Kaplan, 2014; Zhang, Giabbanelli, Arah, & Zimmerman, 2014) serve to highlight the dearth of empirical data available to explore associations between the food environment and health and can underscore and justify priorities for the generation of empirical data, particularly food-related behaviors and preferences. With the collection of additional data, model parameters can be better informed and model processes and outcomes better calibrated. Additionally, they reveal that single interventions are not likely to produce desired impacts in the presence of complex interactions (Giabbanelli & Crutzen, 2017).

Social Environment

The use of ABMs to explore associations between the social conditions of a neighborhood system and health outcomes is much more varied than our previous examples and crosses multiple disciplines and outcomes of interest, including but not limited to drug use (Galea, Hall, & Kaplan, 2009), crime (Yonas et al., 2013), social stigma (Mooney & El-Sayed, 2016), and racial disparities (Orr et al., 2014). Additionally, a key process evaluated in many of these applications is the role of social networks, a topic that this textbook does not cover in depth (El-Sayed et al., 2012). Similar to our previous examples, the applications highlight the benefits of the method in the absence of data available from the application of empirical methods.

In summary, the application of ABM to the study of neighborhoods and health has demonstrated utility in three areas as summarized by Auchincloss (Auchincloss & Diez Roux, 2008).

Conceptual Utility

The interrelated processes that occur between people and their environment are an unavoidable conundrum in the study of neighborhoods. ABMs facilitate a meaningful understanding of *how* these processes may be important in the production of health and disease. Agents can be defined at the multiple levels of influence that are deemed important to these processes (e.g., individual, structural, social, and political).

Methodological Utility

We have aimed to highlight the methodological utility that ABM provides to the study of neighborhoods. To summarize, ABM methods allow for the study of interdependent processes that occur over time and space, as compared to regression methods, which aim to isolate effects, provide summary measures, and ignore feedback and adaptation.

Data Utility

A unique benefit of ABMs, and simulation methods generally, lies in their ability to construct models in the complete absence of empirical data. When empirical data are available, they serve to highlight areas where empirical data, or the quality of the data, are lacking. Furthermore, they can provide estimates of intervention impacts when experimental designs, such as randomized trials, are either unethical or infeasible.

Lastly, despite the fact that ABMs are still relatively new in their applications to neighborhoods and health research, the early development of models alone opens up the field for further and future investigation. Take, for example, the exploratory model of Yang et al. (2011), developed to explore adult walking behaviors within a city. The initial model was built upon to further explore walking differences by socioeconomic status (Yang et al., 2012) based on observations made in the initial model. Additionally, these models laid the necessary groundwork, both methodologically and conceptually, to evaluate walking behaviors of school children (instead of adults) using ABM, and the potential impact of hypothetical interventions (Yang & Diez-Roux, 2013; Yang et al., 2014).

CURRENT LIMITATIONS OF THE AGENT-BASED MODEL

Despite the many and varied benefits of ABMs, they are not without limitation. Here we highlight a few of the limitations that are commonly cited. As with any set of limitations identified in scientific investigations, approaches may be available to minimize their impact or to place bounds on their potential impact on study outcomes. We also review these.

ABMs are well suited for the study of complex processes, as explained. However, the implementation of the model requires some assumptions and simplification of processes. Many of the cited limitations of ABM are a result of this necessary simplification. For example, we previously discussed that ABMs are typically minimalist models, containing only sufficient detail for the intended outcome to be observed. Therefore, models can be very sensitive to the choice of agent behaviors and/or behavioral rules. The use of sensitivity analyses will aid in discussions of this potential limitation.

Additionally, ABMs have often been constructed to observe emergent patterns from lower level interactions regardless of optimization or magnitude of scale. Instead, the focus has been on facilitating understanding of underlying processes. For example, the Schelling model of segregation was initialized with fewer than 100 agents. However, as appreciation for the method has grown and the possibility for optimizing policy interventions, for example, has been realized, the limitations of model scale have increasingly been highlighted. In response to the increasing demands for large-scale ABMs, technical solutions are under development.

Similar to traditional statistical models, conclusions made from model observation and outcomes are contingent on the model assumptions. However, in contrast to the traditional methods, the assumptions of an ABM are explicitly encoded into the model and may subjectively reflect the biases of the modeler. To avoid the latter, model assumptions should be explicitly described and easily defensible given current knowledge.

Parameterization of the model can be limited similarly. ABMs provide opportunities for investigation when traditional methods are unavailable due to a lack of empirical data, or because they are cost prohibitive or unethical, for example. However, the valid parameterization of the model under these circumstances has been called into question. Sensitivity analysis and other model calibration techniques can again be used to place estimates on the bounds of this limitation. Although the identification of data gaps by ABM is highlighted positively, the utility of early models beyond that benefit may inherently be limited by subjective parameter estimation. We would argue, however, that precise parameterization of a model should not be the focus of or the sole reason for dismissing any model.

Lastly, limitations are typically model specific and should be discussed in the presentation of any model.

CONCLUSIONS

Computer simulation does not replace the need for empirical research. It is rather an adjunct that affords an approach to complex systems that cannot be achieved using more traditional analytic methods. As such, there are several areas in which computer simulation, such as ABM, can benefit the future study of neighborhoods and health.

Throughout this book, the authors provide examples of neighborhood-level effects on individual health or health behaviors, the underlying mechanisms of which are not well understood. Early explorations into neighborhood home foreclosures (discussed in Chapter 10) and spatial stigma (discussed in Chapter 11), for example, highlight this opportunity for ABM to be used to develop explanations for *how* neighborhood home foreclosures and spatial stigma may produce negative impacts on health, health behaviors, or other social processes.

This textbook also discusses methods for both qualitative and quantitative data collection that are important to accurately characterizing and operationalizing the neighborhood environment (Chapters 2, 3, and 7). The limited application of ABM to neighborhoods and health research to date has already highlighted the dearth of existing data, particularly spatial data, and the uncertainty with which existing data have been measured. The continued application of ABM in this area can make use of the methodological advancements and improvements to data collection tools for empirical research through better informed model parameters and hypotheses about underlying processes and mechanisms. Additionally, its continued implementation can assist in further refinement of empirical research.

Neighborhood intervention research is also briefly discussed in this book (Chapter 6). Generally, the application of intervention methods to the study of neighborhoods and health is limited for a variety of reasons, but importantly it includes reasons related to the necessity for complex and multilevel interventions—an area that is still under development (Cleary, Gross, Zaslavsky, & Taplin, 2012). ABMs provide a useful laboratory for not only evaluating outcomes of complex interventions but also afford the opportunity to deepen understanding of the dynamics of intervention impact.

We briefly mentioned some of the common software platforms that are used to assist in the development and implementation of ABM. A primary benefit of these software packages is that many of the important and necessary model components and processes are already programmed and only require context- and data-specific adjustments. There exists opportunity to enhance the utility of these packages to neighborhoods and health researchers through the development of software that provides model inputs for common neighborhood domains.

To conclude, traditional population health methods primarily include observation of a population over time through the collection of data, either through observation or abstraction (a simulation model's "inputs"), and subsequently analysis of that data uses statistical models to make inferences about causal pathways operating in the population. Similarly, in intervention research, we subject members of a population to one or more conditions and observe changes to that population over time. In both approaches (i.e., observational and intervention research), our inferences are limited to the information that was collected and the varying conditions that were explicitly studied. In other words, the only answers we can get are the ones in which the data are available to answer them. The application of ABM offers a flexible alternative with unique benefits, useful to the future study of neighborhoods and health.

REFERENCES

Auchincloss, A. H., & Diez Roux, A. V. (2008). A new tool for epidemiology: The usefulness of dynamic-agent models in understanding place effects on health. *American Journal of Epidemiology*, *168*(1), 1–8. doi:10.1093/aje/kwn118

Auchincloss, A. H., & Garcia, L. M. T. (2015). Brief introductory guide to agent-based modeling and an illustration from urban health research. *Cadernos De Saude Publica*, *31*, S65–S78. doi:10.1590/0102-311X00051615

Auchincloss, A. H., Riolo, R. L., Brown, D. G., Cook, J., & Diez Roux, A. V. (2011). An agent-based model of income inequalities in diet in the context of residential segregation. *American Journal of Preventive Medicine, 40*(3), 303–311. doi:10.1016/j.amepre.2010.10.033

Badland, H., White, M., MacAulay, G., Eagleson, S., Mavoa, S., Pettit, C., & Giles-Corti, B. (2013). Using simple agent-based modeling to inform and enhance neighborhood walkability. *International Journal of Health Geographics, 12*. doi:Artn 58 10.1186/1476-072x-12-58

Bonabeau, E. (2002). Agent-based modeling: methods and techniques for simulating human systems. *Proceedings of the National Academy of Sciences USA, 99*(Suppl 3), 7280–7287. doi:10.1073/pnas.082080899

Borshchev, A., & Filippov, A. (2004). *From system dynamics and discrete event to practical agent based modeling: Reasons, techniques, tools.* Paper presented at the the 22nd International Conference of the System Dynamics Society, Oxford, England.

Chalabi, Z., & Lorenc, T. (2013). Using agent-based models to inform evaluation of complex interventions: Examples from the built environment. *Preventive Medicine, 57*(5), 434–435. doi:10.1016/j.ypmed.2013.07.013

Cleary, P. D., Gross, C. P., Zaslavsky, A. M., & Taplin, S. H. (2012). Multilevel interventions: Study design and analysis issues. *Journal of the National Cancer Institute Monographs, 2012*(44), 49–55. doi:10.1093/jncimonographs/lgs010

Conte, R., & Paolucci, M. (2014). On agent-based modeling and computational social science. *Frontiers in Psychology, 5*, 668. doi:10.3389/fpsyg.2014.00668

Diez Roux, A. V. (2007). Integrating social and biologic factors in health research: A systems view. *Annals of Epidemiology, 17*(7), 569–574. doi:10.1016/j.annepidem.2007.03.001

Diez Roux, A. V. (2016). Neighborhoods and health: What do we know? What should we do? *American Journal of Public Health, 106*(3), 430–431. doi:10.2105/AJPH.2016.303064

Diez Roux, A. V., & Auchincloss, A. H. (2009). Understanding the social determinants of behaviours: Can new methods help? *International Journal of Drug Policy, 20*(3), 227–229. doi:10.1016/j.drugpo.2008.11.003

Diez Roux, A. V., & Mair, C. (2010). Neighborhoods and health. *Annals of the NY Academy of Sciences, 1186*, 125–145. doi:10.1111/j.1749-6632.2009.05333.x

El-Sayed, A. M., Scarborough, P., Seemann, L., & Galea, S. (2012). Social network analysis and agent-based modeling in social epidemiology. *Epidemiologic Perspectives and Innovations, 9*(1), 1. doi:10.1186/1742-5573-9-1

Filatova, T., Verburg, P. H., Parker, D. C., & Stannard, C. A. (2013). Spatial agent-based models for socio-ecological systems: Challenges and prospects. *Environmental Modelling & Software, 45*, 1–7. doi:10.1016/j.envsoft.2013.03.017

Galea, S., Hall, C., & Kaplan, G. A. (2009). Social epidemiology and complex system dynamic modelling as applied to health behaviour and drug use research. *International Journal of Drug Policy, 20*(3), 209–216. doi:10.1016/j.drugpo.2008.08.005

Galea, S., Riddle, M., & Kaplan, G. A. (2010). Causal thinking and complex system approaches in epidemiology. *International Journal of Epidemiology, 39*(1), 97–106. doi:10.1093/ije/dyp296

Giabbanelli, P. J., & Crutzen, R. (2017). Using agent-based models to develop public policy about food behaviours: Future directions and recommendations. *Computational and Mathematical Methods in Medicine.* doi:Artn 5742629 10.1155/2017/5742629

Grimm, V., Berger, U., Bastiansen, F., Eliassen, S., Ginot, V., Giske, J., . . . DeAngelis, D. L. (2006). A standard protocol for describing individual-based and agent-based models. *Ecological Modelling, 198*(1–2), 115–126. doi:10.1016/j.ecolmodel.2006.04.023

Hammond, R. A. (2009). Complex systems modeling for obesity research. *Preventing Chronic Disease, 6*(3), A97.

Hammond, R. A., & Dube, L. (2012). A systems science perspective and transdisciplinary models for food and nutrition security. *Proceedings of the National Academy of Sciences USA, 109*(31), 12356–12363. doi:10.1073/pnas.0913003109

Handy, S., Cao, X. Y., & Mokhtarian, P. L. (2006). Self-selection in the relationship between the built environment and walking—Empirical evidence from northern California. *Journal of the American Planning Association, 72*(1), 55–74. doi:10.1080/01944360608976724

Li, Y., Lawley, M. A., Siscovick, D. S., Zhang, D., & Pagan, J. A. (2016). Agent-based modeling of chronic diseases: A narrative review and future research directions. *Preventing Chronic Disease, 13*, E69. doi:10.5888/pcd13.150561

Lovasi, G. S., Grady, S., & Rundle, A. (2012). Steps forward: Review and recommendations for research on walkability, physical activity and cardiovascular health. *Public Health Review, 33*(4), 484–506.

Luke, D. A., & Stamatakis, K. A. (2012). Systems science methods in public health: Dynamics, networks, and agents. *Annual Review of Public Health, 33*, 357–376. doi:10.1146/annurev-publhealth-031210-101222

Mabry, P. L., Milstein, B., Abraido-Lanza, A. F., Livingood, W. C., & Allegrante, J. P. (2013). Opening a window on systems science research in health promotion and public health. *Health Education & Behavior, 40*(1 Suppl), 5S-8S. doi:10.1177/1090198113503343

Macal, C. M., & North, M. J. (2007). Agent-based modeling and simulation: Desktop ABMS. *Proceedings of the 2007 Winter Simulation Conference, Vols 1–5*, 83–94.

Maglio, P. P., & Mabry, P. L. (2011). Agent-based models and systems science approaches to public health. *American Journal of Preventive Medicine, 40*(3), 392–394. doi:10.1016/j.amepre.2010.11.010

Marshall, B. D., & Galea, S. (2015). Formalizing the role of agent-based modeling in causal inference and epidemiology. *American Journal of Epidemiology, 181*(2), 92–99. doi:10.1093/aje/kwu274

McCormack, G. R., & Shiell, A. (2011). In search of causality: A systematic review of the relationship between the built environment and physical activity among adults. *International Journal of Behavioral Nutrition and Physical Activity, 8*. doi:Artn 125 10.1186/1479-5868-8-125

Mooney, S. J., & El-Sayed, A. M. (2016). Stigma and the etiology of depression among the obese: An agent-based exploration. *Social Science & Medicine, 148*, 1–7. doi:10.1016/j.socscimed.2015.11.020

Nianogo, R. A., & Arah, O. A. (2015). Agent-based modeling of noncommunicable diseases: A systematic review. *American Journal of Public Health, 105*(3), e20–e31. doi:10.2105/AJPH.2014.302426

Nikolai, C., & Madey, G. (2009). Tools of the trade: A survey of various agent based modeling platforms. *Jasss—the Journal of Artificial Societies and Social Simulation, 12*(2).

North, M. J., Collier, N. T., Ozik, J., Tatara, E. R., Macal, C. M., Bragen, M., & Sydelko, P. (2013). Complex adaptive systems modeling with repast simphony. *Complex Adaptive Systems Modeling, 1*(3).

Northridge, M. E., Sclar, E. D., & Biswas, P. (2003). Sorting out the connections between the built environment and health: A conceptual framework for navigating pathways and planning healthy cities. *Journal of Urban Health-Bulletin of the New York Academy of Medicine, 80*(4), 556–568. doi:10.1093/jurban/jtg064

Orr, M. G., Galea, S., Riddle, M., & Kaplan, G. A. (2014). Reducing racial disparities in obesity: Simulating the effects of improved education and social network influence on diet behavior. *Annals of Epidemiology, 24*(8), 563–569. doi:10.1016/j.annepidem.2014.05.012

Orr, M. G., Kaplan, G. A., & Galea, S. (2016). Neighbourhood food, physical activity, and educational environments and black/white disparities in obesity: A complex systems simulation analysis. *Journal of Epidemiology and Community Health, 70*(9), 862–867. doi:10.1136/jech-2015-205621

Railsback, S. F., Lytinen, S. L., & Jackson, S. K. (2006). Agent-based simulation platforms: Review and development recommendations. *Simulation-Transactions of the Society for Modeling and Simulation International, 82*(9), 609–623. doi:10.1177/0037549706073695

Rice, K. (2012). The utility of multilevel modeling vs. agent-based modeling in examining spatial disparities in diet and health: The case of food deserts. In A. Desai (Ed.), *Simulation for policy inquiry* (pp. 63–82). New York, NY: Springer Science + Business Media, LLC.

Sargent, R. G. (2013). Verification and validation of simulation models. *Journal of Simulation, 7*(1), 12–24. doi:10.1057/jos.2012.20

Schelling, T. C. (1969). Models of segregation. *American Economic Review, 59*(2), 488–493.

Schelling, T. C. (1971). Dynamic models of segregation. *Journal of Mathematical Sociology, 1*(2), 143–186.

Subramanian, S. V., Jones, K., & Duncan, C. (2003). Multilevel methods for public health research. In I. Kawachi & L. Berkman (Eds.), *Neighborhoods and health* (pp. 65–111). New York, NY: Oxford University Press.

Thiele, J. C., Kurth, W., & Grimm, V. (2014). Facilitating parameter estimation and sensitivity analysis of agent-based models: A cookbook using Net Logo and R. *Jasss—the Journal of Artificial Societies and Social Simulation, 17*(3).

Trochim, W. M., Cabrera, D. A., Milstein, B., Gallagher, R. S., & Leischow, S. J. (2006). Practical challenges of systems thinking and modeling in public health. *American Journal of Public Health, 96*(3), 538–546. doi:10.2105/AJPH.2005.066001

Widener, M. J., Metcalf, S. S., & Bar-Yam, Y. (2013). Agent-based modeling of policies to improve urban food access for low-income populations. *Applied Geography, 40*, 1–10. doi:10.1016/j.apgeog.2013.01.003

Yang, Y., Diez-Roux, A., Evenson, K. R., & Colabianchi, N. (2014). Examining the impact of the walking school bus with an agent-based model. *American Journal of Public Health, 104*(7), 1196–1203. doi:10.2105/AJPH.2014.301896

Yang, Y., & Diez-Roux, A. V. (2013). Using an agent-based model to simulate children's active travel to school. *International Journal of Behavioral Nutrition and Physical Activity, 10*. doi:Unsp 67 10.1186/1479-5868-10-67

Yang, Y., Roux, A. V. D., Auchincloss, A. H., Rodriguez, D. A., & Brown, D. G. (2011). A spatial agent-based model for the simulation of adults' daily walking within a city. *American Journal of Preventive Medicine, 40*(3), 353–361. doi:10.1016/j.amepre.2010.11.017

Yang, Y., Roux, A. V. D., Auchincloss, A. H., Rodriguez, D. A., & Brown, D. G. (2012). Exploring walking differences by socioeconomic status using a spatial agent-based model. *Health & Place, 18*(1), 96–99. doi:10.1016/j.healthplace.2011.08.010

Yonas, M. A., Burke, J. G., Brown, S. T., Borrebach, J. D., Garland, R., Burke, D. S., & Grefenstette, J. J. (2013). Dynamic simulation of crime perpetration and reporting to examine community intervention strategies. *Health Education & Behavior, 40*(1 Suppl), 87S–97S. doi:10.1177/1090198113493090

Zhang, D. L., Giabbanelli, P. J., Arah, O. A., & Zimmerman, F. J. (2014). Impact of different policies on unhealthy dietary behaviors in an urban adult population: An agent-based simulation model. *American Journal of Public Health, 104*(7), 1217–1222. doi:10.2105/Ajph.2014.301934

Zhu, W. M., Nedovic-Budic, Z., Olshansky, R. B., Marti, J., Gao, Y., Park, Y., . . . Chodzko-Zajko, W. (2013). Agent-based modeling of physical activity behavior and environmental correlations: An introduction and illustration. *Journal of Physical Activity & Health, 10*(3), 309–322.

6

EXPERIMENTAL AND QUASI-EXPERIMENTAL DESIGNS IN NEIGHBORHOOD HEALTH EFFECTS RESEARCH

STRENGTHENING CAUSAL INFERENCE AND PROMOTING TRANSLATION

Nicole M. Schmidt, Quynh C. Nguyen, and Theresa L. Osypuk

As discussed in other chapters of this book, neighborhood context may be one of the most important upstream social determinants of health, and causes of health inequity, in the United States and elsewhere. Although the literature examining neighborhood effects on health is vast and continues to grow, as recent reviews have noted, the evidence base remains predominantly descriptive, based on observational studies employing traditional methods that often fail to control for important threats to internal validity and that fail to engage the epidemiological imagination (Arcaya et al., 2016; Oakes, Andrade, Biyoow, & Cowan, 2015). For example, arguably the biggest threat to causal inference in the neighborhood effects literature is residential selection (Oakes, 2004; Sampson, 2008), where people move to certain types of neighborhoods and these moves are also associated with their health. Yet residential selection is seldom actually modeled in neighborhood health effects research. Therefore, among the most important priorities for this area of scholarship is to strengthen causal inference by employing stronger designs at the onset, such as experimental and quasi-experimental designs, to alleviate such threats to validity.

In this chapter, we focus on the application of experimental and quasi-experimental designs for assessing neighborhood effects on health. First, we will define some assumptions for causal inference. Second, we will describe the features of experimental, quasi-experimental, and longitudinal designs, with particular attention to addressing causal inference. Third, we will discuss examples of studies using experimental, quasi-experimental, and longitudinal designs applying a causal framework for neighborhood effects studies. In particular, we will provide a more in-depth empirical look at the largest and most well-known experiment that has examined neighborhood effects on health, the Moving to Opportunity (MTO) Demonstration Project. Lastly, we discuss the implications of experimental, quasi-experimental, and causal longitudinal designs in terms of translation and policy evaluation.

CAUSAL INFERENCE ASSUMPTIONS

Internal validity is defined as the extent to which the cause–effect association is estimated without bias, thereby allowing stronger causal inference. Causal inference generally relies on three primary assumptions: exchangeability, positivity, and consistency. The neighborhood health effects literature poses challenges for each of these assumptions, as we will discuss. First, exchangeability is defined as the lack of confounding; in other words, the exposed and unexposed are exchangeable, and therefore exactly similar as a group, but for the specific exposure under study. Exchangeability is the most well-articulated challenge for causal inference in the neighborhood literature (much like the fields of epidemiology or social science writ large), typically because its literature relies on observational studies that may always be threatened by unmeasured confounding. In other words, one or more unmeasured variables may be common prior causes of both the exposure (neighborhood context) and the health outcome.

The second important inference guiding causal inference is positivity, meaning that the treatment-control contrast is maintained (and units in each condition are present) within each strata of covariates. Conceptually, there is insufficient overlap between the distributions of exposed and unexposed within a third variable. Positivity is a challenging assumption for neighborhood research given the stark inequality in neighborhood environments present in the United States by race and social position (Osypuk & Acevedo-Garcia, 2010). Such inequality has been deemed structural confounding (Oakes, 2006; Oakes & Johnson, 2006) (also discussed in Chapter 12), because some demographic groups do not reside in certain neighborhood environments. The violation of positivity is expressed as distinctly separate distributions of neighborhood quality, for example, by race. Despite that neighborhood context is hypothesized as a strong cause of health disparities, this violation of positivity makes it difficult to understand how strong a cause it is, with methodological rigor at the individual level (Osypuk & Acevedo-Garcia, 2010).

The third assumption for causal inference is consistency, which means that the exposure is defined with enough specificity that different variants of exposure do not have different effects on the outcome (Rehkopf, Glymour, & Osypuk, 2016). For example, consistency may be violated when exposure is defined by a bundled neighborhood exposure, for example by an index of neighborhood socioeconomic status (Rehkopf et al., 2016). The consistency assumption has received very little attention in social epidemiology, including neighborhood effects research, perhaps because the understanding of this assumption has been masked by opaque technical language that has not been specifically digestible for social researchers. However, the assumption is clearly relevant for neighborhood effects research, particularly because clear definitions make it much easier to translate findings and act to intervene on the exposure.

Generalizability is defined as whether the cause–effect association in one population is the same as for another population, or different based on population traits, places, or times (Shadish, Cook, & Campbell, 2002). Generalizability is also called external validity or representativeness: how well results from a study are representative of people and circumstances outside of the particular study population and context. Although generalizability (external validity) is often considered a secondary consideration to causal inference (internal validity), some have taken issue with that characterization. For example, estimating a causal effect in a narrowly defined, non–randomly selected population may not be problematic if treatment effects are homogenous across different subgroups. However, treatment effect heterogeneity across various subgroups may be very common. This heterogeneity may be masked by narrow eligibility criteria in a randomized trial, for example. When such a finding is not replicated in another population subgroup, it may be deemed nongeneralizable. Selection of a representative sample in the first place can be viewed as a core element of the study (Sampson, 2010).

EXPERIMENTAL STUDY DESIGNS

Experimental designs, also called randomized controlled trials (RCTs), are considered the gold standard for identifying cause and effect relationships, across disciplines (Austin, 2011). Experimental designs are characterized by many features that strengthen causal inference, but two features are particularly important: randomization of treatment assignment with at least one comparison group; and investigator manipulation and assignment of study exposure or treatment (Shadish et al., 2002).

Random Assignment

Random assignment is the strongest tool for achieving exchangeability between two groups, by conceptually breaking any possible association between the exposure of interest and any other baseline variable, except for an association that emerges by chance. Thus, randomization of treatment assignment is important for several reasons (Shadish et al., 2002). First, it provides the best guarantee that the control group (i.e., the unexposed or those without the treatment under study) is a valid substitute population for the treatment group. The desired comparison group for the treatment group is the counterfactual, in other words, the treatment group had they not received treatment. Although it is not possible to obtain this counterfactual at the individual level, the RCT design achieves it at the group level. Random assignment also avoids self-selection into treatment, which is an important source of bias.

Second and relatedly, randomization is one of the few methods that controls for characteristics that are unknown and/or unmeasured between populations. Operationally, randomization achieves this group comparability by balancing any possible factor in equal quantities across the treatment groups. This control for unmeasured confounding is particularly transcendent compared to most other methods of confounding control. Health outcomes can be influenced by a variety of factors. Thus, when we study the potential effect of a treatment, we must isolate its effect and control for bias by controlling for any other relevant factor that is a prior common cause of both the exposure and the health outcome. However, methods of controlling for confounding typically require us to identify and measure all potential confounders, or they require us to make assumptions about the pattern of these confounders (e.g., by controlling time-stable confounding in longitudinal models with fixed effect models, which does not control time-varying confounders).

Finally, randomization satisfies the assumption of statistical tests for exogeneity (where the error terms are uncorrelated with the explanatory variables). This allows for the evaluation of the effect of treatment on the outcome. If the errors are exogenous, then the effect estimates are unbiased.

Investigator-Assigned Exposure

Manipulation of the exposure by study investigators means the treatment is clearly defined and measured, which satisfies the consistency criterion for causal inference, thereby more easily facilitating replication. Investigator assignment of exposure also means that the exposure is manipulable (in other words, able to be manipulated), which is not a given for some exposures that have received attention in the social epidemiology literature such as race or social class (Shadish et al., 2002). Moreover, although some exposures may be manipulated in theory, it may be unethical or impractical to manipulate them. For example, researchers may be interested in the effects of child maltreatment on health; however, it is unethical to randomly assign some children to be maltreated and others not. On the contrary, it may be unethical to randomly assign participants to a “no treatment” group if a drug treatment is known to be effective.

Investigator assignment of treatment within a prospective design (where exposure and disease occur in time after the study is initiated) together provide assurance that the exposure precedes disease, thus preserving temporal order for a causal effect. This design element is not specific to experimental designs since other intervention studies and longitudinal designs can also achieve this.

Limitations and Strengths of Experimental Designs

Although experimental designs overcome many limitations of other study designs that hinder causal inference, experiments are not without limitations. First, external validity may be an issue if studies cannot be generalized to other populations and real-world circumstances. This is a particular concern when researchers prioritize compliance to treatment and therefore are willing to trade off narrowing the inclusion criteria (e.g., to enroll more compliant subjects) to improve internal validity. Random assignment substantially strengthens causal inference (i.e., providing assurances for internal validity). However, random assignment is a separate concept from random sampling (Table 6-1)—in which participants are drawn from a population with a known probability of selection. In the case of simple random sampling, participants have an equal chance of being selected from a population. Random sampling allows for broader inferences for how the results will relate to the wider population (strong external validity).

Second, low compliance can bias results, because although one can randomly assign treatment, one cannot force a participant, ethically or practically, to follow the treatment regimen. Low compliance typically waters down the true treatment effect (if everyone had complied) toward the null. Notably, there are methods that can account for low compliance analytically given some additional assumptions, for example, instrumental variable (IV) analysis (Angrist & Imbens, 1995; Angrist, Imbens, & Rubin, 1996; Newhouse & McClellan, 1998). Third, the consistency of treatment implementation (e.g., intervention integrity) may be an issue, particularly

Table 6-1 Random Sampling Versus Random Assignment

	Random Assignment	*No Random Assignment*	
Random sampling	Enables causal inference and generalizations to the population	Correlation statements, generalizable to the population	**Generalizable**
No random sampling	Enables causal inference, only for the study sample	Correlation statements, only for the study sample	**Not generalizable**
	Causation	**Correlation**	

with multisite trials, which would relate to differences in the treatment received and violate the consistency assumption. This could happen, for example, if the treatment was delivered differently at each trial site based on the expertise of the local team implementing the trial. Fourth, experimental designs may be costly and take many years before the effects of treatment on outcomes can be assessed. Fifth, whenever investigators assign a treatment, special ethical procedures must be followed to ensure the protection of human subjects. Sixth, experiments typically answer very narrow research questions, compared to other designs such as prospective cohort studies. Moreover, most traditional experiments are designed to test main effects of treatment on outcomes, which means that in practice they are underpowered to test more complex hypotheses; for example, to identify heterogeneous treatment effects among subgroups (moderation) or to understand the mechanisms through which treatment works (mediation). Lastly, as with any longitudinal design, attrition (study dropout) is a possible source of bias.

There are some features of experimental designs that make them strong for causal inference but, in practice, are difficult to implement for neighborhood effects research, including blinding of the exposure from participants or study staff and use of a placebo. Blinding prevents differential misclassification error that is patterned by either participant or staff expectations of how the treatment should operate to affect the health outcome. Failure to blind participants can lead them to believe a treatment is effective via psychological mechanisms or the placebo effect. Therefore, masking the participant's exposure status from all relevant parties helps provide assurance that measurements and analyses are conducted in an unbiased and fair manner with regard to the outcome.

Specific Types of Experimental Studies

Randomized trials can take a variety of forms. The active treatment or exposure could be (1) a clinical trial, which is a therapeutic drug or device offered to people with some disease or condition to treat or manage that disease or (2) a preventive trial, which is a preventive or prophylactic vaccine, procedure, or intervention (e.g., health education) offered. In the case of neighborhood effects research, the latter is more appropriate for population health, for example, via assignment to live in a particular type of neighborhood or for a particular neighborhood to receive an intervention. Moreover, a randomized trial could involve two or more exposure groups, as long as each group corresponds to a different assigned treatment component. For example, one treatment group could be given health behavior counseling and anti-diabetic medication while another treatment group may only be given the behavior counseling. We discuss specific examples of experimental studies in the neighborhood effects health literature next.

Randomization can also be applied to different types of units, resulting in different types of trials. Although individuals are most commonly randomized for clinical trials, a group randomized trial refers to the random assignment of other relevant contexts within which individuals are nested that would correspond to a natural site for an exposure to act. For example, group randomized trials (also known as community trials) may treat schools, classrooms, physicians, housing developments, or neighborhoods as the unit of assignment. For neighborhood effects research, both levels of units (at the individual and neighborhood level) have been used and proposed, as we discuss further in the next section.

QUASI-EXPERIMENTAL STUDY DESIGNS

Quasi-experimental designs describe the class of studies that are *nonrandomized interventions*. They have some similar features and benefits as experimental designs, for example, including prospective designs to establish temporal order between exposure and disease, as well as a clearly specified, investigator-assigned exposure, but quasi-experimental designs lack random assignment of a treatment intervention. Quasi-experimental designs are utilized when randomization is not feasible or possible, in cases such as when it is unethical to assign or withhold a particular treatment to an individual, or if implementing a randomized experiment would be too difficult and/or costly (Harris et al., 2006). Quasi-experiments are popular in practice-based research. Examples of quasi-experimental studies include pre-post intervention studies, where outcome measurements are compared before and after an intervention; nonrandomized community trials, where communities are selected to receive an intervention but not at random; cross-over interventions, where for example, half of subjects receive an intervention in the first half of the study period, while the second half receives the intervention during the second half of the study period; and natural experiments, where a naturally occurring phenomenon, one not initiated by the investigator him/herself for the primary purpose of research, is treated as the exposure (Handley, Schillinger, & Shiboski, 2011; Harris et al., 2006). Like experiments, quasi-experiments are a relatively rare and underutilized tool for testing neighborhood effects (Oakes et al., 2015).

In quasi-experimental studies, the investigator manipulates the "exposure" but does not randomly assign it (Table 6-2). Since quasi-experimental studies do not involve random treatment assignment, they may provide fewer assurances of internal validity compared to randomized trials, with respect to exchangeability of the

Table 6-2 Categorization of Study Designs, by Study Components

Study Type	*Manipulation of Exposure*	*Randomization*	*Temporal Ordering*
Experimental	Yes	Yes	Yes
Quasi-experimental	Yes	No	Yes
Natural experiments	Yes, but naturally occurring[†]	No	Yes
Observational-longitudinal	No	No	Yes
Observational-cross–sectional	No	No	No

[†] A naturally occurring exposure is one that is outside the investigator's control, such as a natural disaster or the enactment of a new government policy.

exposure groups. Quasi-experiments may also be difficult to replicate, particularly if they leverage a naturally occurring exposure, such as a natural disaster (e.g., flood or hurricane) or the enactment of a new local, state, or national policy.

However, quasi-experimental studies are very popular and widely used in applied research, although they are underutilized for neighborhood-health effects research. Quasi-experiments may contribute to our understanding of neighborhood phenomena, particularly when randomization is not feasible. For example, an investigator may not be allowed to randomly assign treatment in school settings, psychiatric hospitals, or clients of community agencies, given logistical or ethical barriers. On the other hand, since many quasi-experiments are implemented in real-world circumstances, this may increase their external validity.

Quasi-experimental designs encompass a wide variety of study types, including community trials designed for education and behavior change at the group level—for example, comparison of obesity rates in schools given healthy eating interventions versus those who were not given the intervention. Quasi-experimental studies also include pretest-posttest study designs, in which the investigator implements an intervention and compares outcomes before and after the intervention. Pretest-posttest study designs may or may not have a comparison group. If there is not an additional comparison group, then preintervention outcome values are compared against postintervention outcomes values. In this case, the individual serves as his or her own control group. If there is an additional comparison group, pre-post differences are compared among those who received the intervention and those did not. This comparison is called a difference-in-difference study design.

Natural experiments are one subgroup of the quasi-experimental design that leverage a naturally occurring external exposure (one not initiated or controlled by the research investigator) that in our case causes change at the neighborhood level to mimic a pseudo-random intervention. Natural experiments may have strong causal inference because it may be argued that the exposure occurs as if it were random, for example, examining how a natural disaster affects health outcomes by comparing outcomes across populations that were otherwise comparable before the disaster. We discuss specific examples next.

OBSERVATIONAL STUDY DESIGNS: LONGITUDINAL AND CROSS-SECTIONAL STUDIES

Observational studies, including cross-sectional and longitudinal studies, are the most common research designs in the neighborhood health effects literature. Cross-sectional designs in particular, which measure variables at one point in time, are extremely common because they are easy to implement and are cost effective. A recent systematic review of the neighborhood health effects literature noted that over 70% of studies were cross-sectional (Arcaya et al., 2016). Cross-sectional studies can be a valuable tool for providing descriptive information, for example, for estimating the disease burden in a population. Cross-sectional studies also may be valuable to establish preliminary evidence in the early stages of research, as in exploratory studies. However, cross-sectional studies lack many of the features present in stronger designs to facilitate causal inference, including random assignment, investigator-assigned treatment, and preservation of temporal order between exposure and health outcome. Since we focus on causal inference in this chapter, we will not discuss further cross-sectional neighborhood studies on health.

Longitudinal studies are a more powerful design than cross-sectional studies, because they allow ascertaining the temporal order of exposure and disease. The prospective cohort study, a classic longitudinal design in epidemiology, is characterized by enumerating exposure at baseline among a clearly defined population who is free of the disease outcome of interest at baseline, and enumerating if certain respondents develop incident (new cases of) disease, when across time, and how this is patterned by their initial exposure status. Longitudinal studies are also increasingly collecting repeated measurements of exposures, outcomes, and confounders over time. Among the neighborhood health effects literature, longitudinal designs are the second most common design, accounting for over 20% of studies (Arcaya et al., 2016).

Although longitudinal designs do not contain such elements as random assignment or manipulating an exposure, the ability to establish temporal ordering of an exposure of interest and an outcome is a strong design feature. Moreover, if measurements are repeated, longitudinal designs are ideal for analyzing changes or trends in both exposures and outcomes over time (Singer & Willett, 2003). Longitudinal studies may also be more representative than interventions or experiments, particularly if they are drawn from a probability sample in a well-defined population, with high study participation rates, and if attrition is low across time. Longitudinal studies are more flexible than intervention studies (e.g., one can examine a range of exposures or outcomes in a longitudinal design), and therefore they may answer broader research questions than an intervention design. Although longitudinal studies have some beneficial features, they are not without limitations. Longitudinal studies are time consuming, sometimes spanning decades, making them costly and subject to attrition of subjects over time. Moreover, longitudinal studies are observational, meaning that the exposures are naturally occurring, and respondent selected, rather than being assigned. This means that some exposures may not be very specific, or even manipulable. Recent methodological innovations allow strengthened causal inference using longitudinal data. We will discuss a few such methods, including marginal structural models and fixed effects analysis, in a later section of the chapter.

EXPERIMENTAL AND QUASI-EXPERIMENTAL DESIGNS EXAMINING NEIGHBORHOOD EFFECTS ON HEALTH: EXAMPLES FROM THE LITERATURE

We conducted a brief review of the literature, to identify experimental and quasi-experimental studies examining neighborhood effects on health. We conducted a search of the literature in PubMed using combinations of keywords, including neighborhood/neighbourhood, neighborhood/neighbourhood effects, and experiment. We also supplemented our formal search by purposive inclusion of other relevant literature. Our literature search is not meant to be a comprehensive review of the experimental and quasi-experimental neighborhood health effects literature; rather, it is intended merely to illustrate the broad categories and examples of studies identified by our search. Based on the search results, we broadly characterize this literature into five categories: housing mobility and voucher experiments, place-based randomized trials, natural experiments, quasi-experimental neighborhood studies, and longitudinal designs paired with causal analytic methods.

Housing Mobility and Voucher Experiments: Household-Based Randomized Trials

The bulk of experimental research related to neighborhood effects on health comes from housing mobility and voucher studies, where participants or households are randomly assigned a housing voucher enabling them to rent a private market rental apartment in a better neighborhood. This approach uses the move to different types of neighborhoods to make inferences about changes in neighborhood exposures, and as such it may not be capturing a pure neighborhood effect (e.g., neighborhood exposures are bundled with moving) (Ludwig et al., 2008; Sampson, 2008). Moreover, the study population is typically low-income households, so the evidence may not apply to higher income populations. As we will discuss later, the voucher-based design has several practical advantages over neighborhood intervention designs.

Moving to Opportunity

Arguably the most well-known housing mobility experiment contributing to the neighborhood health effects literature is the Moving to Opportunity (MTO) for Fair Housing Demonstration Project. The MTO experiment was designed to combat the effects of very distressed, high-poverty, federally funded housing projects prevalent in the United States by the late 1960s (Briggs, Popkin, & Goering, 2010). The distressed conditions of the housing projects, characterized by drug dealing, gang violence, chronic poverty, and welfare dependency, peaked in the 1980s, and no social programs had successfully mitigated these issues (Briggs et al., 2010). The one exception was the results emerging from the Gautreaux program, a quasi-experimental evaluation of a court-ordered desegregation housing program that followed families across time who moved out of Chicago public housing into different areas of the Chicago metro area. We discuss this study later in the chapter. Although MTO focused on moving families into low-poverty neighborhoods, rather than racially integrated neighborhoods, it became the first large-scale social experiment aimed at battling the devastating effects of concentrated poverty (Briggs et al., 2010).

The MTO study tested whether public housing families who received one of two types of rental housing vouchers would experience improved outcomes, compared to families who remained in public housing. From 1994 through 1997, the US federal government's Department of Housing and Urban Development (HUD) randomly assigned volunteer low-income families with at least one child, who were living in distressed public housing, to one of three treatment groups (Goering et al., 1999). (1) The low poverty treatment group received a Section 8 voucher that could only be used to rent an apartment in neighborhoods where less than 10% of households in the census tract lived below the poverty line, plus they received housing counseling to facilitate the moves. (2) The Section 8 treatment group received a regular Section 8 voucher to subsidize rent of a private market apartment and no other intervention; they did not have any locational constraints on the types of neighborhoods where they could rent an apartment. (3) Finally, the control group did not receive any Section 8 voucher or any intervention, but they continued to remain eligible to live in public housing (an in-place comparison group). A Section 8 voucher, now called a Housing Choice Voucher, works primarily by increasing affordability of rent through government subsidy. Households typically pay 30% of their income toward rent of a private market apartment, and the local housing authority (using federal funds) pays the difference (up to a locally defined rental ceiling) directly to the landlord. The MTO study used random assignment at the household level, and there were two uniform quantitative evaluations across the five different cities where MTO was conducted: at 4–7 years and 10–15 years following baseline. Qualitative interviews with adult and youth participants and site-specific early evaluations were also conducted (Briggs et al., 2010; Clampet-Lundquist, Edin, Kling, & Duncan, 2011; DeLuca & Dayton, 2009; Popkin et al., 2002; Popkin, Leventhal, & Weismann, 2008).

The main goal of MTO was to improve household economic outcomes; however, only very recent work has identified economic benefits among the youngest cohort of children in MTO (Chetty, Hendren, & Katz, 2016). Unexpectedly, the MTO intervention primarily influenced health outcomes. For example, MTO household heads, which were predominately single mothers, experienced improved health outcomes at the interim and final follow-up surveys, including reductions in obesity, diabetes, self-reported physical limitations, psychological distress, and major depression, and increases in feeling calm/peaceful (Ludwig et al., 2011, 2012; Orr et al., 2003; Sanbonmatsu et al., 2011, 2012). Effects of MTO on children's health was strongly modified by child gender, where the health of girls generally benefited, but the health of boys generally did not (or was harmed). For example, interim survey findings (4–7 years after random assignment) identified reductions in treatment group girls' psychological distress, lifetime marijuana use, lifetime smoking, and an index of risky behaviors, compared to the control group who remained in public housing, but increases in treatment group boys' psychological distress, behavior problems, smoking, and risky behaviors compared to controls (Kling, Liebman, & Katz, 2007; Orr et al., 2003; Osypuk, Schmidt, et al., 2012; Osypuk, Tchetgen Tchetgen, et al., 2012). The final survey (10–15 years after random assignment) displayed some similar findings, with reductions in girls' psychological distress, serious behavioral/emotional problems, conduct disorder, and alcohol use, and increases in boys' smoking, depression, conduct disorder, and posttraumatic stress disorder (PTSD) (Kessler et al., 2014; Sanbonmatsu et al., 2011).

Recently, scholars, including the authors of this chapter, have begun unpacking the MTO treatment effects to better understand how and why MTO impacted health. In particular, studies have examined how effects differ by subgroups (moderation), through what mechanisms MTO impacted health (mediation), and when treatment was most influential (life course effects). For example, Osypuk and colleagues have demonstrated that MTO effects on adolescent mental health were modified by baseline family history of health/developmental problems, violent victimization, parental enrollment in school, and teen parenthood (Nguyen, Schmidt, Glymour, Rehkopf, & Osypuk, 2013; Osypuk, Schmidt, et al., 2012; Osypuk, Tchetgen Tchetgen, et al., 2012). Other research using machine learning methods, such as recursive partitioning, are identifying vulnerable subgroups to MTO treatment effects, suggesting there is wide variation in the effects of MTO on mental health identified by cross-classification of multiple simultaneous baseline variables, in lieu of traditional approaches like treatment-by-baseline variable interactions tested one at a time (Nguyen, Rehkopf, Schmidt, & Osypuk, 2016).

Spatial effect modification has also been studied. Graif, Arcaya, and Diez Roux analyzed MTO data and found that escaping concentrated neighborhood disadvantage in both the immediate and surrounding neighborhoods was associated with improvements in composite mental health scores. However, escaping neighborhood disadvantage in only one or the other neighborhoods, but not both, did not improve mental health. Their study results indicate that improving the broader socio-spatial contexts in which people live can significantly improve residents' mental health (Graif, Arcaya, & Diez Roux, 2016).

Schmidt, Glymour, and Osypuk utilized the MTO demonstration study to test life-course hypotheses: to examine if neighborhood mobility has differential impacts on adolescents' risky behaviors depending on the age when children moved from their baseline residence. Their findings were patterned by gender, and they revealed that boys 10 years and older experienced unexpected, adverse consequences on risky behaviors, while MTO was associated with lower substance use among girls 9 years and older (Schmidt, Glymour, & Osypuk, 2016). These findings suggest that *the age at which* children moved through the MTO program makes a difference, to influence different outcomes, as predicted by developmental or life-course models.

Finally, one study leveraged the MTO design to introduce a new form of bias, to advance the methodological literature. Glymour, Nguyen, et al. hypothesized that there might be selective adherence to treatment assignment in MTO—an understudied issue in the literature on experimental studies. Selective adherence may lead to misinterpretations of intent-to-treat analyses of randomized trials (Glymour et al., 2016). Moreover, investigating treatment adherence has policy implications because if individuals choose treatments that benefit them the most, paternalistic policies that mandate such treatment may cause harm. The authors investigated whether MTO household heads selectively chose treatments of greatest anticipated benefit to themselves or their families (meaning: when offered a housing voucher to move, did they use the voucher to move? Or did they fail to use it?). The authors found that patterns differed by child gender, so the story was not straightforward empirically despite the interesting methodological issue. Specifically, instrumental variables analysis suggested that adolescent boys least likely to move experienced the most adverse effects on behavioral problems compared to adolescent boys most likely to move, providing evidence in favor of our hypothesis: that those least likely to move would be least likely to benefit. In contrast, adolescent girls least likely to move experienced the most beneficial effects on psychological distress compared to girls most likely to move, which was evidence against our hypothesis. The gendered patterns are difficult to interpret, but they may have related to the perceived benefits of the move, rather than the actualized benefits that emerged. MTO families (like most extremely low-income households) faced numerous social and economic challenges when deciding to move to different neighborhoods with their voucher, not the least of which were time constraints. As a result, half of MTO families that received housing vouchers did not utilize them. However, these results, as with other MTO evidence, reinforce that an adolescent's gender was one of the most important influences on how the housing intervention affected health. Despite being one of the most important social stratification variables in social science, gender is an understudied dimension of neighborhood health effects literature. Therefore, understanding how social context differs and interacts with gender is an important future direction to consider.

Other Housing Voucher Studies

Although MTO is the most well-known housing voucher experiment, there are a few smaller scale studies that have randomly assigned housing vouchers to enable moves to better neighborhoods and evaluated these voucher studies for health outcomes. These have been reviewed by Osypuk and colleagues (Osypuk, Joshi, Geronimo, & Acevedo-Garcia, 2014), and we provide a brief overview here. HUD partnered with the Department of Veterans Affairs to provide homeless veterans with diagnosed mental health or substance use disorders with a randomly assigned Section 8 voucher, allowing them to find stable housing. This study, called the HUD-VASH Program, did improve housing stability and had positive impacts on addiction and substance use, but it did not affect physical health. Two studies targeted homeless people with HIV/AIDS diagnoses: the Housing Opportunities for Persons with AIDS (HOPWA) and the Chicago Housing for Health Partnership (CHHP) (Osypuk et al., 2014). Both studies randomly assigned homeless HIV/AIDS positive participants a Section 8 voucher (or not), in addition to typical case management. HOPWA showed improvements in depression and stress, while CHHP showed fewer hospitalizations/emergency room visits and improvements in viral loads and immunity, among the voucher groups. One final housing mobility experiment is the Welfare to Work Vouchers (WtW V) study, where the treatment group received usual Temporary Assistance for Needy Families (TANF) benefits plus a Section 8 voucher, social and housing search services, and employment assistance, compared to usual TANF benefits (Osypuk et al., 2014). This study did not affect health outcomes.

As discussed earlier, only a small body of literature has randomized housing vouchers to low-income populations and evaluated their effects on health outcomes, with the most literature coming out of the MTO study. Our review demonstrated that subsidizing cost of housing with vouchers is a promising intervention to improve mental health in clinical and nonclinical populations. However, these housing policies rarely consider health as part of their logic models or design, and the health outcomes that were evaluated were fragmented across studies and often poorly measured. The housing interventions were also quite heterogeneous, in terms of the targeted population and the intervention components (including whether and which health services were included, e.g., among ill populations). Although we identified and reviewed studies that have considered health outcomes, the majority of social and economic policy studies rarely consider health and ignore that these programs could indirectly influence health via the social determinants of health. This is a promising and growing area of recent social epidemiology inquiry (Osypuk et al., 2014).

Place-Based Neighborhood Randomized Trials

Although the bulk of experimental studies are rental voucher experiments, a smaller class of experimental studies have examined whether exposure to neighborhood, or place-based, risks and resources is associated with health outcomes and health behaviors. These studies randomize neighborhoods as the unit to different conditions, called group or neighborhood randomized trials, rather than by randomizing individuals to a given treatment. We discuss a few select examples of this class of methods next.

In a recent review, Oakes and colleagues (2015) discussed a few area-based group randomized trials that targeted disease prevention. Three studies aimed to reduce underage alcohol abuse by offering community-level interventions to change support for alcohol use (e.g., education, parental intervention, changing the neighborhood environment) (Komro et al., 2008; Perry et al., 1996; Wagenaar et al., 2000), and another targeted community understanding and norms to reduce the time between the onset of heart attack symptoms and hospital arrival (Luepker et al., 2000). Overall, these studies showed mixed, and sometimes nonreplicable, effects on the target outcomes (Oakes et al., 2015).

In Catalonia, Spain, Triguero-Mas and colleagues used a randomized case-crossover study to examine individuals' mood and heart rate as a result of traveling to and spending 30 + minutes in a natural outdoor environment characterized as green (a forest with no water), blue (a beach), or urban (a city square) (Triguero-Mas et al., 2017). They found that green environment exposure was associated with lower negative mood, and blue environment exposure favorably changed people's heart rate variability (Triguero-Mas et al., 2017). This may inspire future neighborhood designs to incorporate access to natural outdoor environments. Another study among residents in Chicago public housing found beneficial effects in reducing aggression and violence among women who were randomized to live in public housing units surrounded by more vegetation compared to those with little to no vegetation (Kuo & Sullivan, 2001).

In-Progress Trials

Charles Branas and his team are conducting two active randomized trials that intervene on neighborhood physical disorder to decrease substance abuse and violence. One randomized trial is testing the stabilization of abandoned or vacant lots (the unit of random assignment) as a potential prevention strategy for substance abuse. Outcomes examined include illegal drug trafficking and consumption, drunkenness, and drinking (Branas, Kondo, Murphy, South, & Polsky, 2016). Quasi-experimental evidence from this ongoing study is discussed later in the chapter, but experimental evidence suggests that residents who walked past a vacant lot after receiving randomly assigned greening treatment experienced decreases in heart rate compared to when they walked past the same vacant lot before receiving treatment (South, Kondo, Cheney, & Branas, 2015). The second randomized trial underway by Branas is examining the remediation of abandoned buildings as a strategy to prevent long-standing violence and substance abuse. The abandoned building is the unit of random assignment. The trial consists of the following four treatment arms: full abandoned housing remediation, graffiti and trash clean-up only, trash clean-up only, and no housing remediation or clean-up. Longitudinal outcomes to be measured 18 months before and after treatment include alcohol and drug abuse and violence among residents living near the abandoned building site. The two trials will provide critical information about the impact of physical features of the neighborhood environment on social processes and behaviors.

Natural Experiments

Natural experiments are defined as a naturally occurring event with a comparison condition that does not experience the event (Shadish et al., 2002); they are distinguished from quasi-experiments in that the investigator is not usually involved in generating the exposure for the purposes of research (e.g., a natural disaster, or a new policy is implemented). Natural experiments are a valuable tool for investigating neighborhood effects on health, and they are most useful in circumstances where an intervention is likely to have an important health impact but is unclear exactly how, or how large, effects will be. It may also be valuable if implementing an experiment and randomizing people or other units would be unethical or impractical, but there is nonetheless a potential for the treatment to be replicated, scaled up, or generalized to other situations (Craig et al., 2012). The bulk of natural experiments we found related to the built environment (Chapter 8) or the retail food and alcohol environment (Chapter 9), but we also discuss a few unique natural experiments.

Primarily natural experiments on the built environment revolve around improvements to green space or transportation and how they impact health and health behaviors. For example, installing an urban greenway that connected pedestrian residential neighborhoods to retail shops and schools increased walking, cycling, and total physical activity in Knoxville, Tennessee (Fitzhugh, Bassett, & Evans, 2010). Likewise, improvements to a park in Victoria, Australia, led to increases in walking and vigorous physical activity (Veitch et al., 2012). Studies also suggest that improvements to transportation may impact health positively. Installation of a new light rail transit system in Salt Lake City, Utah, had a positive association with increased physical activity (Miller et al., 2015), while improved transportation connecting the city center to impoverished neighborhoods in Medellin, Colombia, led to declines in homicide rates (Cerdá et al., 2012).

A few studies have examined the impact of grocery store and fast food availability on health. For example, in eight northern California neighborhoods, Zhang and colleagues examined whether living near a new supermarket opening was associated with a favorable change in body mass index (Zhang et al., 2016). They found that new supermarket openings reduced travel distance to the nearest supermarket by 0.7 miles on average, but this was not associated with body mass index changes (Zhang et al., 2016). Dubowitz and colleagues implemented a similar natural experiment design to test how improving food availability for low-income families in Pittsburgh, Pennsylvania (via a new supermarket) impacted obesity and diet for minority neighborhoods. Results have not been straightforward. Although they found positive changes in perceived access to healthy food and measures of overall diet quality, daily calorie and sugar intake, and percentage of calories from fat, sugars, and alcohol, these improvements were not associated with using the new supermarket. They also did not see improvements in consumption of fruits, vegetables, and whole grains, or BMI (Dubowitz et al., 2015). In Victoria, Australia, another group of researchers used a natural experiment study design to explore whether the opening of a new McDonald's restaurant was associated with increased consumption of McDonald's products; they did not find an increase in consumption of McDonald's products (Thornton et al., 2016). A few studies have also examined how alcohol retail outlets impact health. In these innovative studies, the researchers examined the destruction of alcohol retail stores after the 1992 riots in Los Angeles that led to declines in alcohol outlet density. Leveraging this exogenous change, studies found that decreased alcohol outlet availability led to declines in assault rates (Yu, Li, & Scribner, 2009) and gonorrhea (Cohen et al., 2006).

Finally, we mention two additional interesting natural experiments that have leveraged natural occurrences to examine neighborhood effects on health. In one study, researchers tested how the reduction in soil lead levels after flooding in New Orleans was associated with eclampsia (Zahran, Magzamen, Breunig, & Mielke, 2014). Zahran and colleagues found that mothers living in ZIP codes that experienced a reduction in soil lead levels post flooding experienced a significant decline in eclampsia risk, indicating that lead exposure is related to pregnancy outcomes. The other study examined the effects of a refugee dispersal program on diabetes risk in Sweden (White et al., 2016). In Sweden, government policy quasi-randomly assigned refugees to live in particular neighborhoods to ease labor and housing market conditions in populous areas. White and colleagues classified neighborhoods as either high-, moderate-, or low-deprivation neighborhoods and found that being assigned to a high-deprivation neighborhood, compared to a low-deprivation neighborhood, led to increased risk of diabetes.

Instrumental Variable Analysis

Instrumental variable (IV) analysis is a rigorous method that can obtain causal estimates of neighborhoods on health. Randomization inherently creates an instrument that can be leveraged to obtain effects of an experimental exposure on outcomes, but in the absence of randomization, natural experiments may provide a valid estimate of the effect of an exposure on health (Glymour, 2006). In IV analysis, one identifies a variable that is related to the exposure of interest but is not directly related to the outcome (only indirectly through its effect on the exposure) (Angrist et al., 1996). Assuming IV assumptions are met, IV analysis returns a consistent estimate of the causal effect of the exposure on the outcome (Angrist et al., 1996), without necessarily requiring control for individual confounders. In the context of nonexperimental data, it can be very difficult to identify a valid instrument that meets IV assumptions; thus, studies applying instrumental variable analysis to understand neighborhood effects on health are rare. We highlight a few studies here. One study employed a measure of how metropolitan governments encourage residential sorting as an instrument, and it found a causal association between residential segregation and poor birth outcomes among Black women (Ellen, 2000). A few studies, discussed more extensively in Chapter 9, leveraged distance to major highways as an instrument for the effects of eating fast food on obesity, with mixed findings (Anderson & Matsa, 2011; Dunn, Sharkey, & Horel, 2012). Recently Kawachi and colleagues (Kawachi, Ichida, Tampubolon, & Fujiwara, 2013) reviewed several studies examining the effects of neighborhood social capital on health using IV analysis. The chosen instrument varied across studies, for example length of residence in a community or income inequality, but generally the results identified a causal relationship between how an individual perceived social capital in his or her neighborhood and health outcomes (Kawachi et al., 2013).

In-Progress Natural Experiments

In East village, London (formerly the London 2012 Olympic village), Ram and colleagues are utilizing a natural experiment provided by the rapid neighborhood development changes taking place in East Village, as a result of investment prior to and since the Olympics. East Village is being designed to create a mixed-use residential neighborhood with design features—such as access to open space and parks, transportation links, and walking and cycling paths—that encourage physical activity. Their project titled ENABLE London (Examining Neighborhood Activities in Built Living Environments in London) will be examining physical activity and other health behavioral changes among individuals relocating to the East Village compared to a control population living outside of the East Village during a 2-year study. Data collection and processing are currently underway and results are expected to inform urban planning (Ram et al., 2016). Elsewhere, Durand and colleagues are utilizing a major expansion of the light rail lines in Houston, Texas, as a natural experiment to determine if the use of mass transit can increase individuals' physical activity over 4 years. This study is underway, and it aims to inform how transportation projects impact health (Durand et al., 2016).

Quasi-Experimental Neighborhood Interventions

Gautreaux

The Gautreaux Assisted Housing Program was the result of a landmark Supreme Court decision in 1976 (Acevedo-Garcia et al., 2004). Chicago public housing residents brought a class action lawsuit against HUD alleging racial discrimination, resulting in a federal court order requiring HUD to offer Section 8 vouchers to Gautreaux families as a remedy that allowed them to move out of public housing into racially integrated neighborhoods (Acevedo-Garcia et al., 2004; Goering & Feins, 2003). The identification of the effects relied on the allocation of the location of the voucher (in suburban or in central city areas) that the evaluation authors argued were somewhat random, and simply allocated in order of the waiting list. However, later analyses found strong patterns in the preferences that may have influenced the disposition of the location of the voucher that each household received, which may have biased findings (selection bias into treatment condition) (Acevedo-Garcia 2004). Results from the Gautreaux program showed education and economic improvements among children from the Gautreaux families who moved to the suburbs, and they provided a foundation for launching the MTO experiment (Goering & Feins, 2003). There were few explicit health measures included in the evaluation, however, and a review of evidence suggested that Gautreaux families who moved to suburban areas had less access to and less satisfaction with medical care than nonmovers or city movers (Acevedo-Garcia et al., 2004). Although the quasi-experimental design improves on observational evidence, in addition to questions about how household preferences influenced the type of voucher they may have received, the empirical evidence evaluating Gautreaux suffered from some methodological limitations, including attrition, and the lack of an untreated control group (Acevedo-Garcia et al., 2004). A more recent paper did find positive impacts of Gautreaux, with significantly lower all-cause and homicide mortality rates among young males who moved to more advantaged neighborhoods at age 25 or younger (Votruba & Kling, 2009). However, it would be subject to the same selection-into-treatment concerns noted earlier.

HOPE VI/Urban Renewal

HOPE VI is a major federally sponsored urban renewal program financed by HUD that demolished and revitalized deteriorated public housing units in high-poverty neighborhoods in large quantities throughout the United States (Lindberg et al., 2010). As discussed in a recent literature review by Lindberg et al. (2010), the longitudinal HOPE VI Panel Study was designed to track the well-being of 887 public housing residents in five distressed public housing developments that were slated for demolition, across a 4-year period. This study provides a comprehensive source of the health status of the public housing residents, including to document the extremely poor health status of these public housing families at baseline (before demolition), as well as at 2 and 4 years after demolition. HOPE VI public housing residents had higher prevalence of poor self-rated health, chronic health problems (such as obesity, hypertension, arthritis, diabetes, depression, other mental health problems, and work-related disability), and multiple simultaneous health conditions, as well as higher mortality rates compared to both the US population and to the US population of Black women (Manjarrez, Popkin, & Guernsey, 2007). The HOPE VI evaluation has demonstrated not only that health had *not* improved as a result of the housing demolition policy, but that health actually worsened from 2001 to 2005. A subsequent follow-up in 2009 in Chicago showed even worse health problems and mortality rates (Price & Popkin, 2010). Even for the segment of the population that were relocated to better (safer) environments (the group that relocated to private rental units with a housing choice voucher), no health improvements were detected as a result of the policy (Manjarrez et al., 2007). Unfortunately, since the HOPE VI evaluation did not include an untreated comparison group, and since participants reported much worse health at baseline than is seen in US population-based surveys, we cannot separate out aging effects (as health generally worsens with higher age) from effects of the policy. Notably, HOPE VI was an involuntary housing relocation program, and among HOPE VI households, 84% had been relocated between 2001 and 2005, and only a very small number of households were living in their original public housing developments. Among relocated households in 2005, 43% were living in private rental units subsidized by housing vouchers, 22% had moved to other public housing developments, 13% were living unassisted in other rental or owned units, and only 5% had moved to the revitalized HOPE VI sites (Manjarrez et al., 2007). Therefore, few of the HOPE VI households were benefiting from the revitalized housing directly (in terms of housing units) or indirectly (in terms of health benefits) a few years following the demolition. Ultimately, Lindberg et al. concluded that more evaluation was needed to assess HOPE VI effects on health. The literature has advanced in the past 6 years, however, and we discuss more promising quasi-experimental urban renewal efforts next.

In Glasgow, Scotland, Egan, and colleagues evaluated a quasi-experiment of a housing-led urban renewal program in 14 disadvantaged neighborhoods. Repeated cross-sectional household surveys were conducted in 2006 (baseline) and 2011 (follow-up). There were three intervention groups: one consisted of residents living in neighborhoods undergoing demolition; one consisted of residents receiving housing improvements; and the control group consisted of residents residing in neighborhoods where other residents were receiving housing improvements but they were not (Egan et al., 2013). The demolition and control groups had similar mental and physical health, but the housing improvement group reported improved mental health compared to controls (Egan et al., 2013). Researchers further categorized areas depending on the average amount of urban renewal investment they received per household: (i) <£5,000 ("lower" investment), (ii) £5,000–£10,000 ("medium" investment), or (iii) >£10,000 ("higher" investment). Results suggested that more urban renewal investment was associated with greater improvements in mental health, less decline in physical health, and a modest reduction in health inequalities over a 5-year period (Egan et al., 2016).

Vacant Lot/Blight Remediation

Charlie Branas and colleagues examined whether greening of vacant lots reduced crime and promoted health (Branas et al., 2011). Implementing a decades-long intervention study utilizing a difference-in-difference design, treated vacant lots were compared against matched groups of control vacant lots that were eligible to receive the intervention but did not. Across Philadelphia, over 4,400 vacant lots were greened between 1999 and 2008, and the analysis suggested that greening of vacant lots was associated with reductions in gun assault rates. Additionally, subgroup analyses identified that for some sections of the city, greening of vacant lots was also associated with lower stress levels and higher physical activity among residents living nearby (Branas et al., 2011). Branas and colleagues further tested urban blight remediation (i.e., cleaning and repairing abandoned buildings, along with greening of vacant lots) and found that urban blight remediation significantly reduced rates of firearm violence, and that it was cost-effective in having a high return on investment for those living nearby (Branas et al., 2016).

Simulation Models

One very different methodological advancement in the neighborhood health effects literature that has emerged in the past decade is the use of simulation studies, in lieu of strictly empirical studies, to examine how the theoretical manipulation of a neighborhood characteristic may influence health. For example, agent-based models allow one to specify the causal "world" of variables and specify their relationships as inputs. Such models may be better situated to model phenomena when contingency is important, when feedback loops (reverse causality) complicate the estimation, or when there are emergent properties that are impossible to detect with simple, discrete sections of a causal model (Auchincloss & Diez Roux, 2008). A small literature has developed in this line of agent-based neighborhood research that is discussed in Chapter 5.

As mentioned briefly earlier, another way to leverage simulation models is in the context of sensitivity models to inform how realistic or unrealistic our assumptions are about the influence of unmeasured confounding. Such bias sensitivity models have been implemented in the context of mediation models of the MTO treatment on health, to test how unmeasured confounders may bias the indirect (mediation) effects under study (Nguyen, Osypuk, Schmidt, Glymour, & Tchetgen Tchetgen,

2015; Schmidt, Glymour, & Osypuk, 2017). Despite the advent of big data methods and computing power, there has been surprisingly little research in social epidemiology, or neighborhood effects literature, leveraging simulation methods; integrating such methods into empirical analyses could strengthen and bound conclusions about bias from unmeasured confounding (Glymour, Osypuk, & Rehkopf, 2013).

Twin Studies

One final example of a quasi-experimental design to investigate neighborhood health effects on health is twin research. Twin studies may help overcome two fundamental problems in neighborhoods research: selection, where people's choice of neighborhood is shaped by their family or other background context; and reverse causation, where people's health influences their choice of neighborhood, and not neighborhoods influencing their health (Duncan et al., 2014). Since twins have the same genes, background demographic factors, and (typically) family upbringing, any associations found between neighborhood context and health are not attributable to these background factors (Duncan et al., 2014). Duncan and colleagues discuss specific ways that twin studies can overcome these methodological challenges in neighborhoods research, but these studies remain rare. Our search identified one study that tested the effects of neighborhood social deprivation on drug abuse among twins and siblings, and found a positive association over and above the effects of shared genes and background factors (Kendler, Maes, Sundquist, Ohlsson, & Sundquist, 2014).

This last example raises an important point about quasi-experiments that should be made explicit. Researchers using the term *quasi-experiment* may mean one of two things: (1) a specific intervention is manipulated by researchers, albeit in a nonrandom manner; or (2) the study employs strong techniques to control for confounding. The difference is that in the first case, researchers explicitly intervene to compare an "exposed" group to an "unexposed" comparison group, while in the second case there is no clear untreated comparison, just strong control for potential confounding variables. In this chapter, the neighborhood interventions discussed previously are examples of the first case, whereas twin studies and the longitudinal studies discussed in the next section are examples of the second case.

Neighborhood Context as Moderator

Although we do not go into great detail here, it is important to note that neighborhoods, or aspects of neighborhoods (e.g., abandoned lots), do not necessarily need to be the unit of randomization in an experiment in order to affect health outcomes.

Rather, it is possible that neighborhoods may act to modify, or otherwise alter, the effects of an intervention on health. For example, Pruitt and colleagues (Pruitt et al., 2014) found that effects of a randomized behavioral intervention to increase colorectal screening was spatially dependent, meaning that an individual's colorectal screening use was positively associated with that of his or her neighbor's. This highlights the importance of considering potential neighborhood and spatial effects of interventions on health, even when neighborhoods are not the exposure of interest (Pruitt et al., 2014).

LEVERAGING LONGITUDINAL DESIGNS TO STUDY NEIGHBORHOOD EFFECTS ON HEALTH

Another approach to obtaining causal neighborhood effects on health is to leverage longitudinal research designs. Although observational data do not manipulate an exposure or randomly assign treatment, and therefore may fall short with consistency, exchangeability, or positivity assumptions, they do have the advantage of being able to establish temporal ordering to ensure that an exposure precedes the health outcome of interest. Moreover, with advances in causal analytic methods using counterfactual frameworks, analyzing longitudinal designs provides researchers with good opportunities for advancing our understanding of neighborhood effects on health, and such analytic methods may significantly strengthen the internal validity of estimates. Examples of analytic techniques for estimating causal effects with longitudinal data include fixed effects models and marginal structural models (MSMs).

Fixed effects regression models control for unobserved confounders in longitudinal samples with repeat observations by comparing individuals during periods of an exposure to themselves during periods without the exposure (Petersen, 2004). These models, therefore, require repeated observations of individuals and sufficient variability on the observed variables over time, but they are effective in controlling for unobserved time-stable explanatory variables (Petersen, 2004). Airaksinen et al. (2016) used fixed effects regression to examine whether neighborhood socioeconomic status (SES) and urbanization were associated with alcohol use, smoking, exercise, and interest in health. In fixed effects models, they found that urban environments were associated with increased smoking and alcohol use, but also a greater interest in personal health. Neighborhood SES was also associated with a greater interest in personal health. Additionally, Astell-Burt, Feng, Kolt, and Jalaludin (2015) found that within-person variation in an individual's exposure to crime across time was associated with psychological distress. Other studies have applied fixed effects and found associations between the availability of, and proximity to, tobacco outlets and smoking (Pulakka et al., 2016), and alcohol outlets and heavy drinking (Halonen, Kivimaki, Virtanen, et al., 2013), as well as neighborhood disadvantage and smoking (Halonen et al., 2016). Applying this same fixed effects method, Jokela (2014), however, found that associations between neighborhood disadvantage and self-rated health, mental health, physical functioning, smoking, and physical activity among elders were entirely due to between-person differences rather than due to change in neighborhood deprivation within individuals, suggesting that neighborhoods do not influence health. A few other studies examining within-individual change, but applying traditional regression rather than fixed effects methods, have found associations between the distance to, and number of, sports facilities and physical activity (Halonen et al., 2015), wine outlet availability and alcohol consumption (Halonen et al., 2014), and distance to tobacco outlets and smoking cessation (Halonen, Kivimaki, Kouvonen, et al., 2013). As Oakes (2014) points out, pitfalls of studies such as this include that people rarely make moves that cause dramatic changes to their neighborhood environments, so within-person variability is often limited (Lemelin et al., 2009), and it still does not account for the voluntary nature of residential changes (and thus may be limited in generalizability).

Marginal structural models (MSMs), estimated with inverse probability of treatment weights (IPTW), are a class of models that allow for estimating the causal effects of time-varying "treatments" when there are (measured) time-varying confounders that are predicted by prior treatment and also predict subsequent treatment and the outcome (Robins, 1999; Robins, Hernan, & Brumback, 2000). Causal estimates of time-varying treatments are consistent causal estimates of the treatment effect, assuming all time-varying confounders are measured (Robins, 1999; Robins et al., 2000). MSMs have been applied for the identification of causal neighborhood effects on health since approximately 2010. MSMs have identified causal effects of poor and disadvantaged neighborhoods on increased alcohol consumption (Cerdá, Diez-Roux, Tchetgen Tchetgen, Gordon-Larsen, & Kiefe, 2010), worse self-rated health (Glymour, Mujahid, Wu, White, & Tchetgen Tchetgen, 2010; Kravitz-Wirtz, 2016), mortality risk (Do, Wang, & Elliott, 2013), teen parenthood (Wodtke, 2013), and decreased cognitive ability (Sharkey & Elwert, 2011). As with any observational study, studies using MSM analytic methods are subject to bias from unmeasured confounding, and their primary contribution is to model time-varying phenomena, and in the specificity of the temporal exposure (and its confounding) patterns.

CONCLUSIONS AND IMPLICATIONS

The body of literature that we reviewed was not large; however, we found considerable heterogeneity in terms of the type or sector of neighborhood exposure that was tested, the design applied (e.g., the unit of random assignment), and the health outcomes evaluated. These differences make it difficult to summarize substantive conclusions succinctly. Generally, our review found that neighborhood effects were weaker and more mixed among methodologically stronger studies (i.e., the experiments), while results were more consistent for natural experiments and longitudinal designs applying causal methods. This is consistent with findings from other reviews (Oakes et al., 2015). Although results from these diverse studies are not uniform in their conclusions, they do suggest that some neighborhood characteristics—particularly neighborhood aesthetics such as greenness, physical signs of disorder, and neighborhood poverty/disadvantage—can affect a wide range of outcomes, including mental health, substance use, and crime. Neighborhood quality characterized by closeness to amenities, business/economic characteristics, and safety has been connected with mental health, chronic conditions, and mortality. Another promising intervention for improving health is through housing vouchers, such as MTO. Although it is impossible to disentangle the effects of neighborhoods, housing, and mobility in voucher studies, housing voucher studies have demonstrated positive effects on adolescent girls' mental health and mothers' mental and physical health, as well as the mental health of clinical populations. However, the harmful effects on boys' mental health and risky behaviors are not trivial, and they illustrate how neighborhoods may have heterogeneous effects on health for different subgroups of the population.

The take-away message here is that there is ample opportunity to expand the literature, particularly by capitalizing on policy changes or other natural experiments to understand how health may change in response to different area-based exposures. Experiments have long been considered the gold standard of study designs, and in recent decades there has been a dramatic increase in experimental studies across disciplines (Sampson, 2010). However, as Sampson argues, experimental designs are not a panacea and merely require a different set of assumptions than nonexperimental studies. As noted in Table 6-1, both random sampling and random assignment of treatment are needed in order for an experiment to be *causal* and *generalizeable*. Factors limiting causal inference, even in the context of experiments, include nonrandom or selective sampling, low compliance, interference (i.e., the stable unit treatment variance assumption, which is related to consistency discussed earlier), and weak links to theory (Sampson, 2010). More important, just because an experiment may be internally valid, that does not necessarily mean a study is externally valid, and external validity is a critical component of effective policy translation (Sampson, 2010). The translation of evidence into policies and programs that can improve the health of the population is an important goal of public health research. As Sampson points out, many of the most impactful advances in improving public health, such as improving car safety and reducing smoking, were based on observational studies. Although experiments are not required for effective public health policies, combining strong experimental and quasi-experimental methods while focusing on policy translation may be an important step for moving the field forward.

TRANSLATION AND POLICY EVALUATION

Social epidemiology has traditionally engaged in descriptive and etiologic research, while translational research has lagged behind, as might be expected in such a young field. Although much of the neighborhood effects research that we have discussed in this chapter is stronger methodologically than cross-sectional evidence, the degree to which their findings are policy relevant depends on many factors. Internal validity is certainly important for translation, including whether studies meet traditional causal inference assumptions (as we have discussed in some detail here), but generalizeability is also essential; the failure of these assumptions can hamper the translation of etiologic findings to effective policies and programs.

Methodological Issues

Notably, the consistency assumption requires that the exposure be defined unambiguously, for example, in terms of form or dose, very specifically, and doing so is crucial for understanding which aspects of the neighborhood environment can or should be changed through policy or practice (Rehkopf et al., 2016). Often, in observational studies, the exposure is defined too broadly and fails to inform specific intervention efforts. In this way, experimental and quasi-experimental studies have a very large advantage over observational studies: They define a clear exposure that can be manipulated; therefore, exposures are much more policy relevant than those of observational studies. For example, an important feature of MTO is that the treatment aligns with the leading US affordable housing policy, based on voucher subsidies for rental units among low-income families. Policy-relevant exposures, such as MTO, that focus on realistic intervention points (Glymour et al., 2013) are uniquely positioned to translate the identification of causal effects into maximizing population health (Galea, 2013).

A neighborhood exposure that naturally occurs typically is different from the same exposure that might be manipulated by an intervention. For example, consistency is challenged when one operationalizes an exposure as an index, such as neighborhood socioeconomic status, which is often operationalized as a combination of available compositional measures derived from administrative (e.g., Census Bureau) data. The difficulty is that if one achieves different effects on health by changing one dimension of the neighborhood SES index (e.g., % poverty) than by changing another dimension of it (e.g., % low education), then consistency is violated (Rehkopf et al., 2016). However, another side of this argument considers the strong intercorrelation of the specific neighborhood measures that operationalize neighborhood quality since neighborhood quality is difficult to measure. In other words, operationalizing neighborhood quality by multiple dimensions may be more policy relevant, since one can rarely manipulate just one component anyway. Tracking a multidimensional measure of neighborhood quality may better capture the complexity of neighborhood inequality defined by multiple dimensions (Acevedo-Garcia et al., 2014; Osypuk, 2015). For example, neighborhood revitalization efforts famously intervene on multiple factors to improve a neighborhood, including housing, retail, transportation, and services; thus, change is manipulated via a bundled intervention simultaneously.

There is also too little attention to whether the study population matches the target population of a relevant policy, which relates to basic issues such as the study's sampling frame and a given policy's eligibility, but also treatment heterogeneity and generalizability (Osypuk, 2015). The majority of epidemiologic research is focused primarily on internal validity, considering generalizability as a lesser concern. However, as alluded to earlier, policy translation centrally concerns generalizability of findings. Social policies, particularly in the United States, are generally targeted at disadvantaged individuals, and neighborhood interventions (e.g., urban renewal) are generally focused in disadvantaged areas of the inner city. What does it mean if an observational study models the effect of moving from one neighborhood to another, if the sample includes the higher range of socioeconomic status individuals? Are there policies to target higher SES populations to move? If so, these policies would be markedly different than the largest affordable housing policies, which are targeted to low-income households. One might argue that self-selection is more important for higher SES populations, and thus descriptive evidence may be convincing here (Osypuk, 2015). For example, one goal of urban planners is to attract residents to new neighborhoods (Handy, Xinyu, & Mokhtarian, 2006). More important though, heterogeneity is very common in social epidemiology, and it suggests that neighborhood health effects, and the policies that map onto them, may be markedly different for different socioeconomic groups. Therefore, it may not be so relevant whether a given causal effect exists for the entire population, particularly if the exposure relates to a targeted policy; it may be more relevant whether the causal effect exists for the population who is the intended target of a certain policy (Osypuk, 2015).

Policy Translation in Practice

As a recent review of the health effects of experimental studies of housing policy, and of other social and economic policies showed, there are few strong examples of social policy evaluations that measured health outcomes well (Osypuk et al., 2014). The existing small body of literature is fragmented, not only in terms of the policy evaluated but also in terms of the definition of the treatment provided, the context in which the treatment was delivered (e.g., across place/site), and the population target (there was a large divide between programs targeting single men– vs. single mother–headed households with children). Osypuk and colleagues did find that social and economic policies, evaluated within experimental designs, do influence health, but this body of literature is still very young, with the strongest evidence in the housing voucher domain (as summarized earlier). Even these strong designs of social policies have difficulty guiding us on their health effects because few policies outside of the health sector have even considered health in their logic models, never mind as outcomes (Osypuk et al., 2014).

A review of recent federal initiatives around changing neighborhood environments reveals ample opportunity to evaluate such changes for their health effects. The Obama Administration prioritized several place-based neighborhood initiatives, including Promise Neighborhoods and Choice Neighborhoods, which share the goal to offer multisectoral place-based resources and services in disadvantaged areas. Promise Neighborhood implementation grants administered by the US Department of Education support nonprofit organizations, institutions of higher education, and Indian tribes in their efforts to improve the educational and development outcomes of youth living in distressed communities (by, for instance, improving early learning outcomes and transitions to college and a career) (US Department of Education, 2017). Choice Neighborhoods, administered by the US Department of Housing and Urban Development, supports communities with HUD-assisted housing or public housing to transform housing, as well as assets and amenities in the surrounding neighborhood such as schools, safety, and commercial activity (US Department of Housing & Urban Development, 2017). Challenges faced by both programs include (1) working across public and private agencies in order to accomplish a continuum of solutions, (2) building community support and engagement in neighborhood transformative activities, and (3) developing local infrastructure and systems to sustain and scale-up effective transformation efforts. There are some health-related intervention components, such as planned improvements in education and developmental outcomes that have strong impacts on health. Additionally, program components can include community amenities such as outdoor play space and street redesign efforts to increase walkability—both of which can boost physical activity and decrease chronic conditions. Both of these large-scale federal grant programs have supported integrative, transformative change for neighborhoods in cities around the United States.

CONCLUDING THOUGHTS

The objective of this chapter was to discuss the application of experimental and quasi-experimental designs to the study of neighborhood health effects. To do this, we described the features of experimental, quasi-experimental, and longitudinal designs, and then discussed examples from the neighborhood health effects literature, as well as implications for policy and translation. Since 70% of neighborhood-health effects studies are cross-sectional, there is a great opportunity to leverage stronger designs, including experimental, quasi-experimental, and longitudinal designs, to understand how dimensions of the neighborhood context influence health. The features of an experimental study—including random assignment of treatment and manipulation of the treatment—permit a strong foundation for causal inference rather than just greater understanding of correlational structures. Nonetheless, limitations of experimental studies include generalizability of study findings beyond the study population and policy relevance of the study exposure in real-world settings. In this chapter, we additionally discussed that longitudinal study designs are strengthening our understanding of neighborhood effects, particularly by ruling out time-stable confounding in fixed-effects designs. Each study design has merits, and the choice of which to use may be dependent on resources, existing knowledge on the topic, and willingness of study partners, among other factors. Neighborhood effects studies share the common goal of investigating the potential effects of contextual factors on a variety of health outcomes. By leveraging the strengths of each of these study designs, and working to produce rigorous and policy-relevant research, social epidemiology scholars have the potential to contribute to this common goal and to move the neighborhood health effects literature forward.

REFERENCES

Acevedo-Garcia, D., McArdle, N., Hardy, E. F., Crisan, U. I., Romano, B., Norris, D., . . . Reece, J. (2014). The Child Opportunity Index: Improving collaboration between community development and public health. *Health Affairs*, *33*(11), 1948–1957. doi:10.1377/hlthaff.2014.0679

Acevedo-Garcia, D., Osypuk, T. L., Werbel, R. E., Meara, E. R., Cutler, D. M., & Berkman, L. F. (2004). Does housing mobility policy improve health? *Housing Policy Debate*, *15*(1), 49–98.

Airaksinen, J., Hakulinen, C., Pulkki-Raback, L., Lehtimaki, T., Raitakari, O. T., Keltikangas-Jarvinen, L., & Jokela, M. (2016). Neighbourhood effects in health behaviors: A test of social causation with repeat-measurement longitudinal data. *The European Journal of Public Health*, *26*(3), 417–421.

Anderson, M. L., & Matsa, D. A. (2011). Are restaurants really supersizing America? *American Economic Journal: Applied Economics*, *3*(1), 152–188.

Angrist, J. D., & Imbens, G. W. (1995). Two-stage least-squares estimation of average causal effects in models with variable treatment intensity. *Journal of the American Statistical Association*, *90*(430), 431–442.

Angrist, J. D., Imbens, G. W., & Rubin, D. B. (1996). Identification of causal effects using instrumental variables. *Journal of the American Statistical Association*, *91*(434), 444–455.

Arcaya, M. C., Tucker-Seeley, R. D., Kim, R., Schnake-Mahl, A., So, M., & Subramanian, S. V. (2016). Research on neighborhood effects on health in the United States: A systematic review of study characteristics. *Social Science & Medicine*, *168*, 16–29.

Astell-Burt, T., Feng, X., Kolt, G. S., & Jalaludin, B. (2015). Does rising crime lead to increasing distress? Longitudinal analysis of a natural experiment with dynamic objective neighbourhood measures. *Social Science & Medicine*, *138*, 68–73.

Auchincloss, A. H., & Diez Roux, A. V. (2008). A new tool for epidemiology: The usefulness of dynamic-agent models in understanding place effects on health. *American Journal of Epidemiology*, *168*(1), 1–8.

Austin, P. C. (2011). An introduction to propensity score methods for reducing the effects of confounding in observational studies. *Multivariate Behavioral Research*, *46*(3), 399–424.

Branas, C., Cheney, R., MacDonald, J., Tam, V., Jackson, T., & Ten Have, T. (2011). A difference-in-difference analysis of health, safety, and greening vacant urban space. *American Journal of Epidemiology*, *174*(11), 1296–1306.

Branas, C., Kondo, M., Murphy, S., South, E., & Polsky, D. (2016). Urban blight remediation as a cost-beneficial solution to firearm violence. *American Journal of Public Health*, *106*, 1–7.

Briggs, X. d. S., Popkin, S. J., & Goering, J. (2010). *Moving to Opportunity: The story of an American experiment to fight ghetto poverty* New York, NY: Oxford University Press.

Cerdá, M., Diez-Roux, A. V., Tchetgen Tchetgen, E. J., Gordon-Larsen, P., & Kiefe, C. (2010). The relationship between neighborhood poverty and alcohol use: Estimation by marginal structural models. *Epidemiology*, *21*(4), 482–489.

Cerdá, M., Morenoff, J. D., Hansen, B. B., Tessari Hicks, K. J., Duque, L. F., Restrepo, A., & Diez-Roux, A. V. (2012). Reducing violence by transforming neighborhoods: A natural experiment in Medellín, Colombia. *American Journal of Epidemiology*, *175*(10), 1045–1053. doi:10.1093/aje/kwr428

Chetty, R., Hendren, N., & Katz, L. F. (2016). The effects of exposure to better neighborhoods on children: New evidence from the Moving to Opportunity experiment. *American Economic Review*, *106*(4), 855–902.

Clampet-Lundquist, S., Edin, K., Kling, J. R., & Duncan, G. J. (2011). Moving teenagers out of high-risk neighborhoods: How girls fare better than boys. *American Journal of Sociology*, *116*(4), 1154–1189.

Cohen, D. A., Ghosh-Dastidar, B., Scribner, R., Miu, A., Scott, M., Robinson, P., . . . Brown-Taylor, D. (2006). Alcohol outlets, gonorrhea, and the Los Angeles civil unrest: A longitudinal analysis. *Social Science & Medicine*, *62*(12), 3062–3071.

Craig, P., Cooper, C., Gunnell, D., Haw, S., Lawson, K., Macintyre, S., . . . Thompson, S. (2012). Using natural experiments to evaluate population health interventions: New MRC guidelines. *Journal of Epidemiology & Community Health*, *66*(12), 1182–1186.

DeLuca, S., & Dayton, E. (2009). Switching social contexts: The effects of housing mobility and school choice programs on youth outcomes. *Annual Review of Sociology, 35*, 457–491.

Do, D. P., Wang, L., & Elliott, M. R. (2013). Investigating the relationship between neighborhood poverty and mortality risk: A marginal structural modeling approach. *Social Science & Medicine, 91*(0), 58–66. doi:http://dx.doi.org/10.1016/j.socscimed.2013.03.003

Dubowitz, T., Ghosh-Dastidar, M., Cohen, D. A., Beckman, R., Steiner, E. D., Hunter, G. P., . . . Collins, R. L. (2015). Diet and perceptions change with supermarket introduction in a food desert, but not because of supermarket use. *Health Affairs, 34*(11), 1858–1868. doi:10.1377/hlthaff.2015.0667

Duncan, G. E., Mills, B., Strachan, E., Hurvitz, P., Huang, R., Moudon, A. V., & Turkheimer, E. (2014). Stepping towards causation in studies of neighborhood and environmental effects: How twin research can overcome problems of selection and reverse causation. *Health & Place, 27*, 106–111.

Dunn, R., Sharkey, J. R., & Horel, S. (2012). The effect of fast-food availability on fast-food consumption and obesity among rural residents: An analysis by race/ethnicity. *Economics & Human Biology, 10*(1), 1–13.

Durand, C. P., Oluyomi, A. O., Gabriel, K. P., Salvo, D., Sener, I. N., Hoelscher, D. M., . . . Kohl, H. W. (2016). The effect of light rail transit on physical activity: Design and methods of the travel-related activity in neighborhoods study. *Frontiers in Public Health, 4*, 103. doi:10.3389/fpubh.2016.00103

Egan, M., Katikireddi, S. V., Kearns, A., Tannahill, C., Kalacs, M., & Bond, L. (2013). Health effects of neighborhood demolition and housing improvement: A prospective controlled study of two natural experiments in urban renewal. *American Journal of Public Health, 103*, e47–e53.

Egan, M., Kearns, A., Katikireddi, S. V., Curl, A., Lawson, K., & Tannahill, C. (2016). Proportionate universalism in practice? A quasi-experimental study (GoWell) of a UK neighbourhood renewal programme's impact on health inequalities. *Social Science & Medicine, 152*, 41–49. doi:http://dx.doi.org/10.1016/j.socscimed.2016.01.026

Ellen, I. G. (2000). Is segregation bad for your health? The case of low birth weight. In W. G. Gale & J. R. Pack (Eds.), *Brookings-Wharton papers on Urban Affairs 2000* (pp. 203–229). Washington, DC: Brookings Institution Press.

Fitzhugh, E. C., Bassett, D. R., & Evans, M. F. (2010). Urban trails and physical activity: A natural experiment. *American Journal of Preventive Medicine, 39*(3), 259–262.

Galea, S. (2013). Commentary: An argument for consequentialist epidemiology. *American Journal of Epidemiology, 178*(8), 1185–1197. doi:doi:10.1093/aje/kwt172

Glymour, M. M. (2006). Natural experiments and instrumental variable analyses in social epidemiology. In J. M. Oakes & J. S. Kaufman (Eds.), *Social epidemiology* (pp. 429–460). San Francisco, CA: Jossey-Bass.

Glymour, M. M., Mujahid, M., Wu, Q., White, K., & Tchetgen Tchetgen, E. J. (2010). Neighborhood disadvantage and self-assessed health, disability, and depressive symptoms: Longitudinal results from the health and retirement study. *Annals of Epidemiology, 20*, 856–861.

Glymour, M. M., Nguyen, Q. C., Matsouaka, R., Tchetgen Tchetgen, E. J., Schmidt, N. M., & Osypuk, T. L. (2016). Does mother know best? Treatment adherence as a function of anticipated treatment benefit. *Epidemiology, 27*(2), 265–275. doi:10.1097/ede.0000000000000431

Glymour, M. M., Osypuk, T. L., & Rehkopf, D. H. (2013). Invited commentary: Off-roading with social epidemiology—exploration, causation, translation. *American Journal of Epidemiology*, *178*(6), 858–863.

Goering, J., & Feins, J. (2003). *Choosing a better life? Evaluating the Moving to Opportunity social experiment*. Washington, DC: The Urban Institute Press.

Goering, J., Kraft, J., Feins, J., McInnis, D., Holin, M. J., & Elhassan, H. (1999). *Moving to Opportunity for Fair Housing Demonstration Program: Current status and initial findings*. Washington, DC: Office of Policy Development and Research, US Department of Housing and Urban Development

Graif, C., Arcaya, M. C., & Diez Roux, A. V. (2016). Moving to opportunity and mental health: Exploring the spatial context of neighborhood effects. *Social Science & Medicine*, *162*, 50–58. doi:http://dx.doi.org/10.1016/j.socscimed.2016.05.036

Halonen, J. I., Kivimaki, M., Kouvonen, A., Pentti, J., Kawachi, I., Subramanian, S. V., & Vahtera, J. (2013). Proximity to a tobacco store and smoking cessation: A cohort study. *Tobacco Control*, *23*, 146–151.

Halonen, J. I., Kivimaki, M., Pentti, J., Virtanen, M., Subramanian, S. V., Kawachi, I., & Vahtera, J. (2014). Association of the availability of beer, wine, and liquor outlets with beverage-specific alcohol consumption: A cohort study. *Alcoholism: Clinical and Experimental Research*, *38*(4), 1086–1093.

Halonen, J. I., Kivimaki, M., Virtanen, M., Pentti, J., Subramanian, S. V., Kawachi, I., & Vahtera, J. (2013). Proximity of off-premise alcohol outlets and heavy alcohol consumption: A cohort study. *Drug and Alcohol Dependence*, *132*, 295–300.

Halonen, J. I., Pulakka, A., Stenholm, S., Pentti, J., Kawachi, I., Kivimaki, M., & Vahtera, J. (2016). Change in neighborhood disadvantage and change in smoking behaviors in adults: A longitudinal, within-individual study. *Epidemiology*, *27*, 803–809.

Halonen, J. I., Stenholm, S., Kivimaki, M., Pentti, J., Subramanian, S. V., Kawachi, I., & Vahtera, J. (2015). Is change in availability of sports facilities associated with change in physical activity? A prospective cohort study. *Preventive Medicine*, *2015*, 10–14.

Handley, M. A., Schillinger, D., & Shiboski, S. (2011). Quasi-experimental designs in practice-based research settings: Design and implementation considerations. *The Journal of the American Board of Family Medicine*, *24*(5), 589–596. doi:10.3122/jabfm.2011.05.110067

Handy, S., Xinyu, C., & Mokhtarian, P. L. (2006). Self-selection in the relationship between the built environment and walking. *Journal of the American Planning Association*, *72*(1), 55–74. doi:10.1080/01944360608976724

Harris, A. D., McGregor, J. C., Perencevich, E. N., Furuno, J. P., Zhu, J., Peterson, D. E., & Finkelstein, J. (2006). The use and interpretation of quasi-experimental studies in medical informatics. *Journal of the American Medical Informatics Association: JAMIA*, *13*(1), 16–23. doi:10.1197/jamia.M1749

Jokela, M. (2014). Are neighborhood health associations causal? A 10-year prospective cohort study with repeated measurements. *American Journal of Epidemiology*, *180*(8), 776–784.

Kawachi, I., Ichida, Y., Tampubolon, G., & Fujiwara, T. (2013). Causal inference in social capital research. In I. Kawachi, S. Takao, & S. V. Subramanian (Eds.), *Global perspectives on social capital and health*. New York, NY: Springer.

Kendler, K., Maes, H. H., Sundquist, K., Ohlsson, H., & Sundquist, J. (2014). Genetic and family and community environmental effects on drug abuse in adolescence: A Swedish national twin and sibling study. *American Journal of Psychiatry*, *171*(2), 209–217.

Kessler, R. C., Duncan, G., Gennetian, L., Katz, L., Kling, J. R., Sampson, N. A., . . . Ludwig, J. (2014). Associations of housing mobility interventions for children in high-poverty neighborhoods with subsequent mental disorders during adolescence. *JAMA*, *311*(9), 937–947.

Kling, J. R., Liebman, J. B., & Katz, L. F. (2007). Experimental analysis of neighborhood effects. *Econometrica*, *75*(1), 83–119.

Komro, K., Perry, C., Veblen-Mortensen, S., Farbakhsh, K., Toomey, T., Stigler, M., . . . Williams, C. (2008). Outcomes from a randomized controlled trial of a multi-component alcohol use preventive intervention for urban youth: Project Northland Chicago. *Addiction*, *103*(4), 606–618.

Kravitz-Wirtz, N. (2016). Cumulative effects of growing up in separate and unequal neighborhoods on racial disparities in self-rated health in early adulthood. *Journal of Health & Social Behavior*, *57*(4), 453–470.

Kuo, F., & Sullivan, W. (2001). Aggression and violence in the inner city: Effects of environment via mental fatigue. *Environment and Behavior*, *33*(4), 543–571.

Lemelin, E. T., Diez Roux, A. V., Franklin, T. G., Carnethon, M., Lutsey, P. L., Ni, H., . . . Shrager, S. (2009). Life-course socioeconomic positions and subclinical atherosclerosis in the multi-ethnic study of atherosclerosis. *Social Science & Medicine*, *68*(3), 444–451.

Lindberg, R., Shenassa, E., Acevedo-Garcia, D., Popkin, S., Villaveces, A., & Morley, R. L. (2010). Housing interventions at the neighborhood level and health: A review of the evidence. *Journal of Public Health Management and Practice*, *16*(5 E-Supplement), S44–S52.

Ludwig, J., Duncan, G. J., Gennetian, L. A., Katz, L. F., Kessler, R. C., Kling, J. R., & Sanbonmatsu, L. (2012). Neighborhood effects on the long-term well-being of low-income adults. *Science*, *337*(6101), 1505–1510.

Ludwig, J., Liebman, J. B., Kling, J. R., Duncan, G. J., Katz, L. F., Kessler, R. C., & Sanbonmatsu, L. (2008). What can we learn about neighborhood effects from the Moving to Opportunity experiment? A comment on Clampet-Lundquist and Massey. *American Journal of Sociology*, *114*(1), 144–188.

Ludwig, J., Sanbonmatsu, L., Gennetian, L., Adam, E., Duncan, G. J., Katz, L. F., . . . McDade, T. W. (2011). Neighborhoods, obesity, and diabetes—A randomized social experiment. *The New England Journal of Medicine*, *365*(16), 1509–1519.

Luepker, R., Raczynski, J., Osganian, S., Goldberg, R., Finnegan, J. J., Hedges, J., . . . Simons-Morton, D. (2000). Effect of a community intervention on patient delay and emergency medical service use in acute coronary heart disease: The Rapid Early Action for Coronary Treatment (REACT) Trial. *JAMA*, *284*(1), 60–67.

Manjarrez, C. A., Popkin, S. J., & Guernsey, E. (2007). *Poor health: Adding insult to injury for HOPE VI families.* Retrieved from http://www.hartfordinfo.org/Issues/wsd/Housing/gblock/HOPEVI_Health.pdf

Miller, H. J., Tribby, C. P., Brown, B. B., Smith, K. R., Werner, C. M., Wolf, J., . . . SImas Oliveira, M. G. (2015). Public transit generates new physical activity: Evidence from individual GPS and accelerometer data before and after light rail construction in a neighborhood of Salt Lake City, Utah, USA. *Health & Place*, *36*, 8–17.

Newhouse, J., & McClellan, M. (1998). The use of instrumental variables. *Annual Reviews of Public Health*, *19*, 17–34.

Nguyen, Q. C., Osypuk, T. L., Schmidt, N. M., Glymour, M. M., & Tchetgen Tchetgen, E. J. (2015). Practical guide for conducting mediation analysis with multiple mediators using inverse odds ratio weighting. *American Journal of Epidemiology*, *181*(5), 349–356.

Nguyen, Q. C., Rehkopf, D. H., Schmidt, N. M., & Osypuk, T. L. (2016). Heterogeneous effects of housing vouchers on the mental health of US adolescents. *American Journal of Public Health, 106*(4), 755–762.doi: 10.2105/AJPH.2015.303006

Nguyen, Q. C., Schmidt, N. M., Glymour, M. M., Rehkopf, D. H., & Osypuk, T. L. (2013). Were the mental health benefits of a housing mobility intervention larger for adolescents in higher socioeconomic status families? *Health & Place, 23*, 79–88.

Oakes, J. M. (2004). The (mis)estimation of neighborhood effects: Causal inference for a practicable social epidemiology. *Social Science & Medicine, 58*(10), 1929–1952.

Oakes, J. M. (2006). Commentary: Advancing neighbourhood-effects research—selection, inferential support, and structural confounding. *International Journal of Epidemiology, 35*, 643–647.

Oakes, J. M. (2014). Invited commentary: Repeated measures, selection bias, and effect identification in neighborhood effect studies. *American Journal of Epidemiology, 180*(8), 785–787.

Oakes, J. M., Andrade, K. E., Biyoow, I. M., & Cowan, L. T. (2015). Twenty years of neighborhood effect research: An assessment. *Current Epidemiology Reports, 2*, 80–87.

Oakes, J. M., & Johnson, P. J. (2006). Propensity score matching for social epidemiology. In J. M. Oakes & J. S. Kaufman (Eds.), *Methods in social epidemiology* (pp. 370–392). San Francisco, CA: Jossey-Bass, Inc.

Orr, L., Feins, J. D., Jacob, R., Beecroft, E., Sanbonmatsu, L., Katz, L. F., . . . Kling, J. R. (2003). *Moving to Opportunity for Fair Housing Demonstration Program: Interim impacts evaluation.* Washington, DC: Office of Policy Development and Research, US Department of Housing and Urban Development

Osypuk, T. L. (2015). Shifting from policy relevance to policy translation: Do housing and neighborhoods affect children's mental health? *Social Psychiatry and Psychiatric Epidemiology, 50*(2), 215–217. doi:10.1007/s00127-014-0998-6

Osypuk, T. L., & Acevedo-Garcia, D. (2010). Beyond individual neighborhoods: A geography of opportunity perspective for understanding racial/ethnic health disparities. *Health & Place, 16*(6), 1113–1123.

Osypuk, T. L., Joshi, P., Geronimo, K., & Acevedo-Garcia., D. (2014). Do social and economic policies influence health? A review. *Current Epidemiology Reports, 1*(3), 149–164. doi:10.1007/s40471-014-0013-5

Osypuk, T. L., Schmidt, N. M., Bates, L. M., Tchetgen-Tchetgen, E. J., Earls, F. J., & Glymour, M. M. (2012). Gender and crime victimization modify neighborhood effects on adolescent mental health. *Pediatrics, 130*(3), 472–481.

Osypuk, T. L., Tchetgen Tchetgen, E. J., Acevedo-Garcia, D., Earls, F. J., Lincoln, A., Schmidt, N. M., & Glymour, M. M. (2012). Differential mental health effects of neighborhood relocation among youth in vulnerable families. *Archives of General Psychiatry, 69*(12), 1284–1294.

Perry, C., Williams, C., Veblen-Mortensen, S., Toomey, T., Komro, K., Anstine, P., . . . Wolfson, M. (1996). Project Northland: Outcomes of a communitywide alcohol use prevention program during early adolescence. *American Journal of Public Health, 86*(7), 956–965.

Petersen, T. (2004). Analyzing panel data: Fixed- and random-effects models. In M. Hardy & A. Bryman (Eds.), *Handbook of data analysis* (pp. 331–345). London, UK: Sage.

Popkin, S. J., Harris, L. E., Cunningham, M. K., Bradley, J., Graham, A., & Comey, J. (2002). *Families in transition: A qualitative analysis of the MTO experience. Final Report.* Retrieved from http://www.huduser.org/Publications/pdf/mtoqualf.pdf

Popkin, S. J., Leventhal, T., & Weismann, G. (2008). *Girls in the 'hood: The importance of feeling safe*. Retrieved from http://www.urban.org/UploadedPDF/411636_girls_in_the_hood.pdf

Price, D., & Popkin, S. (2010). *The health crisis for CHA families*. Retrieved from https://www.urban.org/sites/default/files/publication/29016/412184-The-Health-Crisis-for-CHA-Families.PDF.

Pruitt, S. L., Leonard, T., Murdoch, J., Hughes, A., McQueen, A., & Gupta, S. (2014). Neighborhood effects in a behavioral randomized controlled trial. *Health & Place, 30*, 293–300.

Pulakka, A., Halonen, J. I., Kawachi, I., Pentti, J., Stenholm, S., Jokela, M., . . . Kivimaki, M. (2016). Association between distance from home to tobacco outlet and smoking cessation and relapse. *JAMA Internal Medicine, 176*(10), 1512–1519.

Ram, B., Nightingale, C. M., Hudda, M. T., Kapetanakis, V. V., Ellaway, A., Cooper, A. R., . . . Owen, C. G. (2016). Cohort profile: Examining neighbourhood activities in built living environments in London: The ENABLE London—Olympic Park cohort. *BMJ Open, 6*(10). doi:10.1136/bmjopen-2016-012643

Rehkopf, D. H., Glymour, M. M., & Osypuk, T. L. (2016). The consistency assumption for causal inference in social epidemiology: When a rose is not a rose. *Current Epidemiology Reports, 3*(1), 63–71.

Robins, J. M. (1999). Association, causation, and marginal structural models. *Synthese, 121*(1/2), 151–179.

Robins, J. M., Hernan, M. A., & Brumback, B. (2000). Marginal structural models and causal inference in epidemiology. *Epidemiology, 11*(5), 550–560.

Sampson, R. J. (2008). Moving to Inequality: Neighborhood effects and experiments meet social structure. *American Journal of Sociology, 114*(1), 189–231.

Sampson, R. J. (2010). Gold standard myths: Observations on the experimental turn in quantitative criminology. *Journal of Quantitative Criminology, 26*, 489–500.

Sanbonmatsu, L., Ludwig, J., Katz, L. F., Gennetian, L. A., Duncan, G. J., Kessler, R. C., . . . Lindau, S. T. (2011). *Moving to Opportunity for Fair Housing Demonstration Program: Final impacts evaluation*. Retrieved from https://www.huduser.gov/publications/pdf/mtofhd_fullreport_v2.pdf

Sanbonmatsu, L., Marvakov, J., Potter, N., Yang, F., Adam, E., Congdon, W. J., . . . McDade, T. W. (2012). The long-term effects of Moving to Opportunity on adult health and economic self-sufficiency. *Cityscape: A Journal of Policy Development and Research, 14*(2), 109–136.

Schmidt, N. M., Glymour, M. M., & Osypuk, T. L. (2016). Adolescence is a sensitive period for housing mobility to influence risky behaviors: An experimental design. *Journal of Adolescent Health*. doi:http://dx.doi.org/10.1016/j.jadohealth.2016.10.022

Schmidt, N. M., Glymour, M. M., & Osypuk, T. L. (2017). Housing mobility and adolescent mental health: The role of substance use, social networks, and family mental health in the Moving to Opportunity Study. *SSM—Population Health, 3*, 318–325.

Shadish, W. R., Cook, T. D., & Campbell, D. T. (2002). *Experimental and quasi-experimental designs for generalized causal inference*. New York, NY: Houghton Mifflin.

Sharkey, P., & Elwert, F. (2011). The legacy of disadvantage: Multigenerational neighborhood effects on cognitive ability. *American Journal of Sociology, 116*(6), 1934–1981. doi:10.1086/660009

Singer, J. D., & Willett, J. B. (2003). *Applied longitudinal data analysis: Modeling change and event occurrence*. New York, NY: Oxford University Press.

South, E., Kondo, M., Cheney, R., & Branas, C. (2015). Neighborhood blight, stress, and health: A walking trial of urban greening and ambulatory heart rate. *American Journal of Public Health, 205*, 909–913.

Thornton, L. E., Ball, K., Lamb, K. E., McCann, J., Parker, K., & Crawford, D. A. (2016). The impact of a new McDonald's restaurant on eating behaviours and perceptions of local residents: A natural experiment using repeated cross-sectional data. *Health & Place, 39*, 86–91. doi:http://dx.doi.org/10.1016/j.healthplace.2016.03.005

Triguero-Mas, M., Gidlow, C. J., Martínez, D., de Bont, J., Carrasco-Turigas, G., Martínez-Íñiguez, T., . . . Nieuwenhuijsen, M. J. (2017). The effect of randomised exposure to different types of natural outdoor environments compared to exposure to an urban environment on people with indications of psychological distress in Catalonia. *PLoS ONE, 12*(3), e0172200. doi:10.1371/journal.pone.0172200

US Department of Education. (2017). Promise Neighborhoods 2017. Retrieved from https://www2.ed.gov/programs/promiseneighborhoods/index.html

US Department of Housing & Urban Development. (2017). Choice Neighborhoods. Retrieved from https://portal.hud.gov/hudportal/HUD?src=/program_offices/public_indian_housing/programs/ph/cn

Veitch, J., Ball, K., Crawford, D., Abbott, G. R., Psych, G. D., & Salmon, J. (2012). Park improvements and park activity: A natural experiment. *American Journal of Preventive Medicine, 42*(6), 616–619.

Votruba, M. E., & Kling, J. R. (2009). Effects of neighborhood characteristics on the mortality of black male youth: Evidence from Gautreaux, Chicago. *Social Science & Medicine, 68*(5), 814–823.

Wagenaar, A. C., Murray, D., Gehan, J., Wolfson, M., Forster, J., Toomey, T., . . . Jones-Webb, R. (2000). Communities mobilizing for change on alcohol: Outcomes from a randomized community trial. *Journal of Alcohol Studies, 61*(1), 85–94.

White, J. S., Hamad, R., Li, X., Basu, S., Ohlsson, H., Sundquist, J., & Sundquist, K. (2016). Long-term effects of neighbourhood deprivation on diabetes risk: Quasi-experimental evidence from a refugee dispersal policy in Sweden. *The Lancet Diabetes and Endocrinology, 4*(6), 517–524.

Wodtke, G. (2013). Duration and timing of exposure to neighborhood poverty and the risk of adolescent parenthood. *Demography, 50*(5), 1765–1788.

Yu, Q., Li, B., & Scribner, R. A. (2009). Hierarchical additive modeling of nonlinear associations with spatial correlations: An application to relate alcohol outlet density and neighborhood assault rates. *Statistics in Medicine, 28*, 1896–1912.

Zahran, S., Magzamen, S., Breunig, I. M., & Mielke, H. W. (2014). Maternal exposure to neighborhood soil Pb and eclampsia risk in New Orleans, Louisiana (USA): Evidence from a natural experiment in flooding. *Environmental Research, 133*, 274–281.

Zhang, Y. T., Laraia, B. A., Mujahid, M. S., Blanchard, S. D., Warton, E. M., Moffet, H. H., & Karter, A. J. (2016). Is a reduction in distance to nearest supermarket associated with BMI change among type 2 diabetes patients? *Health & Place, 40*, 15–20. doi:http://dx.doi.org/10.1016/j.healthplace.2016.04.008

7

QUALITATIVE METHODS AND NEIGHBORHOOD HEALTH RESEARCH

Danya E. Keene

The vast majority of research examining the relationships between neighborhoods and health has relied on quantitative methods. However, qualitative methods such as interviews, focus groups, and observations, offer an important contribution to this literature. While qualitative methods, and in particular, ethnography, have long been used by social scientists to examine place and neighborhoods as social phenomena (Anderson, 1999; Bourgois, 1995; Deener, 2012; Desmond, 2016; Gans, 1962; Pattillo, 2007, for example), more recently these methods have been applied by scholars across the social sciences to examine the intersections of place and health (Frohlich, Potvin, Chabot, & Corin, 2002; Fullilove, 2004; Keene & Ruel, 2013; Keene & Padilla, 2010; Klinenberg, 2001; Mullings & Wali, 1999; Popay et al., 2003; Walton, 2014, for example).

Quantitative methods are particularly well suited for examining the extent to which certain characteristics of neighborhoods, or certain processes of neighborhood change, are associated with health outcomes. However, qualitative methods can help to explain why neighborhoods matters for health. By drawing on resident perspectives and observations of daily life to illuminate complex and often previously unknown processes, these methods can help to shed light on how places shape health behavior, how place affects access to health risks and resources, or how experiences of place may get under the skin to affect health. These methods can also provide insight into the agency of residents who actively engage with the structural features of their environment. Furthermore, qualitative research that occurs in collaboration with neighborhood residents can give voice to local concerns and inform policy and programmatic action.

Qualitative studies can stand on their own by providing in-depth and holistic descriptions of what neighborhoods are like, how neighborhoods are experienced and navigated by their residents, and what neighborhood characteristics mean to those who encounter them. Qualitative methods can also accompany quantitative studies of neighborhoods and health to illuminate the processes and mechanisms that underlie quantitative associations between neighborhood characteristics and health outcomes. Qualitative research can also serve as formative work for future quantitative studies by employing open-ended questioning and an inductive approach to uncover new concepts. This formative work can help researchers to develop survey questions that are fielded with larger samples, or hypotheses that are tested with existing survey data.

This chapter describes some of the ways that qualitative research has contributed to our understanding of how neighborhoods affect health. The first section describes some shared characteristics of qualitative methods. The second and third sections briefly describe various approaches to qualitative data collection and analysis. The last section of the chapter uses examples from qualitative studies to illustrate some of the unique contributions of qualitative research to the study of neighborhoods and health.

SHARED CHARACTERISTICS OF QUALITATIVE RESEARCH

The term "qualitative research" encompasses a broad diversity of theoretical orientations, study designs, and modes of data collection and analysis (Bradley, Curry, & Devers, 2007; Corbin & Strauss, 2014). Qualitative approaches include, but are not limited to, grounded theory, phenomenology, ethnography, narrative analysis, comparative historical analysis, and hybrids of these approaches (Corbin & Strauss, 2014). It is beyond the scope of this chapter to fully describe this breadth, but this section describes some characteristics of qualitative approaches that are shared across many qualitative traditions.

First, qualitative research is generally inductive. Qualitative research questions are typically framed in an open-ended manner, allowing the researcher to engage in broad discovery, rather than specific hypothesis testing. For example, while a quantitative study might ask about how the presence of grocery stores is quantitatively associated with measures of obesity, a qualitative researcher interested in the neighborhood determinants of obesity may explore more broadly how neighborhood residents obtain food (Cannuscio, Weiss, & Asch, 2010; Zenk et al., 2011). Though qualitative researchers may test their data and interpretations against existing theoretical frameworks, or test their own emerging hypotheses against their data, this deductive thinking typically occurs alongside inductive analysis.

The inductive nature of qualitative work allows researchers to refine their research questions and the direction of their inquiry according to what they are learning, and to ask questions that they may not have known to ask without this grounding. In keeping with this inductive approach, qualitative researchers often iterate between data collection and analysis, and between deductive and inductive thinking. This inductive, flexible, and iterative approach also allows for the possibility to identify concepts that are not contained in existing neighborhood surveys and to think about the relationship between place and health in new ways. For example, a researcher studying neighborhood food environment may discover that perceptions of safety shape the journeys that residents take to shop for food, leading to new questions about the relationship between perceived neighborhood safety and nutrition (Zenk et al., 2011).

Second, qualitative research is often holistic and contextualized. Quantitative models often seek to control for the effect of context, in order to isolate particular relationships or variables of interest. In contrast, qualitative methods seek to understand phenomena in context and to capture the full range of complex and often multidirectional relationships that can be difficult to incorporate in quantitative models. This holistic nature of qualitative work is particularly relevant to neighborhood research, given that neighborhoods contain many complex and multidimensional features, which may interact with a broad array of individual characteristics to affect health (Macintyre & Ellaway, 2003).

Third, qualitative research often operates in a social constructivist tradition that considers knowledge to be socially constructed and context dependent (Corbin & Strauss, 2014). This tradition recognizes the importance of subjective experiences, meanings, and perceptions in shaping actions and behaviors that matter for health and well-being. Administrative and survey data are well suited for documenting the structural features of neighborhoods such as the number and location of parks, abandoned buildings, grocery stores, hospitals, or streets with sidewalks. But understanding how individuals perceive and respond to these structural features can provide a fuller understanding of how these neighborhood features are linked to health (Frohlich et al., 2002; Popay et al., 2003).

Finally, qualitative research can give voice to neighborhood residents themselves. As O'Campo and Caughy (2006) note, the largely quantitative literature on neighborhoods and health, "has almost exclusively been conducted without input from those who reside in these community settings" (p. 202). In contrast, their participatory concept mapping approach involves neighborhood residents in the research process through qualitative data collection that provides an opportunity for residents to share their experiences and perspectives (O'Campo & Caughy, 2006; O'Campo et al., 2009). Qualitative research can give voice to individuals and communities by telling the stories of how their residents experience place, what meanings they attach to place, and what actions they take to navigate aspects of their environment.

Qualitative research that occurs in a participatory tradition, where researchers and neighborhood residents work together to determine how the research will be conducted and what questions it seeks to answer, can also give voice to neighborhood communities by prioritizing issues that are salient to them and using findings to address neighborhood needs (Farquhar, Parker, Schulz, & Israel, 2006; Mullings & Wali, 1999; Wang, 2006).

COLLECTING QUALITATIVE DATA ON NEIGHBORHOODS AND HEALTH

Qualitative research encompasses a range of well-established data collection methods. For example, neighborhood researchers have used qualitative interviews that allow participants to narrate their own perceptions and experiences of place in response to open-ended questions (Clampet-Lundquist, Kling, Edin, & Duncan, 2011; Frye et al., 2014; Keene & Ruel, 2013, for example). Qualitative interviews provide an opportunity for participants to tell their own story and to discuss the issues that they deem relevant to the research question. In contrast to a survey, where a participant responds to set questions that are determined in advance, qualitative interviews are a partnership between the participant and the researcher who are both working toward the common goal of knowledge production (Weiss, 1998). Qualitative interviews can range from structured sets of open-ended questions to unstructured conversations (Corbin & Strauss, 2014). In a semistructured interview, a common form of interviews used in qualitative studies of neighborhoods and health, the researcher has a predetermined set of topics to be covered during the interview, but does not necessarily ask questions in a particular order or limit the interview to these questions. This allows the participant to lead the conversation and raise new topics that are relevant to the research question.

Other researchers have employed focus groups, where groups of 6–12 participants, led by a facilitator, come together to discuss aspects of their neighborhoods and their health (Eriksson & Emmelin, 2013; Farquhar et al., 2006; Weathers et al., 2011). Focus groups provide an opportunity to examine shared experiences and shared norms that emerge through group discussion (Morgan, 1993). By bringing groups of neighborhood residents together, they can also empower individuals to speak on topics that they may be reluctant to bring up in individual interviews (Morgan, 1993). On the other hand, focus groups are less able to capture individual experiences in depth (Braun & Clarke, 2013). Focus groups can also be challenging to moderate, and careful attention must be paid to group composition and dynamics (Braun & Clarke, 2013).

Others have employed ethnographic methods of observation, spending extended periods of time in neighborhoods, observing and participating in daily life (Mullings & Wali, 1999). Observations provide a unique opportunity to understand how residents interact with features of their environment to affect their health, a process that is often difficult to capture in an interview. By documenting actions, observations can also capture things that participants are unable to articulate. Additionally, ethnographers who spend extended periods of time in a neighborhood often build a rapport with residents that facilitates unique insights into neighborhood life.

In addition to the use of these more common methods, scholars have developed unique qualitative approaches to data collection that are designed for, are particularly well suited for, the study of health and place. For example, the go-along interview (Carpiano, 2009; Evans & Jones, 2011; Garcia, Eisenberg, Frerich, Lechner, & Lust, 2012; Kusenbach, 2003; Walton, 2014) combines features of interviews and observations to allow the researcher to "walk through" the lived experience of place. In the go-along interview, participants take the researcher on a walk through the spaces that are salient to them, while also narrating their experiences of place. The go-along interview addresses some of the limitations of both observations and interviews. For example, observations can document what the surrounding environment is like, but they are often insufficient for capturing how residents perceive and interact with place. Likewise, sit-down interviews provide useful tools for examining individual perceptions and biographies, but they are less well suited for capturing contextual information, in part because participants are not primed to think about how context affects their lives (Carpiano, 2009; Kusenbach, 2003). Carpiano (2009) notes that the go-along interview, as a hybrid of observation and interview, provides an opportunity for the researcher to be led through a "spatialized journey" and to learn "about the local area via the interplay of the respondent's ideas and the researcher's own experience of the respondent's environment" (p. 267).

Photovoice is another qualitative data collection approach that, like the go-along interview, can bring environmental cues to the interview context (Haines-Saah, Oliffe, White, & Bottorff, 2013; Nykiforuk, Vallianatos, & Nieuwendyk, 2011; Wang, Morrel-Samuels, Mutchison, Bell, & Pestronk, 2004). Photovoice is a participatory research method that employs photography as a way for residents to represent their communities (Catalani & Minkler, 2010). Participants are given cameras and asked to document salient features of their daily lives and the places where they spend time. The photos then serve as prompts for focus group discussions or interviews, providing contextual cues in a similar manner to the walks or rides that occur in the go-along interview. The photovoice methodology is also action oriented: participants document their communities through photography and photo narratives, and use these tools to engage in critical dialogue with policy makers and other agents of change (Wang, 2006).

Participatory photo mapping builds on photovoice methodology, employing participant-generated maps, photos, drawings, and narrative interpretations of these artifacts to "actively and methodically interpret people's experience through representations that they share with [the researchers]" (Dennis, Gaulocher, Carpiano, & Brown, 2009). It also incorporates an emerging field of qualitative geographic information systems (GIS) which uses GIS software (see Chapter 3) to map qualitative data onto geographic coordinates (Boschmann & Cubbon, 2014; Keddem et al., 2015; Matthews, Detwiler, & Burton, 2005).

These data collection approaches, summarized in Table 7-1, all share some common features. In particular, they can capture residents' experience of place, offering

Table 7-1 Approaches to Qualitative Data Collection

Approach	*Examples From Neighborhoods and Health Literature*
	Common qualitative data collection methods
Interviews	Clampet-Lundquist, S., Kling, J. R., Edin, K., & Duncan, G. J. (2011). Moving teenagers out of high-risk neighborhoods: How girls fare better than boys. *American Journal of Sociology, 116*(4), 1154–1189
Focus groups	Frohlich, K. L., Potvin, L., Chabot, P., & Corin, E. (2002). A theoretical and empirical analysis of context: Neighborhoods, smoking, and youth. *Social Science & Medicine, 54*, 1401–1417.
Observations	Mullings, L., & Wali, A. (1999). *Stress and resilience: The social context of reproduction in Central Harlem*. New York, NY: Kluwer Academic/Plenum.
	Qualitative data collection methods uniquely suited for the study of neighborhoods and health
Go-along interview	Carpiano, R. M. (2009). Come take a walk with me: The "go-along" interview as a novel method for studying the implications of place for health and well-being. *Health & Place, 15*(1), 263–272.
Photovoice	Wang, C., Morrel-Samuels, S., Mutchison, P., Bell, L., & Pestronk, R. (2004). Flint Photovoice-community building among youth, adults and policymakers. *American Journal of Public Health, 94*(6), 911–916.
Participatory photomapping	Dennis, S. F., Gaulocher, S., Carpiano, R. M., & Brown, D. (2009). Participatory photo mapping (PPM): Exploring an integrated method for health and place research with young people. *Health and Place, 15*(2), 466–473.

rich descriptions, and providing insights into the many complex processes through which neighborhoods affect health. Additionally, the open-ended nature of these data collection approaches allows for a process of discovery through inductive analysis.

A BRIEF OVERVIEW OF QUALITATIVE ANALYSIS

It is beyond the scope of this chapter to fully describe the numerous and varied approaches to qualitative analysis, a subject that many qualitative methods textbooks and articles address (Braun & Clark, 2013; Charmaz, 2014; Corbin & Strauss, 2014; Miles & Huberman, 1994; Timmermans & Tavory, 2012, for example). However, this section briefly describes some general features of qualitative analysis that are shared across many qualitative methodologies.

In the most general terms, qualitative analysis involves ascribing meaning to raw data through a process of interpretation (Corbin & Strauss, 2014; Denzin, 1998). As Denzin notes, "meaning is not in the text," but rather produced through an active process of interpretation and representation. Qualitative researchers are often conscious of how their own perspectives, experiences, subjectivity, and theoretical orientations affect their interpretation of the data (Corbin & Strauss, 2014).

The process of qualitative analysis typically involves transcribing, reading, coding, and displaying the data. In the first step, interview audio files are typically transcribed into written transcripts (see Braun & Clarke, 2013) or jottings from field observations are transcribed into field notes (see Emerson, Fritz, & Shaw, 1995). Qualitative researchers read and reread these textual files to gain an overall impression of the data and to begin identifying patterns and emergent themes. Coding, a process of developing concepts and applying them to pieces of data, is typically conducted throughout the process of data collection and analysis. In later stages of analysis, coding also allows researchers to systematically sort data according to identified concepts (Bradley, Curry, & Devers, 2007; Corbin & Strauss, 2014; Miles & Huberman, 1994). This coding can be done by hand or with qualitative coding software (for example, Atlas-Ti, NVIVO, or Dedoose). Qualitative researchers typically record the thought process that accompanies coding and analysis in memos that describe the data, make comparisons, develop concepts, or relate concepts to each other (Corbin & Strauss, 2014).

As illustrated in the section that follows, qualitative analysis can have multiple goals. In some cases, it can be used to provide rich descriptions, showing for example, how residents experience and navigate their neighborhoods. In other cases, concepts developed from qualitative research are used to develop theories that explain the pathways and processes connecting neighborhoods to health.

CONTRIBUTIONS OF QUALITATIVE RESEARCH TO NEIGHBORHOOD AND HEALTH RESEARCH

Explanatory Potential of Qualitative Methods: Identifying Mechanisms and Processes

Qualitative methods are uniquely suited to illuminate what is often a black box of complex and multidirectional mechanisms that underlie quantitative associations between neighborhood characteristics and health (Table 7-2). Developing an understanding of mechanisms and processes is considered to be a critical priority for neighborhood effects research. As O'Campo and colleagues (2009) note, "Identification of the pathways by which neighborhoods affect well-being is critical to moving the field forward toward a more complete understanding of the complex relationships between residential environments and well-being" (p. 57). Additionally, an understanding of these mechanisms is important for designing effective community-based interventions, and informing policies that affect neighborhood environments (Edin & Pirog, 2014; O'Campo, Salmon, & Burke, 2009).

The well-known experimental Moving to Opportunity (MTO) study (see Chapter 6) provides many examples of this explanatory potential of qualitative methods. MTO sought to understand the effects of neighborhood poverty on well-being through a randomized, controlled study that provided vouchers for public housing residents to relocate to lower poverty neighborhoods. The 4,600 MTO participants from five cities were randomly selected into three groups: a control group, a group that received a standard Section 8 rental voucher, and a group that received a Section 8 rental voucher that could only be used in a lower poverty neighborhoods (Orr et al., 2003). Researchers compared these three groups across a range of outcomes, including mental, physical, and behavioral health (Leventhal & Brooks-Gunn, 2003a, 2003b; Sanbonmatsu et al., 2011). They also conducted repeated qualitative interviews with MTO families and observations in MTO neighborhoods (Kling, Liebman, & Katz, 1994). These qualitative data had a profound effect on the interpretation of quantitative findings from the MTO program and on the design of surveys in subsequent waves. As Kling and colleagues note in regard to the qualitative interviews and observations, "For many of the things we learned, it is hard to imagine any other data collection strategy that would have led us to these insights" (p. 3).

Table 7-2 Contributions of Qualitative Research to the Study of Neighborhood Effects

Contribution	*Example*
Explaining pathways	Clampet-Lundquist, S., Kling, J. R., Edin, K., & Duncan, G. J. (2011). Moving teenagers out of high-risk neighborhoods: How girls fare better than boys. *American Journal of Sociology, 116*(4), 1154–1189.
Developing hypotheses, concepts, and theory	Frohlich, K. L., Potvin, L., Chabot, P., & Corin, E. (2002). A theoretical and empirical analysis of context: neighborhoods, smoking, and youth. *Social Science & Medicine, 54*, 1401–1417.
Examining the meaning of place	Popay, J., Thomas, C., Williams, G., Bennett, S., Gatrell, A., & Bostock, L. (2003). A proper place to live: Health inequalities, agency and the normative dimensions of space. *Social Science & Medicine (1982), 57*(1), 55–69.
Examining the navigation of place	Frye, V., Egan, J. E., Tieu, H. Van, Cerdá, M., Ompad, D., & Koblin, B. A. (2014). "I didn't think I could get out of the fucking park." Gay men's retrospective accounts of neighborhood space, emerging sexuality and migrations. *Social Science and Medicine, 104*, 6–14.
Providing a holistic account	Mullings, L., & Wali, A. (1999). *Stress and resilience: The social context of reproduction in Central Harlem.* New York, NY: Kluwer Academic/Plenum.
Giving voice to inform action	Wang, C., Morrel-Samuels, S., Mutchison, P., Bell, L., & Pestronk, R. (2004). Flint Photovoice- community building among youth, adults and policymakers. *American Journal of Public Health, 94*(6), 911–916.

In the MTO study, qualitative research provided important insight into the processes that contributed to health outcomes among MTO families. The interviews provided movers with an opportunity to tell their own story of what it was like to move with a voucher, revealing both the positive changes that they experienced and also the challenges that they encountered. For example, qualitative interviews with experimental group families revealed significant reduction in stressors associated with moving to lower poverty neighborhoods. Participants described the impact that exposure to violence had on their day-to-day lives, their parenting, and their feelings of safety in their old neighborhoods (Kling et al., 1994). On the other hand, participants in the experimental group also described stress associated with paying utility bills in voucher-subsidized apartments (an expense that was covered in public housing), challenges in accessing healthcare as they moved further from urban centers, and more experiences with racism in their new neighborhoods (Kling, Liebman, Katz, & Sanbonmatsu, 2004). These stressors and challenges may have limited the ability of MTO participants to benefit from moves to lower poverty neighborhoods, and they may explain why some of the early health outcomes for MTO movers were not universally positive (Kling, Liebman, & Katz, 2007).

The qualitative MTO data also helped to explain unexpected group differences uncovered in the quantitative analysis of MTO survey data. For example, the survey found that while adolescent girls in both experimental groups experienced improvements across indicators of mental health and health behaviors, male adolescents in the experimental groups experienced significant increases in risky behavior and injuries compared to the control group (Kling & Liebman, 2004). Clampet-Lundquist and colleagues (2011) analyzed interview data with MTO participants to uncover multiple ways that the experience of moving with a voucher differed by gender. For example, they found that boys in the experimental group faced increased levels of monitoring relative to those in the control group, in part because they brought gendered patterns of socializing into neighborhoods where these behaviors were more heavily scrutinized. Additionally, the authors found that boys developed several strategies for navigating the risks of high-poverty neighborhoods, and that that these strategies could be lost with relocation to a lower poverty neighborhood. This loss could then have negative consequences when boys moved back to high-poverty neighborhoods, as was the case with a significant portion of MTO families. In contrast, the authors found that girls' leisure patterns that involved spending more time indoors rendered such neighborhood knowledge less consequential for their well-being. The predetermined MTO survey questions could not have captured these nuanced gendered experiences.

Qualitative data from MTO were also useful for explaining how the program actually played out in people's lives, thus providing an important process evaluation (Edin, Deluca, & Owene, 2012). For example, Rosenblatt and Deluca (2012) used qualitative interviews with Baltimore MTO participants to examine the decision-making processes associated with housing searches among MTO families, and to better understand why so many MTO families who initially moved to lower poverty neighborhoods eventually returned to high-poverty ones. They found that when voucher holders needed to move a second time, many prioritized dwelling quality over neighborhood. They also found that residents' prior experiences in high-poverty neighborhoods, and the strategies that they had developed to navigate these neighborhoods gave them confidence that they could handle the consequences of this trade-off. Here, qualitative data provided an opportunity to observe how residents responded to the MTO program, thus offering insights that can inform future policy and program design.

The Exploratory Potential of Qualitative Methods: Developing New Hypotheses, Concepts, and Theory

The ability of qualitative methods to identify the unexpected or unintended is another important contribution of qualitative research to the study of neighborhoods and health. Qualitative researchers often frame their research questions in broad terms, allowing them to discover and develop new concepts which, as illustrated in the previous examples, are often absent from administrative surveys. These new concepts have helped to refine existing neighborhood surveys, given rise to new hypotheses that can be tested with new or existing data, contributed to new research questions and new domains of neighborhood research, and helped to develop theories for explaining the relationships between neighborhoods and health.

The concept of spatial stigma is one example of a concept that was developed through qualitative research and subsequently tested as a determinant of health in quantitative studies (see Chapter 10). Specifically, ethnographic and interview based studies describe how residents who reside in, or relocate from, economically or socially marginalized neighborhoods experience stigma and discrimination associated with the negative reputation of these areas (Castro & Lindbladh, 2004; Garbin & Millington, 2011; Keene & Padilla, 2010; Macintyre & Ellaway, 2003; Wacquant, 2007; Warr, 2005). This qualitative literature shows how spatial stigma can affect access to jobs, healthcare, and other resources and can serve as a source of health-demoting stress. The qualitative literature also describes the practices that are employed to manage and resist spatial stigma and the potential health implications of these strategies. Drawing on this qualitative literature, researchers have begun to operationalize the concept of spatial stigma in neighborhood surveys (Duncan et al., 2016; Pearce, 2012; Tabuchi, Fukuhara, & Iso, 2012) and have found associations between measures of spatial stigma and poor health.

New concepts that emerge from qualitative analysis can serve as the building blocks of theory, generating new models for explaining the relationship between neighborhoods and health, or refining old ones. For example, Frohlich and colleagues (2002) drew on qualitative data to develop the theory of "collective lifestyles," an explanation for geographically patterned health behaviors that considers an interaction of social practice (agency) and social structure (place). Specifically, drawing on focus groups conducted with youth in 32 Quebec communities, the authors observed how the meanings that participants ascribed to features of their environment shaped their smoking behaviors. The authors note that quantitative research relying on surveys and administrative data can fall short of explaining the contextual determinants of health, because context is "neither just the reflection of the distribution of characteristics nor just the attributes of the area but also the significance that these characteristics hold for people" (p. 1413). Qualitative data allowed them to observe these complex interactions by providing insight into the reasoning behind human actions. The theory of collective lifestyles has been applied beyond this particular setting, to understand the contextual determinants of smoking and health behaviors more broadly (Cummins, Curtis, Diez-Roux, & Macintyre, 2007; Haines-Saah et al., 2013).

Examining the Meanings of Place

As described in the previous example, the meanings that residents ascribe to their neighborhoods, and to specific features of their neighborhoods, are important determinants of their behaviors and of their health. As Popay et al. (2003) note, "The meanings people attach to the experience of places and how these shape social action may provide another link in the complex, causal pathways generating inequalities in health". Page 56 for example, Popay and colleagues (2003) draw on qualitative interviews with residents of high- and low-income neighborhoods to examine the normative dimensions of place as they relate to residents' identities, social actions, and health behaviors. First, they use these interview data to describe residents' understandings of a "proper place" to live. They then describe varying degrees of discordance between residents' definitions of a "proper place" and their actual lived experiences of place. They also describe how individuals constructed positive identities despite living in improper places, through actions that often have implications for health and well-being. Ultimately, their work suggests that the dissonance between one's lived experience of place and one's definition of a proper place is one of the routes through which disadvantaged neighborhoods can contribute to health inequality. They also show that lay knowledge, collected through qualitative methods, has an important role to play in enhancing our understanding of the ways that material conditions, meaning, and action intersect to produce health inequalities (Popay et al., 2003).

As another example of the meanings that places hold, qualitative research has described the strong attachment or sense rootedness that can connect residents to their homes and neighborhoods (Fullilove, 2004; Keene et al., 2010). For example, drawing on ethnographic data collected over 4 years in Boston, Chicago, and San Antonio, Burton and Clark (2005) describe the role that geographically anchored "homeplaces" play in providing a sense of belonging, empowerment, and well-being for working-class African American families in the context of marginalizing forces.

Relatedly, drawing on fieldwork and oral history interviews conducted in five cities, Fullilove (2004) shows how disruptions in these place attachments, as a result of urban renewal programs, played an important role in the ecology of disease. Fullilove (2004) describes the health consequences of urban renewal as rooted not only in the initial trauma of displacement, but also in the loss of health-protective community resources such as locally owned businesses, locally situated social networks of exchange and support, and political institutions that had been growing in number and in effectiveness prior to renewal. The life stories of those individuals who had lived through the renewal era revealed that many of these resources had not been recreated, even a generation later. This work illustrates the power of narrative data in capturing the relationships between place and individual biographies (Fullilove, 1996).

Examining the Navigation of Place

The meanings that residents ascribe to their neighborhoods shape their actions; thus, meaning and agency are interrelated (Frohlich et al., 2002). Qualitative data can reveal the role of human agency in navigating various risks and resources that exist both within and beyond neighborhood spaces.

One area where qualitative research has described the navigation of place is in the study of mobility and health among gay and bisexual men. Quantitative studies have described pronounced geographic variation in sexual minority stigma that predict a range of health outcomes and health behaviors among gay and bisexual men (Hatzenbuehler et al., 2014). Quantitative research has also described health risks and benefits associated with mobility across this geography of stigma (Egan et al., 2011; Pachankis, Eldahan, & Golub, 2016). Complementing these studies, a body of qualitative research has also examined how gay and bisexual men navigate geographic variation in stigma with implications for their physical and mental health (Frye et al., 2014; Kobrak, Ponce, & Zielony, 2015; Lewis, 2014b; Valentine & Skelton, 2003).

In particular, research describes migration to well-established gay enclaves as a quest for identity affirming communities, visible gay spaces, opportunities for socializing and sexualizing, and greater anonymity (Bruce & Harper, 2011; Egan et al., 2011; Kobrak et al., 2015; Lewis, 2014a; Valentine & Skelton, 2003; Waitt & Gorman-Murray, 2011). Building on this literature, in a recent study, my colleagues and I drew on qualitative interview data to examine the intersections of stigma, mobility, and health, in the relatively understudied environment of the small city (Keene, Eldahan, White Hughto, & Pachankis, 2016). We found that the small cities where our study took place served as both destinations and points of departure for our participants. These cities attracted gay and bisexual men from surrounding suburbs and rural areas where sexual minority stigma was more prevalent and where there were fewer spaces and opportunities for gay life. Conversely, participants noted that these small cities did not contain the same identity-affirming communities as urban gay enclaves. Participants described small-city gay spaces as "safe zones," but outside of these spaces, many minimized or concealed their sexual identities. This atmosphere of limited acceptance motivated movement from small cities to larger ones, as men sought places where they could "let my hair down" or "be yourself." Some discussed plans to move to large gay enclaves, and others engaged in regular travel, back and forth between small cities and larger ones.

The qualitative and open-ended nature of this study allowed us to observe not only these patterns of movement but also the motivations, meanings, and lived experiences that accompanied them. Participants narratives also allowed us to consider the multifaceted ways that mobility across place was related to health. For example, men described a sense of safety associated with gay enclaves where their identities were affirmed but also substance use and potentially risky sexual activity that sometimes accompanied their travel.

In another qualitative study, Frye and colleagues examined the racialized and classed nature of mobility among gay and bisexual men across New York City neighborhoods. They conducted interviews with 20 gay and bisexual men who were recruited from five different New York neighborhoods, including a traditionally gay associated neighborhood (Chelsea), emerging gay spaces (Washington Heights, Fort Greene) and not traditionally gay-associated places (Harlem). They collected accounts of how participants experienced and navigated both sexual and racial identities in their natal and current neighborhoods. They found that across race and class, men described feeling trapped by heteronormative environments of natal neighborhoods, but that lower socioeconomic status and racial minority men had fewer opportunities to leave these neighborhoods, both as youth and as adults. The authors found that some were also reluctant to move to gay neighborhoods that were predominantly White. Others chose to stay in natal neighborhoods where they had strong family ties, despite the heterosexism and sexual marginalization that they experienced. By illustrating the intersection of race, sexuality, and the navigation of place through qualitative interviews, the study provided a nuanced understanding of how young gay, bisexual, and other MSM navigated geographically determined risks and resources.

Capturing a Holistic Perspective on Neighborhoods and Health Through Ethnographic Engagement

In their ability to capture the complex interactions between structure, meaning, social practices, and behaviors, qualitative research can generate holistic models of place and health that are unavailable by other methods. These holistic methods can produce answers to questions about place and health that speak to the roles of multiple actors and multiple processes. They can reveal the intersection between the natural, the material, the social, and the political dimensions of place.

One place where the holistic capabilities of qualitative research are particularly evident is in the example of prolonged ethnographic work that is situated within one community (Anderson, 1999; Bourgois, 1995; Deener, 2012; Desmond, 2016; Gans, 1962; Pattillo, 2007, for example). One example where this long-term ethnography has been used to understand the relationship between neighborhoods and health is the work of the Harlem Birthright Project, as described in Mullings and Wali's ethnography, *Stress and Reslience.* The project was designed to identify the broad social context of pregnancy outcomes among African American women in Harlem in an effort to understand and address persistent and large racial disparities. The study sought to move beyond the single-factor predictor models of quantitative studies that had limited capacity to explain the complex contextual determinants of pregnancy outcomes. The project also sought to engage the local community in the efforts to understand the determinants of pregnancy outcomes using a participatory approach. The project team included a community advisory board and community dialogue groups comprised of neighborhood residents.

The Harlem Birthright Project drew on data from a number of sources collected at 10 Harlem fields sites including (1) ethnographic field research that included participant observations and repeated interviews and observations conducted with 22 longitudinal participants, (2) an ethnographic questionnaire that included closed and open-ended questions and was administered to 100 randomly selected neighborhood women, and (3) 11 focus groups that discussed specific issues related to the context of infant mortality in Harlem. This in-depth study of one geographic area, Harlem, New York City, and the multiple subneighborhoods within this area, provided numerous insights into the ways that both the conditions that women lived in and their attempts to ameliorate these conditions served as stressors that could affect pregnancy outcomes. For example, participants described the stressors associated with inadequate housing but also the stress and labor of managing these housing challenges through, landlord negotiations, visits to housing court, or collective housing activism.

Their ethnographic work also revealed the complexity of what it meant to live in a Black community. On the one hand, participants almost universally valued living in a Black community and described this as a source of resilience. They described strong attachments to their community, with one participant reporting that even if she won the lottery, she would keep her house in Harlem. However, despite their own positive sentiments about Harlem, participants were aware of

Harlem's negative reputation, which they attributed to racism. Residents also articulated the way that this reputation affected their access to services and, ultimately, their birth outcomes. For example, one respondent, who lost a baby in childbirth after a long ambulance wait and mismanagement upon finally arriving at the hospital, attributed her inadequate care to negative perceptions of her neighborhood (see Chapter 10).

This ethnographic account provided a holistic understanding of the contextual determinants of birth and pregnancy outcomes. It also informed policy and programmatic interventions. As the authors note, "This study suggests that listening carefully to the voices of women, speaking directly through their words and their experiences, gives the scientific and the policy community an opportunity to design interventions that make sense to the people they are supposed to benefit" (Mullings & Wali, 1999, p. 165).

Another example of the holistic capability of qualitative work is Eric Klinenberg's use of ethnography to explain how a Chicago heatwave in the 1995 resulted in an unexpectedly large number of deaths (Klinenberg, 1999, 2002). Drawing on field work, interviews, statistical data, cartographical analysis, and historical studies of Chicago, Klinenberg's analysis revealed the social, political, and economic causes of the heatwave's mortality, illustrating that this disaster was not entirely a "natural" one. In particular, his ethnographic work conducted among social workers and residents in economically marginalized Chicago neighborhoods revealed how "literal social isolation" contributed to heat-related deaths among the elderly. In public and political discourse surrounding the heatwave, these elderly residents were blamed for not heeding warnings to seek assistance, but the ground-level accounts of everyday life in the city's most disadvantaged neighborhoods revealed that many considered it too risky to leave their apartments as a result of perceived violence in their surrounding neighborhood. Klinenberg found that many of these older adults barricaded themselves in their homes and "used their walls to protect them from the threatening world around them" (p. 260). His rich account gives texture to these fears, describing, for example, seniors who created makeshift alarm systems, such as electrified door handles, in order to protect themselves from the world outside.

By contextualizing this ethnographic field work within the local political and policy context, Klinenberg also shows that the "literal isolation" of the city's most disadvantaged and elderly population proved particularly deadly, given the new "empowerment era" of city government that emphasized the need for citizens to help themselves and required them to master a new system of social welfare services. As Klineberg notes, "Many of the Chicagoans who died or required emergency care during the heat wave were no doubt among those who, failing to master the system, became, in the state's logic, their own victims." Klineberg's holistic and complex "social autopsy" of this unnatural disaster would not have been possible without qualitative methods that allowed him to observe what life was like on the ground for those who died during the heatwave, including an examination of how they experienced shifts in government services.

Giving Voice to Resident Experiences and Concerns

As noted earlier, in the example of the Harlem Birthright Project, qualitative research that occurs in a participatory tradition can give voice to neighborhood residents, allowing them to develop research that is in sync with community priorities and to participate in the documentation of their community needs and strengths. Qualitative research, conducted with community partners, has also been used in the planning and evaluation of neighborhood interventions (Dennis et al., 2009; Farquhar et al., 2006; Wang et al., 2006). For example, Farquhar and colleagues (2006) describe the way that qualitative methods, including focus groups and qualitative interviews, were utilized by the East Side Village Health Worker Partnership, in Detroit, Michigan (ESVHWP), an academic and community collaboration that was founded with the goal of understanding and improving the social determinants of health for women and families on the east side of Detroit. The project used qualitative methods to identify community needs, develop intervention goals, design programs, and determine how best to implement them. The team also used qualitative methods to evaluate the process and impact of these programs. The authors note that "Programs and interventions that are informed by qualitative methods and include the opinions, experiences and perspectives of the community involved, are more likely to be tailored to the community concerns and less likely to be based solely on health promoters' assumption" (p. 240).

As discussed earlier, photovoice is also a participatory qualitative method that can give voice to and address resident concerns. As one example, the Flint Photovoice project used the photovoice method to understand and address the challenges that Flint faced in the wake of deindustrialization (Wang et al., 2004). The impetus for the project came from the leadership of the Flint Neighborhood Violence Prevention Collaborative, a coalition of 265 neighborhood clubs and groups. Eight local facilitators and 11 professional photographers led focus group workshops with Flint residents who produced photo narratives. These narratives were analyzed through group discussions to produce themes that were then presented to policy makers, the media, community leaders, and the general public. The findings from this work were instrumental in securing CDC funding for Flint's Youth Violence Prevention Center

(Wang et al., 2004). Beyond this center, the Flint Photovoice project helped to build relationships between residents and community leaders, providing a foundation for future collective action. As noted by Wang et al. (2004), "By documenting their own worlds, and critically discussing with the policymakers, the images they produce, community people can initiate grassroots social change" (p. 911).

By giving voice to the lived experiences of neighborhood residents, qualitative research can also play an important role in reaching policy-making audiences. Patton (2002) argues that qualitative accounts have "face validity and credibility" (p. 20) that can be difficult to dismiss, even by those who might disagree with them. Additionally, by giving voice to the experience of neighborhood residents, qualitative research can highlight their agency as they navigate structural constraints and opportunities. This attention to agency can be powerfully humanizing and may be able to combat stigma that has historically been attached to marginalized neighborhoods and those who reside in them (see Chapter 10).

CONCLUSIONS

This chapter has described some of the contributions of qualitative methods such as observations, interviews, focus groups, and photovoice to the literature on neighborhoods and health. In some of these examples, qualitative approaches are used in combination with other methods, and in other cases they are employed on their own. The studies described herein provide knowledge that would not have been attainable through quantitative methods, and they push the field of neighborhood and health research forward in important ways. In particular, they help to identify the complex and multifaceted processes that link neighborhoods and various characteristics of neighborhoods to the health of their residents. An understanding of these mechanisms is valuable for advancing theory, as well as policy and practice. Studies employing qualitative methods have also identified new concepts related to neighborhoods and health, through a process of inductive exploration, and without the constraints of prestructured surveys and administrative data. These new concepts have produced hypotheses for future testing and have led to the design of new survey instruments.

The overview presented in this chapter speaks both to potential consumers and potential producers of qualitative research on neighborhoods and health. In terms of the former, this chapter suggests the many ways that epidemiologists and other quantitative neighborhood researchers can draw on qualitative work to inform study design, statistical models, and interpretation of their findings. Even qualitative work that is not explicitly about health may be valuable for advancing both theory and practice related to neighborhood health. Additionally, given the valuable contributions of existing qualitative research, the overview presented in this chapter suggests a need for more qualitative, ethnographic, and mixed-methods studies that examine the intersection of neighborhoods and health. Such studies are vital to further developing theory regarding the relationships between neighborhoods and health and for informing future urban and neighborhood policy.

REFERENCES

Anderson, E. (1999). *Code of the street*. New York, NY: Norton.

Boschmann, E. E., & Cubbon, E. (2014). Sketch maps and qualitative GIS: Using cartographies of individual spatial narratives in geographic research. *The Professional Geographer*, *66*(2), 236–248.

Bourgois, P. (1995). *In search of respect: Selling crack in El Barrio*. New York, NY: Cambridge University Press.

Bradley, E. H., Curry, L. A., & Devers, K. J. (2007). Qualitative data analysis for health services research: Developing taxonomy, themes, and theory. *Health Services Research*, *42*(4), 1758–1772.

Braun, V., & Clarke, V. (2013). *Successful qualitative research*. Thousand Oaks, CA: Sage.

Bruce, D., & Harper, G. W. (2011). Operating without a safety net: Gay male adolescents and emerging adults' experiences of marginalization and migration, and implications for theory of syndemic production of health disparities. *Health Education & Behavior: The Official Publication of the Society for Public Health Education*, *38*(4), 367–378.

Burton, L. M., & Clark, S. L. (2005). Homeplace and housing in the lives of urban African Americans. In V. MacLoyd, N. Hill, & K. Dodge (Eds.), *African American family life* (pp. 166–206). New York, NY: Guilford Press.

Cannuscio, C. C., Weiss, E. E., & Asch, D. A. (2010). The contribution of urban foodways to health disparities. *Journal of Urban Health*, *87*(3), 381–393.

Carpiano, R. M. (2009). Come take a walk with me: The "go-along" interview as a novel method for studying the implications of place for health and well-being. *Health & Place*, *15*(1), 263–272.

Castro, P. B., & Lindbladh, E. (2004). Place, discourse and vulnerability—a qualitative study of young adults living in a Swedish urban poverty zone. *Health & Place*, *10*(3), 259–272.

Catalani, C., & Minkler, M. (2010). Photovoice: A review of the literature in health and public health. *Health Education & Behavior: The Official Publication of the Society for Public Health Education*, *37*(3), 424–451.

Charmaz, K. (2014). *Constructing grounded theory*. Thousand Oaks, CA: Sage.

Clampet-Lundquist, S., Kling, J. R., Edin, K., & Duncan, G. J. (2011). Moving teenagers out of high-risk neighborhoods: How girls fare better than boys. *American Journal of Sociology*, *116*(4), 1154–1189.

Corbin, J., & Strauss, A. (2014). *The basics of qualitative research*. Thousand Oaks, CA: Sage.

Cummins, S., Curtis, S., Diez-Roux, A. V, & Macintyre, S. (2007). Understanding and representing "place" in health research: A relational approach. *Social Science & Medicine*, *65*(9), 1825–1838.

Deener, A. (2012). *Venice: A contested bohemia in Los Angeles*. Chicago, IL: University of Chicago Press.

Dennis, S. F., Gaulocher, S., Carpiano, R. M., & Brown, D. (2009). Participatory photo mapping (PPM): Exploring an integrated method for health and place research with young people. *Health & Place*, *15*(2), 466–473.

Denzin, N. K., & Lincoln, Y. S. (1998). The art of interpretation, evaluation, and presentation. In N. Denzin & Y. Lincoln (Eds.), *Handbook of qualitative research* (pp. 313–371). Thousand Oaks, CA: Sage.

Desmond, M. (2016). *Evicted: Poverty and profit in the American city*. New York, NY: Crown.

Duncan, D. T., Ruff, R. R., Chaix, B., Regan, S. D., Williams, J. H., Ravenell, J., . . . York, N. (2016). Perceived spatial stigma, body mass index and blood pressure: A global positioning system study among low-income housing residents in New York City. *Geospatial Health*, *11*, 1–4

Edin, K., DeLuca, S., & Owens, A. (2012). Constrained compliance: Solving the puzzle of MTO's lease-up rates and why mobility matters. *Cityscape*, *14*(2), 181–194.

Edin, K., & Pirog, M. A. (2014). Special symposium on qualitative and mixed-methods for policy analysis. *Journal of Policy Analysis and Management*, *33*(2), 345–349.

Egan, J. E., Frye, V., Kurtz, S. P., Latkin, C., Chen, M., Tobin, K., . . . Koblin, B. A. (2011). Migration, neighborhoods, and networks: Approaches to understanding how urban environmental conditions affect syndemic adverse health outcomes among gay, bisexual and other men who have sex with men. *AIDS and Behaviora*, *15*(Suppl 1), 35–50.

Emerson, R. M., Fretz, R. I., & Shaw, L. L. (1995). *Writing ethnographic fieldnotes*. Chicago, IL: University of Chicago Press.

Eriksson, M., & Emmelin, M. (2013). What constitutes a health-enabling neighborhood? A grounded theory situational analysis addressing the significance of social capital and gender. *Social Science and Medicine*, *97*, 112–123.

Evans, J., & Jones, P. (2011). The walking interview: Methodology, mobility and place. *Applied Geography*, *31*(2), 849–858.

Farquhar, S. A., Parker, E. A., Schulz, A. J., & Israel, B. A. (2006). Application of qualitative methods in program planning for health promotion interventions. *Health Promotion Practice*, *7*(2), 234–242.

Frohlich, K. L., Potvin, L., Chabot, P., & Corin, E. (2002). A theoretical and empirical analysis of context: Neighborhoods, smoking, and youth. *Social Science & Medicine*, *54*, 1401–1417.

Frye, V., Egan, J. E., Tieu, H. Van, Cerdá, M., Ompad, D., & Koblin, B. A. (2014). "I didn't think I could get out of the fucking park." Gay men's retrospective accounts of neighborhood space, emerging sexuality and migrations. *Social Science and Medicine*, *104*, 6–14.

Fullilove, M. (1996). Psychiatric implications of displacement: Contributions from the psychology of place. *American Journal of Psychiatry*, *153*(12), 1516–1523.

Fullilove, M. (2004). *Root shock: How tearing up city neighborhoods hurts America and what we can do about it*. New York, NY: Balantine Books.

Gans, H. (1962). *The urban villagers: Group and class in the life of Italian Americans*. New York, NY: Free Press.

Garbin, D., & Millington, G. (2011). Territorial stigma and the politics of resistance in a Parisian banlieue: La Courneuve and Beyond. *Urban Studies*, *49*(10), 2067–2083.

Garcia, C. M., Eisenberg, M. E., Frerich, E. a., Lechner, K. E., & Lust, K. (2012). Conducting go-along interviews to understand context and promote health. *Qualitative Health Research, 22*(10), 1395–1403.

Haines-Saah, R. J., Oliffe, J. L., White, C. F., & Bottorff, J. L. (2013). "It is just not part of the culture here": Young adults' photo-narratives about smoking, quitting, and healthy lifestyles in Vancouver, Canada. *Health and Place, 22*, 19–28.

Hatzenbuehler, M. L., Bellatorre, A., Lee, Y., Finch, B. K., Muennig, P., & Fiscella, K. (2014). Structural stigma and all-cause mortality in sexual minority populations. *Social Science and Medicine, 103*, 33–41.

Keddem, S., Barg, F. K., Glanz, K., Jackson, T., Green, S., & George, M. (2015). Mapping the urban asthma experience: Using qualitative GIS to understand contextual factors affecting asthma control. *Social Science & Medicine, 140*, 9–17.

Keene, D. E., Eldahan, A. I., White Hughto, J. M., & Pachankis, J. E. (2016). "The big ole gay express": Sexual minority stigma, mobility and health in the small city. *Culture, Health & Sexuality, 1058*(October), 1–14.

Keene, D. E., & Padilla, M. B. (2014). Spatial stigma and health inequality. *Critical Public Health, 1596*(July), 1–13.

Keene, D. E., & Ruel, E. (2013). "Everyone called me grandma": Public housing demolition and relocation among older adults in Atlanta. *Cities, 35*, 359–364.

Keene, D., & Padilla, M. (2010). Race, class and the stigma of place: Moving to "opportunity" in Eastern Iowa. *Health & Place, 16*(6), 1216–1223.

Keene, D., Padilla, M., & Geronimus, A. (2010). Leaving Chicago for Iowa's "fields of opportunity": Community dispossession, rootlessness and the quest for somewhere to "Be Ok." *Human Organization, 69*(3), 275–284.

Klinenberg, E. (1999). Denaturalizing disaster: A social autopsy of the 1995 Chicago heat wave. *Theory and Society, 28*(2), 239–295.

Klinenberg, E. (2001). Dying alone: The social production of urban isolation. *Ethnography, 2*(4), 501–531.

Klinenberg, E. (2002). Heat wave: A social autopsy of disaster in Chicago. Chicago, IL: University of Chicago Press.

Kling, J., & Liebman, J. (2004). *Experimental analysis of neighborhood effects on youth*. Boston, MA: National Bureau of Economic Research.

Kling, J., Liebman, J., & Katz, L. (1994). Bullets don't got no name: Consequences of fear in the ghetto. In Thomas S. Weisner (Ed.), *Discovering successful pathways in children's development: Mixed methods in the study of childhood and family life* (pp. 243–282). Chicago: The University of Chicago Press.

Kling, J. R., Liebman, J. B., & Katz, L. F. (2007). Experimental analysis of neighborhood effects. *Econometrica, 75*(1), 83–119.

Kling, J. R., Liebman, J. B., Katz, L. F., & Sanbonmatsu, L. (2004). Moving to opportunity and tranquility: Neighborhood effects on adult economic self-sufficiency and health from a randomized housing voucher experiment. *KSG Working Paper No. RWP04-035*. Available at https://papers.ssrn.com/sol3/papers.cfm?abstract_id=588942.

Klinenberg, E. (1999). Denaturalizing disaster: a social autopsy of the 1995 Chicago heat wave. *Theory and Society,28*(2), 239–295.

Kobrak, P., Ponce, R., & Zielony, R. (2015). New arrivals to New York City: Vulnerability to HIV among urban migrant young gay men. *Archives of Sexual Behavior, 44*(7), 2041–2053.

Kusenbach, M. (2003). Street phenomenology. *Ethnography*, *4*(3), 455–485.

Leventhal, T., & Brooks-Gunn, J. (2003a). Moving to opportunity: An experimental study of neighborhood effects on mental health. *American Journal of Public Health*, *93*(9), 1576–1582.

Leventhal, T., & Brooks-Gunn, J. (2003b). The early impacts of Moving to Opportunity on children and youth in New York. In J. Goering & J. Feins (Eds.), *Choosing a better life: Evaluation of the Moving to Opportunity social experiment.* Washington, DC: The Urban Institute Press. Available at https://scholar.harvard.edu/lkatz/publications/moving-opportunity-interim-impacts-evaluation

Lewis, N. M. (2014a). Moving "out," moving on: Gay men's migrations through the life course. *Annals of the Association of American Geographers*, *104*(2), 225–233.

Lewis, N. M. (2014b). Rupture, resilience, and risk: relationships between mental health and migration among gay-identified men in North America. *Health & Place*, *27*, 212–219.

Macintyre, S., & Ellaway, A. (2003). An overview. In I. Kawachi & L. F. Berkman (Eds.), *Neighborhoods and health* (pp. 20–45). Cambridge, UK: Oxford University Press.

Matthews, S. A., Detwiler, J. E., & Burton, L. M. (2005). Geo-ethnography: Coupling Geographic Information Analysis techniques with ethnographic methods in urban research. *Cartographica: The International Journal for Geographic Information and Geovisualization*, *40*(4), 75–90.

Miles, M. B., & Huberman, A. M. (1994). *Qualitative data analysis: A sourcebook.* Beverly Hills, CA: Sage.

Morgan, P. (1993). *Successful focus groups: Advancing the state of the art.* Newbury Park, CA: Sage.

Mullings, L., & Wali, A. (1999). *Stress and resilience: The social context of reproduction in Central Harlem.* New York, NY: Kluwer Academic/Plenum.

Nykiforuk, C. I. J., Vallianatos, H., & Nieuwendyk, L. (2011). Photovoice as a nethod for revealing community perceptions of the built and social environment. *International Journal of Qualitative Methods*, *10*, 103–125.

O'Campo, P., & Caughy, M. O. (2006). Measures of residential community context. In M. J. Oakes & J. Kauffman (Eds.), *Methods in social epidemiology* (pp. 193–208). San Francisco, CA: Jossey Bass.

O'Campo, P., Salmon, C., & Burke, J. (2009). Neighbourhoods and mental well-being: What are the pathways? *Health and Place*, *15*(1), 56–68.

Orr, L., Feins, J., Jacob, R., Beecroft, E., Sanbonmatsu, L., Katz, L. F., Liebman, J. B., Kling, J. R. (2003). *Moving to Opportunity for Fair Housing Demonstration Program: Interim impacts evaluation.* Retrieved from http://www.huduser/org/publications/fairhsg/mtofinal.html

Pachankis, J. E., Eldahan, A. I., & Golub, S. A. (2016). New to New York: Ecological and psychological predictors of health among recently arrived young adult gay and bisexual urban migrants. *Annals of Behavioral Medicine*, *50*(5), 692–703.

Pattillo, M. (2007). *Black on the block: The politics of race and class in the city.* Chicago, IL: University of Chicago.

Patton, M. (2002). *Qualitative research & evaluation methods.* Thousand Oakes, CA: Sage.

Pearce, J. (2012). The "blemish of place": Stigma, geography and health inequalities. A commentary on Tabuchi, Fukuhara & Iso. *Social Science & Medicine (1982)*, *75*(11), 1921–1924.

Popay, J., Thomas, C., Williams, G., Bennett, S., Gatrell, A., & Bostock, L. (2003). A proper place to live: Health inequalities, agency and the normative dimensions of space. *Social Science & Medicine (1982)*, *57*(1), 55–69.

Rosenblatt, P., & Deluca, S. (2012). We don't live outside, we live in here": Neighborhood and residential mobility decisions among low-income families. *City and Community, 11*(3), 254–284.

Sanbonmatsu, L., Ludwig, J., Katz, L., Gennetian, L., Duncan, G., Kessler, R., Adam, E., McDade, T., & Tessler Lindau, T. (2011). *Moving to Opportunity for Fair Housing Demonstration Program: Final impacts evaluation*. Retrieved from www.huduser.org/publications/pdf/MTOFHD_fullreport_v2.pdf

Tabuchi, T., Fukuhara, H., & Iso, H. (2012). Geographically-based discrimination is a social determinant of mental health in a deprived or stigmatized area in Japan: A cross-sectional study. *Social Science & Medicine, 75*(6), 1015–1021.

Timmermans, S., & Tavory, I. (2012). Theory construction in qualitative research: From grounded theory to abductive analysis. *Sociological Theory, 30*(3), 167–186.

Valentine, G., & Skelton, T. (2003). Finding oneself, losing oneself: The lesbian and gay "scene" as a paradoxical space. *International Journal of Urban and Regional Research, 27*(December), 849–866.

Wacquant, L. (2007). Territorial stigmatization in the age of advanced marginality. *Thesis Eleven, 91*(1), 66–77.

Waitt, G., & Gorman-Murray, A. (2011). "It's about time you came out": Sexualities, mobility and home. *Antipode*, *43*(4), 1380–1403.

Walton, E. (2014). Vital places: Facilitators of behavioral and social health mechanisms in low-income neighborhoods. *Social Science & Medicine, 122*, 1–12.

Wang, C. C. (2006). Youth participation in photovoice as a strategy for community change. *Journal of Community Practice, 14*(1–2), 147–161.

Wang, C., Morrel-Samuels, S., Mutchison, P., Bell, L., & Pestronk, R. (2004). Flint Photovoice-community building among youth, adults and policymakers. *American Journal of Public Health, 94*(6), 911–916.

Warr, D. J. (2005). Social networks in a "discredited" neighbourhood. *Journal of Sociology, 41*(3), 285–308.

Weathers, B., Barg, F. K., Bowman, M., Briggs, V., Delmoor, E., Kumanyika, S., . . . Halbert, C. H. (2011). Using a mixed-methods approach to identify health concerns in an African American community. *American Journal of Public Health, 101*(11), 2087–2092.

Weiss, R. (1998). *Learning from strangers*. New York, NY: Simon & Schuster.

Zenk, S. N., Odoms-Young, A. M., Dallas, C., Hardy, E., Watkins, A., Hoskins-Wroten, J., & Holland, L. (2011). "You have to hunt for the fruits, the vegetables": Environmental barriers and adaptive strategies to acquire food in a low-income African American neighborhood. *Health Education & Behavior, 38*(3), 282–292.

PART II

Connecting Neighborhoods and Health Outcomes

8

DESIGNING HEALTHIER BUILT ENVIRONMENTS

Pedro Gullón and Gina S. Lovasi

Look out your window. What did you see? You probably saw things that people make.
—Hope Jahren, *Lab Girl*, prologue

The "built environment" is comprised of human-made structures and systems that include, among other features, access to and attractiveness of walkable destinations (e.g., retail stores, parks) and community design features (e.g., street connectivity, sidewalk access). Note that this can include "natural" aspects of the neighborhood environment that are sited, delimited, and maintained by people, such as urban green spaces and street trees. Neighborhood-scale built environment characteristics are potentially modifiable, and redesigning built environments to support health has the potential to reach all members of a local community and have an enduring influence. In this chapter, we will discuss the concept of built environment, its implication for population health, and emerging research directions and priorities for moving the field forward.

THE BUILT ENVIRONMENT EFFECTS ON HEALTH CAN BE WEAK OR STRONG, POSITIVE OR NEGATIVE

Despite the seemingly subtle effects of the built environment on health, such population-based approaches have potential importance when applied across entire populations (Lieberman, Golden, & Earp, 2013; Mozaffarian et al., 2012). Certainly, if taken to an extreme, the built environment can curtail our choices, though often the influence is subtler. For example, some environments provide little support for pedestrian convenience and safety, making personal vehicles a much more normative and easy choice. Individual education efforts that emphasize choice and responsibility for health have had limited success, and adherence to such recommendations may depend on the local context (Feathers et al., 2015). Individuals are not the only actors whose choices are relevant to the built environment. The choices of business and government leaders affect everything from what we breathe to temptations faced throughout the day (James, Hart, & Laden, 2015).

A dual focus on both potentially beneficial and harmful aspects of the built environment may best allow us to tackle pressing population health concerns in a balanced way. Distinguishing between these aspects may not always be simple. For example, urban green spaces and landscape elements such as parks or street tree plantings may support mental health (Bowler, Buyung-Ali, Knight, & Pullin, 2010) and physical activity (Almanza, Jerrett, Dunton, Seto, & Pentz, 2012; G. S. Lovasi et al., 2011), but they may not be uniformly safe (Weiss et al., 2011) and can even contribute to problems such as pollen allergy and related asthma exacerbations (Jariwala et al., 2011; G. S. Lovasi et al., 2013).

Over time, the health issues faced within the United States and globally have expanded beyond traditional concerns linked to infectious diseases and toxic environmental exposures to encompass built environment and contextual strategies relevant to chronic diseases prevention such as improving diets and active lifestyles. While we all make decisions that matter for infectious and chronic disease risk, to make healthy choices we need to have those options feasibly within reach given our physical, financial, and time limitations (Tranter, 2010).

DEFINITIONS AND FRAMEWORKS FOR UNDERSTANDING THE ROLE OF THE BUILT ENVIRONMENT

The definitions and frameworks for delimiting the scope of built environment research vary across the scientific literature. For the purpose of this chapter, we will include in the built environment relatively stable aspects of the human-made or modified environment, such as buildings, transportation systems, architectural and urban design features, landscape elements, and cultivated green spaces (G. S. Lovasi, 2012) (Figure 8-1). In the interest of providing a concise orientation to research on the neighborhood built environment and health, we will not give central attention to all topics that interconnect with current research on the built environment, but note here several aspects of neighborhood context that are aptly studied in conjunction with the built environment. The structures that make up the built environment affect physical exposures within the local environment (e.g., air quality, pollutants, water quality, climate) and the social environment (e.g., social capital, social interaction). Although local commercial outlets that provide opportunities to purchase food are important for health and sometimes fall under the umbrella of the built environment, we will largely defer discussion of the food environment to Chapter 9, where this important topic is given focused attention.

The concept of the built environment has to be differentiated from other similar terms as "urban design" or "land use" (Handy, Boarnet, Ewing, & Killingsworth, 2002). "Urban design" usually refers to the design of the city and the physical elements within it, including both their arrangement and their appearance, and is concerned with the function and appeal of public spaces. "Land use" typically refers to the distribution of activities across space, including the proximity and density of different activities (usually using relatively coarse categories, such as residential, commercial, office, industrial, and other). The "built environment," as we define it, is modifiable, subject to regulation and zoning changes, urban design, and investments in the transportation system. The actions of government feature prominently in the literature on built environment, but a range of other actors can be engaged, from local retail to community organizations.

Frameworks evoking the idea of the neighborhood built environment influencing health frequently point to causes and consequences of built environment characteristics at multiple nested levels, from national to individual. Frameworks that include the built environment have differed in emphasis, in part because of the varied characteristics and pathways to health that researchers have studied (see Box 8-1). A variety of ecological frameworks informed by the social ecological theory (Sallis, Owen, & Fisher, 2008; Stokols, 1996) emphasize the multiple levels of contextual influence on individual behavior and health. Several of the frameworks are tailored to the goals of observational and interventional research in different behavioral domains (Sallis et al., 2008). Drawing on previously used frameworks that highlight the role of the built environment (Northridge, Sclar, & Biswas, 2003a), we can classify potential levers to change the built environment (Figure 8-1), distinguishing between the following: (1) land use (e.g., mixed use, residential, industrial); (2) transportations systems (e.g., street network design, public transportation infrastructure); (3) services (e.g., facilities, shopping areas, banking); (4) public resources (e.g., parks, open areas, cultural amenities); (5) zoning regulations (e.g., restricting commercial or residential uses); and (6) buildings (e.g., housing, offices, educational facilities). Moreover, it is important to keep in mind that the built environment is influenced by the socioeconomic and political context (Borrell, Malmusi, & Muntaner, 2017) and that there are individual characteristics (notably socioeconomic position and preferences that influence decisions on where to live) that may confound, interact with, or otherwise complicate observed associations along the pathways between built environment and health outcomes.

Box 8-1 Possible Mechanisms Between Built Environment and Health

Environmental toxins

- Use of chemicals to maintain environment (e.g., pesticides with neurotoxic effects)
- Proximity to sources of toxins (e.g., traffic-related pollution exposures structured by local street network)
- History of accumulated toxins (e.g., past industrial uses with an ongoing legacy of ground or water contamination)

Behavioral

- Constrain options (e.g., if transit unavailable, depend on private vehicles for transportation and accumulate less physical activity)
- Make healthy options easier (e.g., having park or gym closer to home may make regular exercise easier to incorporate into daily living)
- Signal norms that in turn shape behavior (e.g., sidewalks are well maintained, signaling that walking is acceptable and expected)

Psychosocial

- Chronic stressors (e.g., streetscape with limited buffer between pedestrians and vehicle traffic may make daily travel more stressful, particularly for those "captive walkers" without access to a private vehicle or other alternative to walking)
- Stress reduction/recovery (e.g., views of or activity within green space appears to decrease cortisol, etc.)
- Social interaction opportunities (e.g., social destinations/services and depression symptoms)

EMERGING INTEREST IN BUILT ENVIRONMENT WITHIN THE HEALTH SCIENCES

The notion that where you live has consequences for your health is not new. Decisions about city planning, from sanitation to zoning, have at times factored in the likely implications of these decisions for population health (Hirschhorn, 2004; Silver, 2012). From Engels's studies on mortality in suburban areas in Liverpool (Krieger, 2001), to the concept of the "walkable neighborhood," research on built environment has evolved in many ways. However, in recent years, measurement of place-based characteristics, including features of the built environment in the health sciences, is becoming more prominent (Prasad, Gray, Ross, & Kano, 2016).

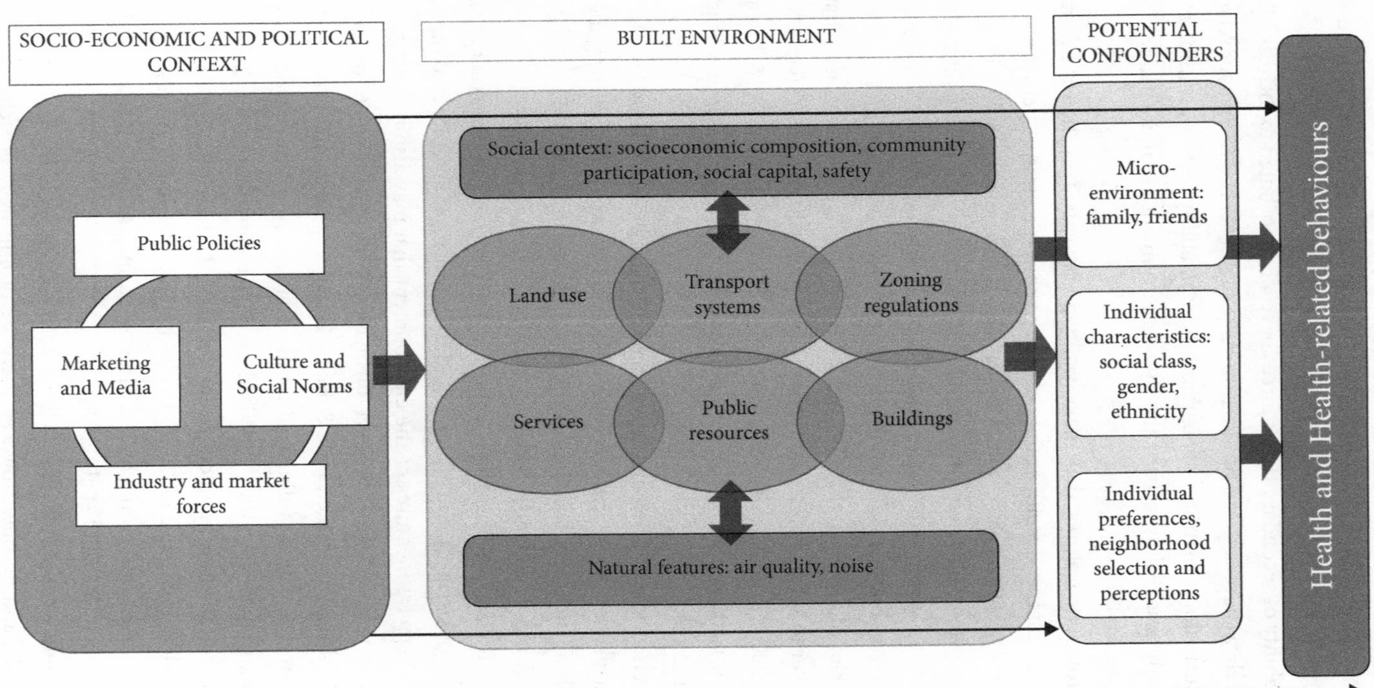

FIGURE 8-1 **Framework to study built environment and health.**

A search on PubMed for the term "built environment" gives 58 scientific paper results published in the year 2000, and 1,005 for the year 2016. Tools such as geographic information systems (GIS) (Vine, Degnan, & Hanchette, 1997) (discussed in Chapter 3) and multilevel modeling (Diez Roux, 2000) (discussed in Chapter 4), and the availability of secondary data sources have all contributed to the feasibility of such research, as have targeted funding efforts (Sallis et al., 2009). Perhaps related to these funding efforts, metrics of neighborhood walkability have been among the most commonly assessed aspects of the built environment (Leal & Chaix, 2011; Saelens & Glanz, 2009).

Built environment features that make walking convenient include residential density, land use mix, and well-connected transportation or transit networks. For example, the SMARTRAQ study found that a GIS-based index of walkability was associated with greater objectively measured physical activity for both youth (Kerr, Frank, Sallis, & Chapman, 2007) and adults (Frank, Schmid, Sallis, Chapman, & Saelens, 2005). As concepts such as neighborhood walkability (Frank et al., 2005; Kerr et al., 2006; Moudon et al., 2006) have become more prominent, they have increasing power to shape policy discussions (Ashe, Jernigan, Kline, & Galaz, 2003; Ottoson et al., 2009), real estate markets (Burchell & Mukherji, 2003; Song & Knaap, 2003; Van Dyck, Cardon, Deforche, & De Bourdeaudhuij, 2011), and thus the neighborhood environment.

Other aspects of the built environment may encourage or discourage walking. Examples that play a role in the perceived safety and attractiveness of neighborhoods for walking include sidewalk width (Cervero & Kockelman, 1997) or quality (Boehmer, Hoehner, Deshpande, Brennan Ramirez, & Brownson, 2007), the presence of natural features such as trees (Larsen et al., 2009), or human-scale architectural features of streetscapes (Ewing, Handy, Brownson, Clemente, & Winston, 2006). More ephemeral measures of the environment that may also be relevant to walking behavior include litter (Shenassa, Liebhaber, & Ezeamama, 2006) or physical disorder (Molnar, Gortmaker, Bull, & Buka, 2004). The range of behaviors and health outcomes that may be influenced by the built environment is broad, from smoking (Chuang, Cubbin, Ahn, & Winkleby, 2005; Giovenco et al., 2016) to depression (Berke, Gottlieb, Moudon, & Larson, 2007; Duncan et al., 2013; James, Hart, Banay, Laden, & Signorello, 2017) to obesity (Zick et al., 2009). In addition, new approaches for understanding built environment, such as liveability, are arising in academic research (Badland et al., 2014).

Most of the built environment research has been conducted in the United States, Canada, Australia, and Europe. However, there are promising approaches for specific features of the built environment that might impact health in different contexts, such as Latin America (Gomez et al., 2015) or South Africa (Malambo, Kengne,

Lambert, De Villers, & Puoane, 2017); despite this, more context-specific research is needed in low- and middle-income countries.

CONTRIBUTIONS AND CONNECTIONS BEYOND THE HEALTH SCIENCES

An astute observer of cities, Jane Jacobs was one of the early writers to discuss how the built environment influences how people navigate their neighborhood. As an activist and author, she described, as an ideal, city planning that features "a most intricate and close grained diversity of uses that give each other constant mutual support, both economically and socially" (1961); thus, she advocated for designs that would mix uses, attract pedestrians to urban centers, and consequently improve the safety of a city by providing informal surveillance or "eyes on the street" (Jacobs, 1961). To do so, she noted that urban planning should encourage a diversity of destinations that would attract visitors throughout the day and night, and recognize the importance of often-used gathering spaces, such as parks prominently located in lively neighborhoods. Jacobs offered examples of successful neighborhoods, including Manhattan's Lower East Side, Boston's North End, and Philadelphia's Rittenhouse Square, all characterized by vibrant public spaces that engaged residents of all ages throughout the daytime and evening hours. Thus, when viewed through a public health lens, this early work and the efforts it inspired across multiple disciplines highlighted the relevance of the built environment to creating safe and attractive spaces for pedestrians to engage in daily physical activity and social interaction.

The abundance of research available as a foundation for understanding the built environment and behavior from beyond the health sciences provides a groundwork for interdisciplinary and cross-sectoral collaborations. It is important to keep in mind that the built environment is influenced by the surrounding macro-environment, and that built environment only represents a part of the complex determinants of health. Understanding the upstream determinants of built environment characteristics and their implications for health means drawing data and expertise from a variety of sectors with expertise in city planning, laws and regulations, education, employment, housing, and other social and economic phenomena. Moreover, for research on the built environment and health to be relevant to current information needs, investigators should elicit and take seriously questions posed by communities, policy makers, and other local stakeholders.

Strategies are needed for working with professionals and community members who can transform aspects of the local built environment with relevance to health, including those from a range of research, design, and practice backgrounds. Crucial to successful collaborations will be overcoming reliance on jargon, understanding fundamentals of other professions, and articulating the distinct characteristics and potential contributions of the health sciences to heterogeneous teams. Several efforts are emerging to connect networks of health researchers and their partners, including the National Neighborhood Indicators Partnership and the American Institute of Architecture consortia in the United States, as well as global efforts such as those led by the World Health Organization and the International Society for Urban Health.

THE RELEVANCE OF THE BUILT ENVIRONMENT TO HEALTH ACROSS BOTH URBAN AND RURAL CONTEXTS

The changes within many sectors and systems that can have measurable impacts on both the built environment and population health have gained particular attention within urban settings (W. T. Caiaffa et al., 2008; Wizemann, 2014). An increasing majority of the world's population now lives in urban areas (Seto, Güneralp, & Hutyra, 2012), and thus our lives and our health are shaped by the design of buildings, transportation systems, and the availability of recreational amenities within urban contexts.

The concentration of urban populations provides an opportunity for localized strategies to protect the health of entire communities. Local action to invest in the built environment can protect the health of more people within a smaller distance because of urbanization. Thus, much work in the field has focused on the urban built environment, using "urban" to describe the geographies where people's homes are concentrated. These same urban areas are often enlivened by a concentration of workplaces and gathering spaces, which provide key contexts for the habits of daily life. We note that cities are prominent in discussions of urban health (Rydin et al., 2012) but also that the definition of urban areas is often inclusive of areas adjacent to cities as well as smaller townships (Caiaffa et al., 2008). The precise threshold for defining an area as urban varies greatly across the world. Recognizing the importance and potential of urban areas should not create blinders or barriers to collaboration. Indeed, urban areas depend crucially on and are connected to rural communities.

There are promising examples of work on health implications of built environments for rural populations (Boehmer, Lovegreen, Haire-Joshu, & Brownson, 2006; Casey et al., 2008; Deshpande, Baker, Lovegreen, & Brownson, 2005; Wilcox, Bopp, Oberrecht, Kammermann, & McElmurray, 2003), though more work is needed. Several studies have directly investigated how the built environment characteristics most salient and influential on behavior differ for rural versus urban contexts. In rural environments, the availability of trails and feeling protected from traffic may be particularly salient, as contrasted with an urban focus on convenience of destinations and safety as signaled by a lack of physical disorder (Doescher et al., 2016; Messing et al., 2015; O. T. Stewart et al., 2016). Importantly, there does appear to be sufficient available data on built environments in rural contexts for this area of investigation to continue developing, with due care taken to ensure consistency and validity (O. T. Stewart et al., 2015).

SCALE EFFECT AND OPTIONS FOR MEASUREMENT OF THE LOCAL BUILT ENVIRONMENT

The built environment can be conceptualized and measured at specific geographic scales, most often highly local areas, variously defined (G. S. Lovasi, Grady, & Rundle, 2012), and labeled as neighborhoods. Boundary issues that arise more generally in defining neighborhoods may be particularly problematic for built environment research, as the very streets and parks and other features of interest lie along administrative area boundaries. In the United States, for example, census tracts are a common neighborhood unit of analysis (as discussed in Chapter 2) and are often bounded by arterial streets, and resources such as transit stops and retail establishments cluster along these boundaries. A small distance beyond the edge of the census tract may include several important features of the built environment, making decisions on where to draw the line consequential.

Built environment research has often focused on measurement of the residential neighborhood, where neighborhood is a socially salient and highly local area near one's home. However, the most relevant scale for measurement of the built environment may depend on whether the surrounding context is typically navigated by car or on foot. For example, if car ownership is low, having destinations such as parks within walking distance may be particularly important, whereas in a low-density environment with higher car ownership, a practical driving distance may be the more relevant scale of measurement. An option in larger scale studies that span environments with different predominant transportation modes may be to develop schemes for weighting these alternative versions of the built environment measure of interest appropriate to those with or without access to a car (Thornton, Pearce, Macdonald, Lamb, & Ellaway, 2012).

Within public health, the focus is often on how features of the neighborhood shape residents' health. However, the built environment may affect population health at both coarser and finer scales as well. Some characteristics of cities may be influenced by national or regional mass influences, and they will therefore not be discoverable with studies comparing neighborhood characteristics within a single city (all under the same mass influence). For example, transit systems facilitate mobility at the level of the metropolitan area. Following Geoffrey Rose's population approach, in order to uncover these mass influences, we must study and compare entire populations (e.g., cities) as well as variation within each population (Rose, 1985).

Focal features of neighborhood built environments to be measured can include community or neighborhood design features (e.g., regional bicycle networks [Winters, Teschke, Brauer, & Fuller, 2016] and community zoning), building site selection and design (e.g., the location and siting of new school buildings), building/facility design (e.g., square footage for physical activity), and element design (e.g., width and lighting of stairwell).

MEASUREMENT APPROACHES FOR BUILT ENVIRONMENT MEASUREMENT

The development of reliable methods and tools to audit the qualities of the urban environment that likely impact physical activity remains an ongoing challenge for public health researchers, urban planners, and policy makers. Some researchers classify these tools into *subjective* (questionnaires and interviews) and *objective* tools (direct observation with checklists, official dataset, etc.) (Diez Roux, 2007). Table 8-1 provides a summary of the different options for measuring the built environment. Built environment characteristics can be gathered from large-scale GIS data sets. Secondary GIS data, while seldom free of error, have the advantage of being independent of behavior or health assessments, avoiding same-source bias (Gullon, Bilal, & Franco, 2014). Such GIS data are, however, often limited in their coverage of features relevant to the pathway of interest. Direct observation is another type of objective measurement, whereby trained observers undertake audits or checklists, which assess different aspects of the neighborhood environment. These observations can include focused measurement of one characteristic of the environment (e.g., the presence of crosswalks); integrative information about the environment (e.g., density of buildings or traffic; Chow et al., 2009); or multifaceted assessments multiple items that represent different aspects of the environment (e.g., indicators of aesthetics or physical disorder; Hoehner, Ivy, Brennan Ramirez, Meriwether, & Brownson, 2006). However, virtual audits are emerging as an option for independent assessment of the local built environment, tailored to the research questions of interest (Gullon et al., 2015; Mooney et al., 2016; A. G. Rundle, Bader, Richards, Neckerman, & Teitler, 2011), as briefly described in Chapter 3. For logistical reasons, especially for studies in large geographic areas, there has been increasing interest for virtually measuring attributes of the built environment thought to be associated with health. Such virtual audits avoid travel time and related expenses, and leverage open-access mapping technologies and stored image repositories, such as Google Street View. Compared

Table 8-1 Options and Technologies to Measure the Built Environment

Measurement Modalities		*Example Measures*	*Useful References*
Secondary data		Walkability index (residential density, land use, destinations, connectivity), access to parks and recreation facilities, public transport	(Sallis et al., 2016 Creatore et al., 2016)
Direct observation	In-field	Single characteristic of a street/block (e.g., the presence of crosswalks); integrative information about the environment (e.g., density of buildings or traffic); or multifaceted assessments	(Evenson, Jones, Holliday, Cohen, & McKenzie, 2016; McGrath et al., 2016)
	Virtual imagery	multiple items that represent different aspects of the urban environment (e.g., indicators of physical disorder)	(Gullon et al., 2015; Mooney et al., 2016)
Mobile devices		Ecological momentary assessment: perceptions of the environment and transient outcomes such as mood at multiple locations and over time	(Dunton et al., 2011; Shiffman et al., 2008)
Questionnaires	Self-report Ecometric	Perceptions of access to destinations or outlets, distance to public transportation, safety, aesthetics	(Kerr et al., 2016; Mujahid et al., 2007)

with physical audits, virtual audits may provide a faster, easier, cheaper, safer, and more reliable method to assess the urban environment (Charreire et al., 2013).

Objective measures of the built environment are even more useful when complemented by perceptions reported by the residents whose health is in question. Associations of self-reported neighborhood characteristics with behavioral or health outcomes may not reflect the true causal association if reporting errors for both environment and outcome are correlated (Gullon et al., 2014; Shenassa et al., 2006). Although concerns about information bias are often raised when built environment characteristics are reported by study subjects, the perspectives and perceptions of residents are important to understand, especially for psychosocial or behaviorally mediated pathways (Blacksher & Lovasi, 2012). Ecometric approaches (Mujahid, Diez Roux, Morenoff, & Raghunathan, 2007) and audits conducted by community members (Hoehner et al., 2006) are promising in that they incorporate perspectives of nearby residents, capturing aspects of the lived experience that may be missed by objective measures alone while avoiding reliance on the same person for reporting on the environment and outcome. Another intriguing new direction is to use mobile devices for ecological momentary assessments (Dunton, Liao, Intille, Spruijt-Metz, & Pentz, 2011; Shiffman, Stone, & Hufford, 2008); by capturing perceptions of the environment and transient outcomes such as mood at multiple locations and over time, this strategy creates opportunities for within-person comparisons (further information on the use of mobile devices for neighborhood health research is provided in Chapter 3).

BUILDING PARTNERSHIPS AND POLICY CHANGE

Health researchers have a growing range of tools for finding the answers to questions about how the built environment affects health, using both existing and newly available data. This dynamic area of research continues developing innovative data and dissemination strategies to meet local needs. Yet even local efforts embedded in unique histories of a given place can be viewed with an eye to what lessons we can share with other communities. Building partnerships and multicity collaborations shows promise for spreading widely the ideas and information that can make healthier lives possible for all.

Using evidence to inform policy and practice is challenging, especially in built environment and health research, where policy changes are outside of the health sector and not necessarily "health directed" (Lieberman et al., 2013). Influencing public policy and practice is an explicit goal for applied built environment and health research. However, the gap between research and policy is in fact increased by a poor fit between academic research and the needs of policy makers and practitioners. To optimize "policy-relevant" research in built environment, Billie Giles-Corti et al. (2015) proposed 10 strategies: (1) understand the "policy world" we are attempting to shift; (2) establish links with policy makers and practitioners; (3) work with knowledge brokers, advocates, and lobbyists; (4) establish research agendas jointly with policy makers and practitioners; (5) undertake interdisciplinary collaborative research; (6) study the health-economic impacts of active living infrastructure; (7) evaluate policy reform through natural experiments; (8) conduct research focusing on community needs and preferences; (9) highlight specific policy implications; and (10) create interdisciplinary built environment and health training programs.

VARIATION IN THE EFFECTS OF THE BUILT ENVIRONMENT ACROSS POPULATION GROUPS

Some features of the local environment that support or undermine health may have a parallel influence on all youth and adult age groups, or across other demographic groupings, but attention to heterogeneity may uncover opportunities to tailor-build environment strategies to specific populations. The potential importance of attending to the different ways that populations use the built environment can be illustrated from the literature on environmental determinants of physical activity.

Research to date on how the built environment shapes outcomes such as physical activity and obesity has been reviewed from a variety of perspectives, including a focus on different population groups (Duncan et al., 2014; Ewing, 2005; Frank & Engelke, 2001; Handy et al., 2002; Hoehner, Brennan, Brownson, Handy, & Killingsworth, 2003; Lee & Moudon, 2004; G. S. Lovasi, Hutson, Guerra, & Neckerman, 2009; Moudon & Lee, 2003; Northridge, Sclar, & Biswas, 2003b; Papas et al., 2007; Perdue, Stone, & Gostin, 2003; Pikora, Giles-Corti, Bull, Jamrozik, & Donovan, 2003; TRB, 2005; Williamson, 2002).

First, consider the potential for built environment effects on outcomes such as physical activity and obesity to vary by age. Childhood physical activity and obesity are correlated with parental physical activity and weight (Davey Smith, Steer, Leary, & Ness, 2007; Fogelholm, Nuutinen, Pasanen, Myohanen, & Saatela, 1999; Lake, Power, & Cole, 1997; Perusse, Tremblay, Leblanc, & Bouchard, 1989; J. F. Sallis, Prochaska, & Taylor, 2000). This may reflect genetic heritability, but it appears to be due in large part to a shared environment (Perusse et al., 1989) as well as parents' behaviors as gatekeepers and role models (Ritchie, Welk, Styne, Gerstein, & Crawford, 2005). With this in mind, interventions have successfully been designed to target children and their parents simultaneously (Beech et al., 2003) (Epstein, Valoski, Wing, & McCurley, 1994; Escobar-Chaves et al., 2010; Golan & Crow, 2004; Sacher et al., 2010). Changes to the local built environment may likewise prove effective in supporting childhood behavior change and obesity prevention because of the simultaneous consequences for both children and the adults in their lives. Among youth, particular attention has been given to the commute to school (Fulton, Shisler, Yore, & Caspersen, 2005; Metcalf, Voss, Jeffery, Perkins, & Wilkin, 2004). While walking or biking to school (labeled "active commuting") in itself represents a regular physical activity opportunity for some children, its consequences appear to extend beyond the duration of the commute because children appear to be more active upon reaching their destination if they walk to get there (Mackett, Lucas, Paskins, & Turbin, 2005), a tendency that may be stronger for boys (Cooper, Page, Foster, & Qahwaji, 2003). In addition to the proximity of home and school, neighborhood or path characteristics have been found to correlate with an active commute (Kerr et al., 2006; McDonald, 2008). Adults who have children walk more if they live near schools (Cerin, Leslie, du Toit, Owen, & Frank, 2007), suggesting that some built environment influences on youth and adult physical activity may be parallel.

Despite the parallels of the available literature on built environment characteristics relevant to youth and adults, there is reason to expect that the strength of observed associations may differ across the life course. As children age and their mobility independence increases, the effect of the neighborhood environment appears to increase. Very young children may be responsive to the home environment, for example the number of rooms in the home (A. Rundle et al., 2009), while adolescents are able to take advantage of neighborhood physical activity facilities (Evenson, Scott, Cohen, & Voorhees, 2007; Gordon-Larsen, Nelson, Page, & Popkin, 2006). However, results appear consistent across age for adolescents and young to middle-aged adults (Papas et al., 2007). The elderly may be more sensitive than younger adults to the effects of the neighborhood environment (Beard et al., 2009; Kubzansky et al., 2005), perhaps due to increased dependence on the accessibility of the local environment following driving restrictions or other reductions in mobility. In addition, different associations by age might be expected for the effects of physical activity venues, such as playgrounds, gyms, and walking trails, since the types of activities favored differ by age. Yet the research findings for youth and adults have often been studied and reviewed separately rather than being systematically juxtaposed (Bancroft et al., 2015).

The effect of built environment on health outcomes may also vary by socioeconomic status or race. For instance, lower socioeconomic status (SES) and high-minority neighborhoods tend to have greater density and destinations (King & Clarke, 2015), whereas their residents report more concerns about aesthetics and safety (Sugiyama et al., 2015); thus, accessible open spaces in these communities may be underutilized for physical activity, due to objectively detectable and perceived threats to safety within these areas (Richardson et al., 2017). Moreover, the socio-spatial correlation between race and SES suggests that it might be difficult to isolate the effect on specific populations (Gaskin et al., 2013).

Beyond the preceding illustration on how SES, race, or age modifies the effect of built environments on physical activity, a range of potential demographic or other population groups can be defined at the population or neighborhood levels. However, there is a risk of treating any specific population as disconnected from the overall distribution of the population as a whole (Frohlich & Potvin, 2008). An alternative approach is to consider vulnerable populations (e.g., minorities, low-income populations) as integral to understanding the distribution of risk factors and therefore affected by the shape and central tendency of this distribution (Frohlich, 2014). For instance, highway subsidies in the United States and other policies associated with urban sprawl tended to promote the use of cars and the creation of low-density residential areas, with health and well-being consequences (Ewing, Meakins, Hamidi, & Nelson, 2014; Mackenbach et al., 2014; Savitch, 2003), while low-density sprawl has been less consequential in European cities due to different urban policies (Kasanko et al., 2006). Given mass influences, studying average neighborhoods in the densest part of the social distribution may be a valuable strategy to uncover mass influences that affect the built environment in different cities, improving the health of the entire population.

CHALLENGES TO MAKING CAUSAL CLAIMS ABOUT HOW THE BUILT ENVIRONMENT AFFECTS HEALTH

Most built environment and health studies use observational and cross-sectional designs (Sarkar & Webster, 2017). However, neighborhoods and cities are not static entities: They are dynamic places that constantly change in terms of their composition, definition, and relationships with the surrounding environment. Although some neighborhoods change very little in their physical, social, and demographic composition over decades, others may change significantly in the course of a few years. Some neighborhoods change very quickly as the result of single or multiple external shocks, such as large-scale neighborhood demolition and rebuilding, gentrification, and other rapid changes in the housing market, or if employment shifts suddenly alter the patterns of residential mobility change. Understanding neighborhood built environments and their role in the surrounding context is crucial in developing a better understanding of how patterns within and among the neighborhoods that we study develop, replicate, and change over time.

There are numerous lenses that can be used to understand the dynamics of neighborhoods (van Ham, Manley, Bailey, Simpson, & Maclennan, 2012). In broad terms, we can group the causes of neighborhood change into three categories. The first set (neighborhood selection) places household behavior as central. Residents "choose" (considering that the choices of household are highly constrained) to live in (or leave) certain neighborhoods and their decisions collectively alter the population composition of neighborhoods. A second set (internal changes) deals with demographic and socioeconomic change of neighborhood residents (the nonmovers). The third relates to external shock to the neighborhoods, including natural disasters, structural changes to the labor market, and large-scale regeneration or reinvestment. In recent years, some studies have explored the effect of these changes in the relationship between built environment, social inequalities, and health. Hirsch et al. (2016) found that, in seven US cities, walking destinations are increasing; however, the unequal distribution across neighborhood sociodemographic characteristics suggests that there is a need for attention to social inequalities when designing healthier built environments. For instance, Koschinski and Talen (2015) has found that the increasing housing prices in walkable neighborhoods play a role in displacing low-SES people to less walkable neighborhoods.

Given these challenges, there is particular need for the field of built environment and health research to draw on a range of study designs and approaches (including complex systems modeling strategies such as agent-based models highlighted in Chapter 5) because most of the studies have been observational, and frequently, cross-sectional. Despite this, some new promising approaches are arising. For example, fixed effects regressions that model changes in health outcomes on changes on built environment have the ability to difference out time-invariant confounders, such as residents' preference for living in healthy neighborhoods (Halonen et al., 2014, 2015). Another approach to take into account residents' preference is to measure neighborhood preference and then stratify the results on those preferences (Frank, Saelens, Powell, & Chapman, 2007). The extent to which common prior causes such as residential preferences explain some of or all of the observed built environment and health associations remains under investigation.

Randomized trials have been recommended as an approach to tackle the difficulties for causality in studies of place and health (Allen, Barn, & Lanphear, 2015; Macintyre, 2011). However, there are ethical and methodological issues that arise when designing trials that investigate how the built environment and other aspects of place affect public health (Allen et al., 2015). Trials that leverage small changes to the built environment may help to clarify causal relationships without the formidable costs and inflexibility of large-scale place-based trials (Lovasi, Mooney, Muennig, & DiMaggio, 2016). An alternative to controlled trials is to measure the impact of natural experiments (Franco, Bilal, & Diez-Roux, 2014), as discussed more extensively in Chapter 6. As an example, from the neighborhood built environment literature, the evaluation of the Neighborhoods Law in Catalonia (Spain) evaluated the effects on health and health inequalities of a renewal project in Barcelona (Mehdipanah et al., 2014). Another key example investigated the effects of new light rail transit on physical activity (MacDonald, Stokes, Cohen, Kofner, & Ridgeway, 2010). It is important to note that the effect of neighborhood built environment change might be stronger as more time passes; longer term follow-up is required to fully capture the impact on residents (Billie Giles-Corti et al., 2013). Despite this promising alternative, it has been argued that the methodological problems and risk of bias pose threats to natural experiments designs (Benton, Anderson, Hunter, & French, 2016).

Another key opportunity is to bring resident perspectives and knowledge into the research process (Blacksher & Lovasi, 2012). Insights from qualitative and mixed methods particularly can be crucial to avoiding harms and refining strategies to maximize health and health equity benefits (Chapter 7). Mixed-methods (Creswell, Klassen, Plano Clark, & Smith, 2011) studies combine and synthesize methods, triangulating among the nuanced subjective perspectives drawn out by qualitative approaches and the quantitative data approaches that often allow for larger sample sizes. Mixed-method designs incorporate and integrate both qualitative and quantitative methods. Quantitative and qualitative methods come from different philosophical and epistemological paradigms. Mixed methods are also key to illuminating complex research problems such as health disparities and perceptions of the built environment (Amaratunga, Baldry, Sarshar, & Newton, 2002); therefore, the use of this methodological approach has been increasing to understand public health issues. Some recent examples can be found in the built environment literature using mixed methods (Bilal et al., 2016; Gomez et al., 2015; Teschke, Dennis, Reynolds, Winters, & Harris, 2016; Willenberg et al., 2010); for example, Willenberg and colleagues used both environmental measures and child perceptions to study school playground and physical activity (Willenberg et al., 2010). Another approach was used by Gomez and colleagues, who combined systematic reviews of the quantitative evidence with a documentary analysis of the sociopolitical barriers and facilitators for urban interventions linked with active living in Latin America (Gomez et al., 2015). However, there is still a need to incorporate mixed-methods approaches starting with the very early steps of the research, and to further integrate both quantitative and qualitative philosophies to better understand the effect of built environment on health.

Overall, the diversity of tools for investigating the built environment makes navigating the literature complicated, but it also offers strengths through triangulation that would not be possible if there were universal use of any single method. Triangulation is premised on the reasoning that no single method ever adequately solves the problem of rival explanations, and that the weakness in a single method will be compensated by the counterbalancing strengths of another (Razum & Gerhardus, 1999). The benefits of triangulation include converging or corroborating findings; opportunities to dispel or support alternative explanations for conclusions drawn from research data; elucidating divergent aspects of a phenomenon; and obtaining a more accurate and comprehensive perspective of participants' experiences (Stewart, Makwarimba, Barnfather, Letourneau, & Neufeld, 2008).

CONCLUSION

Research on how built environments influence health has been strong and growing, with several exciting directions emerging. However, evidence is limited in several critical areas. Assessing consistency of results and explaining inconsistencies has been hampered by different spatial scales and methods used to measure environmental features. In addition to strengthening the work, there are opportunities to expand research on the built environment to new settings globally. Objective and perceived aspects of the built environment have seldom been applied in low- and middle-income countries; yet many of the largest urbanized areas are in the developing world (Tanner & Harpham, 2014), and generalizability of research from high-income countries cannot be assumed.

REFERENCES

Allen, R. W., Barn, P. K., & Lanphear, B. P. (2015). Randomized controlled trials in environmental health research: Unethical or underutilized? *PLoS Medicine, 12*(1), e1001775. doi:10.1371/journal.pmed.1001775

Almanza, E., Jerrett, M., Dunton, G., Seto, E., & Pentz, M. A. (2012). A study of community design, greenness, and physical activity in children using satellite, GPS and accelerometer data. *Health & Place, 18*(1), 46–54. doi:S1353-8292(11)00164-X [pii] 10.1016/j.healthplace.2011.09.003

Amaratunga, D., Baldry, D., Sarshar, M., & Newton, R. (2002). Quantitative and qualitative research in the built environment: Application of "mixed" research approach. *Work Study, 51*(1), 17–31. doi:10.1108/00438020210415488

Ashe, M., Jernigan, D., Kline, R., & Galaz, R. (2003). Land use planning and the control of alcohol, tobacco, firearms, and fast food restaurants. *American Journal of Public Health, 93*(9), 1404–1408.

Badland, H., Whitzman, C., Lowe, M., Davern, M., Aye, L., Butterworth, I., . . . Giles-Corti, B. (2014). Urban liveability: Emerging lessons from Australia for exploring the potential for indicators to measure the social determinants of health. *Social Sciences & Medicine, 111*, 64–73. doi:10.1016/j.socscimed.2014.04.003

Bancroft, C., Joshi, S., Rundle, A., Hutson, M., Chong, C., Weiss, C. C., . . . Lovasi, G. (2015). Association of proximity and density of parks and objectively measured physical activity in the United States: A systematic review. *Social Sciences & Medicine, 138*, 22–30. doi:10.1016/j.socscimed.2015.05.034

Beard, J. R., Blaney, S., Cerda, M., Frye, V., Lovasi, G. S., Ompad, D., . . . Vlahov, D. (2009). Neighborhood characteristics and disability in older adults. *Journal of Gerontology B Psychological Sciences and Social Sciences, 64*(2), 252–257. doi:gbn018 [pii] 10.1093/geronb/gbn018

Beech, B. M., Klesges, R. C., Kumanyika, S. K., Murray, D. M., Klesges, L., McClanahan, B., . . . Pree-Cary, J. (2003). Child- and parent-targeted interventions: The Memphis GEMS pilot study. *Ethnicity & Disease, 13*(1 Suppl 1), S40–S53.

Benton, J. S., Anderson, J., Hunter, R. F., & French, D. P. (2016). The effect of changing the built environment on physical activity: A quantitative review of the risk of bias in natural experiments. *International Journal of Behavior, Nutrition, and Physical Activity, 13*(1), 107. doi:10.1186/s12966-016-0433-3

Berke, E. M., Gottlieb, L. M., Moudon, A. V., & Larson, E. B. (2007). Protective association between neighborhood walkability and depression in older men. *Journal of the American Geriatric Society, 55*(4), 526–533.

Bilal, U., Diez, J., Alfayate, S., Gullon, P., Del Cura, I., Escobar, F., . . . Franco, M. (2016). Population cardiovascular health and urban environments: The Heart Healthy Hoods exploratory study in Madrid, Spain. *BMC Medical Research Methodology, 16*, 104. doi:10.1186/s12874-016-0213-4

Blacksher, E., & Lovasi, G. S. (2012). Place-focused physical activity research, human agency, and social justice in public health: Taking agency seriously in studies of the built environment. *Health Place, 18*(2), 172–179. doi:S1353-8292(11)00159-6 [pii] 10.1016/j.healthplace.2011.08.019

Boehmer, T. K., Hoehner, C. M., Deshpande, A. D., Brennan Ramirez, L. K., & Brownson, R. C. (2007). Perceived and observed neighborhood indicators of obesity among urban adults. *International Journal of Obesity (Lond), 31*(6), 968–977.

Boehmer, T. K., Lovegreen, S. L., Haire-Joshu, D., & Brownson, R. C. (2006). What constitutes an obesogenic environment in rural communities? *American Journal of Health Promotion, 20*(6), 411–421.

Borrell, C., Malmusi, D., & Muntaner, C. (2017). Introduction to the "Evaluating the Impact of Structural Policies on Health Inequalities and Their Social Determinants and Fostering Change" (SOPHIE) Project. *International Journal of Health Services, 47*(1), 10–17. doi:10.1177/0020731416681891

Bowler, D. E., Buyung-Ali, L. M., Knight, T. M., & Pullin, A. S. (2010). A systematic review of evidence for the added benefits to health of exposure to natural environments. *BMC Public Health, 10*, 456. doi:10.1186/1471-2458-10-456

Burchell, R. W., & Mukherji, S. (2003). Conventional development versus managed growth: The costs of sprawl. *American Journal of Public Health, 93*(9), 1534–1540.

Caiaffa, W. T., Ferreira, F. R., Ferreira, A. D., Oliveira, C. D., Camargos, V. P., & Proietti, F. A. (2008). Urban health: "The city is a strange lady, smiling today, devouring you tomorrow." *Cien Saude Colet, 13*(6), 1785–1796.

Caiaffa, W. T., Ferreira, F. R., Ferreira, A. D., Oliveira, C., Di Lorenzo, C., Vitor. P., & Proietti, F. A. (2008). Saúde urbana: "A cidade é uma estranha senhora, que hoje sorri e amanhã te devora." *Ciênc Saúde Coletiva, 13*(6), 1785–1796.

Casey, A. A., Elliott, M., Glanz, K., Haire-Joshu, D., Lovegreen, S. L., Saelens, B. E., . . . Brownson, R. C. (2008). Impact of the food environment and physical activity environment on behaviors and weight status in rural U.S. communities. *Preventive Medicine, 47*(6), 600–604. doi:10.1016/j.ypmed.2008.10.001

Cerin, E., Leslie, E., du Toit, L., Owen, N., & Frank, L. D. (2007). Destinations that matter: Associations with walking for transport. *Health & Place, 13*(3), 713–724.

Cervero, R., & Kockelman, K. (1997). Travel demand and the 3Ds: Density, diversity, and design. *Transportation Research-D., 2*(3), 199–219.

Cooper, A. R., Page, A. S., Foster, L. J., & Qahwaji, D. (2003). Commuting to school: Are children who walk more physically active? *American Journal of Preventive Medicine, 25*(4), 273–276. doi:S0749379703002058

Creatore, M. I., Glazier, R. H., Moineddin, R., Fazli, G. S., Johns, A., Gozdyra, P., . . . Booth, G. L. (2016). Association of neighborhood walkability with change in overweight, obesity, and diabetes. *JAMA, 315*(20), 2211–2220. doi:10.1001/jama.2016.5898

Creswell, J. W., Klassen, Carroll, A., Clark, P., Vicki, L., & Smith, K. C.. (2011). *Best practices for mixed methods research in the health sciences.* Bethesda, MD: National Institutes of Health.

Charreire, H., Mackenbach, J. D., Ouasti, M., Lakerveld, J., Compernolle, S., Ben-Rebah, M., . . . Oppert, J. M. (2013). Using remote sensing to define environmental characteristics related to physical activity and dietary behaviours: A systematic review (the SPOTLIGHT project). *Health & Place, 25C*, 1–9. doi:10.1016/j.healthplace.2013.09.017

Chow, C. K., Lock, K., Teo, K., Subramanian, S. V., McKee, M., & Yusuf, S. (2009). Environmental and societal influences acting on cardiovascular risk factors and disease at a population level: A review. *International Journal of Epidemiology*, *38*(6), 1580–1594. doi:10.1093/ije/dyn258

Chuang, Y. C., Cubbin, C., Ahn, D., & Winkleby, M. A. (2005). Effects of neighbourhood socioeconomic status and convenience store concentration on individual level smoking. *Journal of Epidemiology and Community Health*, *59*(7), 568–573.

Davey Smith, G., Steer, C., Leary, S., & Ness, A. (2007). Is there an intrauterine influence on obesity? Evidence from parent child associations in the Avon Longitudinal Study of Parents and Children (ALSPAC). *Archives of Disease in Childhood*, *92*(10), 876–880. doi:adc.2006.104869 [pii] 10.1136/adc.2006.104869

Deshpande, A. D., Baker, E. A., Lovegreen, S. L., & Brownson, R. C. (2005). Environmental correlates of physical activity among individuals with diabetes in the rural midwest. *Diabetes Care*, *28*(5), 1012–1018.

Diez Roux, A. V. (2000). Multilevel analysis in public health research. *Annual Review of Public Health*, *21*, 171–192.

Diez Roux, A. V. (2007). Neighborhoods and health: Where are we and were do we go from here? *La Revue d'épidémiologie Sante Publique*, *55*(1), 13–21. doi:10.1016/j.respe.2006.12.003

Doescher, M. P., Lee, C., Saelens, B. E., Lee, C., Berke, E. M., Adachi-Mejia, A. M., . . . Moudon, A. V. (2016). Utilitarian and recreational walking among Spanish- and English-speaking Latino adults in micropolitan US towns. *Journal of Immigrant and Minority Health*. doi:10.1007/s10903-016-0383-5

Duncan, D. T., Piras, G., Dunn, E. C., Johnson, R. M., Melly, S. J., & Molnar, B. E. (2013). The built environment and depressive symptoms among urban youth: A spatial regression study. *Spatial and Spatiotemporal Epidemiology*, *5*, 11–25. doi:10.1016/j.sste.2013.03.001

Duncan, D. T., Sharifi, M., Melly, S. J., Marshall, R., Sequist, T. D., Rifas-Shiman, S. L., & Taveras, E. M. (2014). Characteristics of walkable built environments and BMI z-scores in children: Evidence from a large electronic health record database. *Environmental Health Perspectives*, *122*(12), 1359–1365. doi:10.1289/ehp.1307704

Dunton, G. F., Liao, Y., Intille, S. S., Spruijt-Metz, D., & Pentz, M. (2011). Investigating children's physical activity and sedentary behavior using ecological momentary assessment with mobile phones. *Obesity (Silver Spring)*, *19*(6), 1205–1212. doi:oby2010302 [pii] 10.1038/oby.2010.302

Epstein, L. H., Valoski, A., Wing, R. R., & McCurley, J. (1994). Ten-year outcomes of behavioral family-based treatment for childhood obesity. *Health Psychology*, *13*(5), 373–383.

Escobar-Chaves, S. L., Markham, C. M., Addy, R. C., Greisinger, A., Murray, N. G., & Brehm, B. (2010). The Fun Families Study: Intervention to reduce children's TV viewing. *Obesity (Silver Spring)*, *18 Suppl 1*, S99–S101. doi:oby2009438 [pii] 10.1038/oby.2009.438

Evenson, K. R., Jones, S. A., Holliday, K. M., Cohen, D. A., & McKenzie, T. L. (2016). Park characteristics, use, and physical activity: A review of studies using SOPARC (System for Observing Play and Recreation in Communities). *Preventive Medicine*, *86*, 153–166. doi:10.1016/j.ypmed.2016.02.029

Evenson, K. R., Scott, M. M., Cohen, D. A., & Voorhees, C. C. (2007). Girls' perception of neighborhood factors on physical activity, sedentary behavior, and BMI. *Obesity (Silver Spring)*, *15*(2), 430–445.

Ewing, R. (2005). Can the physical environment determine physical activity levels? *Exercise and Sport Sciences Review*, *33*(2), 69–75.

Ewing, R., Handy, S., Brownson, R. C., Clemente, O., & Winston, E. (2006). Identifying and measuring urban design qualities related to walkability. *Journal of Physical Activity and Health, 3*(1), S223–S240.

Ewing, R., Meakins, G., Hamidi, S., & Nelson, A. C. (2014). Relationship between urban sprawl and physical activity, obesity, and morbidity—update and refinement. *Health & Place, 26*, 118–126. doi:10.1016/j.healthplace.2013.12.008

Feathers, A., Aycinena, A. C., Lovasi, G. S., Rundle, A., Gaffney, A. O., Richardson, J., . . . Greenlee, H. (2015). Food environments are relevant to recruitment and adherence in dietary modification trials. *Nutrition Research, 35*(6), 480–488. doi: 10.1016/j.nutres.2015.04.007

Fogelholm, M., Nuutinen, O., Pasanen, M., Myohanen, E., & Saatela, T. (1999). Parent-child relationship of physical activity patterns and obesity. *International Journal of Obesity Related Metabolic Disorders, 23*(12), 1262–1268.

Franco, M., Bilal, U., & Diez-Roux, A. V. (2014). Preventing non-communicable diseases through structural changes in urban environments. *Journal of Epidemiology and Community Health*. doi:10.1136/jech-2014-203865

Frank, L. D., & Engelke, P. O. (2001). The built environment and human activity patterns: Exploring the impacts of urban form on public health. *Journal of Planning Literature, 16*(2), 202–218.

Frank, L. D., Saelens, B. E., Powell, K. E., & Chapman, J. E. (2007). Stepping towards causation: Do built environments or neighborhood and travel preferences explain physical activity, driving, and obesity? *Social Sciences & Medicine, 65*(9), 1898–1914. doi:10.1016/j.socscimed.2007.05.053

Frank, L. D., Schmid, T. L., Sallis, J. F., Chapman, J., & Saelens, B. E. (2005). Linking objectively measured physical activity with objectively measured urban form: Findings from SMARTRAQ. *American Journal of Preventive Medicine, 28*(2 Suppl), 117–125.

Frohlich, K. L. (2014). Commentary: What is a population-based intervention? Returning to Geoffrey Rose. *International Journal of Epidemiology, 43*(4), 1292–1293. doi: 10.1093/ije/dyu111xx.

Frohlich, K. L., & Potvin, L. (2008). Transcending the known in public health practice: the inequality paradox: The population approach and vulnerable populations. *American Journal of Public Health, 98*(2), 216–221.

Fulton, J. E., Shisler, J. L., Yore, M. M., & Caspersen, C. J. (2005). Active transportation to school: Findings from a national survey. *Research Quarterly for Exercise and Sport, 76*(3), 352–357.

Gaskin, D. J., Thorpe, R. J., McGinty, E. E., Bower, K., Rohde, C., Young, J. H., . . . Dubay, L.. (2013). Disparities in diabetes: The nexus of race, poverty, and place. *American Journal of Public Health, 104*(11), 2147–2155. doi:10.2105/AJPH.2013.301420

Giles-Corti, B., Sallis, J. F., Sugiyama, T., Frank, L. D., Lowe, M., & Owen, N. (2015). Translating active living research into policy and practice: One important pathway to chronic disease prevention. *Journal of Public Health Policy, 36*(2), 231–243. doi:10.1057/jphp.2014.53

Giles-Corti, B., Bull, F., Knuiman, M., McCormack, G., Van Niel, K., Timperio, A.. . . Boruff, B. (2013). The influence of urban design on neighbourhood walking following residential relocation: Longitudinal results from the RESIDE study. *Social Science & Medicine, 77*, 20–30. doi:10.1016/j.socscimed.2012.10.016

Giovenco, D. P., Casseus, M., Duncan, D. T., Coups, E. J., Lewis, M. J., & Delnevo, C. D. (2016). Association between electronic cigarette marketing near schools and e-cigarette use among youth. *Journal of Adolescent Health, 59*(6), 627–634. doi:10.1016/j.jadohealth.2016.08.007

Golan, M., & Crow, S. (2004). Targeting parents exclusively in the treatment of childhood obesity: Long-term results. *Obesity, 12*(2), 357–361.

Gomez, L. F., Sarmiento, R., Ordonez, M. F., Pardo, C. F., de Sa, T. H., Mallarino, C. H., . . . Quistberg, D. A. (2015). Urban environment interventions linked to the promotion of physical activity: A mixed methods study applied to the urban context of Latin America. *Social Sciences & Medicine, 131*, 18–30. doi:10.1016/j.socscimed.2015.02.042

Gordon-Larsen, P., Nelson, M. C., Page, P., & Popkin, B. M. (2006). Inequality in the built environment underlies key health disparities in physical activity and obesity. *Pediatrics, 117*(2), 417–424.

Gullon, P., Badland, H. M., Alfayate, S., Bilal, U., Escobar, F., Cebrecos, A., . . . Franco, M. (2015). Assessing walking and cycling environments in the streets of Madrid: Comparing on-field and virtual audits. *Journal of Urban Health*. doi:10.1007/s11524-015-9982-z

Gullon, P., Bilal, U., & Franco, M. (2014). Physical activity environment measurement and same source bias. *Gaceta Sanitaria*. doi:10.1016/j.gaceta.2013.12.011

Halonen, J. I., Kivimaki, M., Pentti, J., Stenholm, S., Kawachi, I., Subramanian, S. V., & Vahtera, J. (2014). Green and blue areas as predictors of overweight and obesity in an 8-year follow-up study. *Obesity (Silver Spring), 22*(8), 1910–1917. doi:10.1002/oby.20772

Halonen, J. I., Stenholm, S., Kivimaki, M., Pentti, J., Subramanian, S. V., Kawachi, I., & Vahtera, J. (2015). Is change in availability of sports facilities associated with change in physical activity? A prospective cohort study. *Preventive Medicine, 73*, 10–14. doi:10.1016/j.ypmed.2015.01.012

Handy, S. L., Boarnet, M. G., Ewing, R., & Killingsworth, R. E. (2002). How the built environment affects physical activity: Views from urban planning. *American Journal of Preventive Medicine, 23*(2 Suppl), 64–73.

Hirsch, J. A., Grengs, J., Schulz, A., Adar, S. D., Rodriguez, D. A., Brines, S. J., & Diez Roux, A. V. (2016). How much are built environments changing, and where?: Patterns of change by neighborhood sociodemographic characteristics across seven U.S. metropolitan areas. *Social Science & Medicine, 169*, 97–105. doi:10.1016/j.socscimed.2016.09.032

Hirschhorn, J. S. (2004). Zoning should promote public health. *American Journal of Health Promotion, 18*(3), 258–260.

Hoehner, C. M., Brennan, L. K., Brownson, R. C., Handy, S. L., & Killingsworth, R. (2003). Opportunities for integrating public health and urban planning approaches to promote active community environments. *American Journal of Health Promotion, 18*(1), 14–20.

Hoehner, C. M., Ivy, A., Brennan Ramirez, L., Meriwether, B., & Brownson, R. C. (2006). How reliably do community members audit the neighborhood environment for its support of physical activity? Implications for participatory research. *Journal of Public Health Management Practices, 12*(3), 270–277.

Jacobs, J. (1961). *The death and life of great American cities*. New York, NY: Random House.

James, P., Hart, J. E., Banay, R. F., Laden, F., & Signorello, L. B. (2017). Built environment and depression in low-income African Americans and whites. *American Journal of Preventive Medicine, 52*(1), 74–84. doi:10.1016/j.amepre.2016.08.022

James, P., Hart, J. E., & Laden, F. (2015). Neighborhood walkability and particulate air pollution in a nationwide cohort of women. *Environmental Research, 142*, 703–711. doi:10.1016/j.envres.2015.09.005

Jariwala, S. P., Kurada, S., Moday, H., Thanjan, A., Bastone, L., Khananashvili, M., . . . Rosenstreich, D. (2011). Association between tree pollen counts and asthma ED visits in a high-density urban center. *Journal of Asthma*, *48*(5), 442–448. doi:10.3109/02770903.2011.567427

Kasanko, M., Barredo, J. I., Lavalle, C., McCormick, N., Demicheli, L., Sagris, V., & Brezger, A. (2006). Are European cities becoming dispersed?: A comparative analysis of 15 European urban areas. *Landscape and Urban Planning*, *77*(1–2), 111–130. doi:http://dx.doi.org/10.1016/j.landurbplan.2005.02.003

Kerr, J., Emond, J. A., Badland, H., Reis, R., Sarmiento, O., Carlson, J., . . . Natarajan, L. (2016). Perceived neighborhood environmental attributes associated with walking and cycling for transport among adult residents of 17 cities in 12 countries: The IPEN study. *Environmental Health Perspectives*, *124*(3), 290–298. doi:10.1289/ehp.1409466

Kerr, J., Frank, L., Sallis, J. F., & Chapman, J. (2007). Urban form correlates of pedestrian travel in youth: Differences by gender, race-ethnicity and household attributes. *Transportation Research Part D*, *12*(3), 177–182.

Kerr, J., Rosenberg, D., Sallis, J. F., Saelens, B. E., Frank, L. D., & Conway, T. L. (2006). Active commuting to school: Associations with environment and parental concerns. *Medicine and Science in Sports and Exercise*, *38*(4), 787–794.

King, K. E., & Clarke, P. J. (2015). A disadvantaged advantage in walkability: Findings from socioeconomic and geographical analysis of national built environment data in the United States. *American Journal of Epidemiology*, *181*(1), 17–25. doi:10.1093/aje/kwu310

Koschinsky, J., & Talen, E. (2015). Affordable housing and walkable neighborhoods: A national urban analysis. *Cityscape*, *17*(2), 13.

Krieger, N. (2001). Historical roots of social epidemiology: Socioeconomic gradients in health and contextual analysis. *International Journal of Epidemiology*, *30*(4), 899–900.

Kubzansky, L. D., Subramanian, S. V., Kawachi, I., Fay, M. E., Soobader, M. J., & Berkman, L. F. (2005). Neighborhood contextual influences on depressive symptoms in the elderly. *American Journal of Epidemiology*, *162*(3), 253–260.

Lake, J. K., Power, C., & Cole, T. J. (1997). Child to adult body mass index in the 1958 British birth cohort: Associations with parental obesity. *Archives of Disease in Childhood*, *77*(5), 376–381.

Larsen, K., Gilliland, J., Hess, P., Tucker, P., Irwin, J., & He, M. (2009). The influence of the physical environment and sociodemographic characteristics on children's mode of travel to and from school. *American Journal of Public Health*, *99*(3), 520–526. doi:AJPH.2008.135319 [pii] 10.2105/AJPH.2008.135319

Leal, C., & Chaix, B. (2011). The influence of geographic life environments on cardiometabolic risk factors: A systematic review, a methodological assessment and a research agenda. *Obesity Review*, *12*(3), 217–230. doi:10.1111/j.1467-789X.2010.00726.x

Lee, C., & Moudon, A. V. (2004). Physical activity and environment research in the health field: Implications for urban and transportation planning practice and research. *Journal of Planning Literature*, *19*(2), 147–181.

Lieberman, L., Golden, S. D., & Earp, J. A. (2013). Structural approaches to health promotion: What do we need to know about policy and environmental change? *Health Education & Behavior*, *40*(5), 520–525. doi:10.1177/1090198113503342

Lovasi, G. S. (2012). Built environment and health. In J. M. Rippe (Ed.), *Encyclopedia of lifestyle medicine and health* (pp. 165–168). Thousand Oaks, CA: Sage.

Lovasi, G. S., Grady, S., & Rundle, A. (2012). Steps forward: Review and recommendations for research on walkability, physical activity and cardiovascular health. *Public Health Reviews*, *33*(2), 484–506.

Lovasi, G. S., Hutson, M. A., Guerra, M., & Neckerman, K. M. (2009). Built environments and obesity in disadvantaged populations. *Epidemiology Review*, *31*, 7–20. doi:mxp005 [pii] 10.1093/epirev/mxp005

Lovasi, G. S., Jacobson, J. S., Quinn, J. W., Neckerman, K. M., Ashby-Thompson, M. N., & Rundle, A. (2011). Is the environment near home and school associated with physical activity and adiposity of urban preschool children? *Journal of Urban Health*, *88*(6), 1143–1157. doi:10.1007/s11524-011-9604-3

Lovasi, G. S., Mooney, S. J., Muennig, P., & DiMaggio, C. (2016). Cause and context: Place-based approaches to investigate how environments affect mental health. *Social Psychiatry and Psychiatric Epidemiology*, *51*(12), 1571–1579.

Lovasi, G. S., O'Neil-Dunne, J. P., Lu, J. W., Sheehan, D., Perzanowski, M. S., Macfaden, S. W., . . . Rundle, A. (2013). Urban tree canopy and asthma, wheeze, rhinitis, and allergic sensitization to tree pollen in a New York City birth cohort. *Environmental Health Perspectives*, *121*(4), 494–500, 500e491–496. doi:10.1289/ehp.1205513

MacDonald, J. M., Stokes, R. J., Cohen, D. A., Kofner, A., & Ridgeway, G. K. (2010). The effect of light rail transit on body mass index and physical activity. *American Journal of Preventive Medicine*, *39*(2), 105–112. doi:10.1016/j.amepre.2010.03.016

Macintyre, S. (2011). Good intentions and received wisdom are not good enough: the need for controlled trials in public health. *Journal of Epidemiology and Community Health*, *65*(7), 564–567. doi:10.1136/jech.2010.124198

Mackenbach, J. D., Rutter, H., Compernolle, S., Glonti, K., Oppert, J. M., Charreire, H., . . . Lakerveld, J. (2014). Obesogenic environments: A systematic review of the association between the physical environment and adult weight status, the SPOTLIGHT project. *BMC Public Health*, *14*, 233. doi:10.1186/1471-2458-14-233

Mackett, R. L., Lucas, L., Paskins, J., & Turbin, J. (2005). The therapeutic value of children's everyday travel. *Transportation Research Part A*, *39*(2–3), 205–219.

Malambo, Pasmore, Kengne, Andre P., Lambert, Estelle V., De Villers, Anniza, & Puoane, Thandi. (2017). Association between perceived built environmental attributes and physical activity among adults in South Africa. *BMC Public Health*, *17*(1), 213. doi:10.1186/s12889-017-4128-8

McDonald, N. C. (2008). Critical factors for active transportation to school among low-income and minority students. Evidence from the 2001 National Household Travel Survey. *American Journal of Preventive Medicine*, *34*(4), 341–344. doi:S0749-3797(08)00005-6 [pii] 10.1016/j.amepre.2008.01.004 [doi]

McGrath, L. J., Hinckson, E. A., Hopkins, W. G., Mavoa, S., Witten, K., & Schofield, G. (2016). Associations between the neighborhood environment and moderate-to-vigorous walking in New Zealand children: Findings from the URBAN study. *Sports Medicine*, *46*(7), 1003–1017. doi:10.1007/s40279-016-0533-x

Mehdipanah, R., Rodriguez-Sanz, M., Malmusi, D., Muntaner, C., Diez, E., Bartoll, X., & Borrell, C. (2014). The effects of an urban renewal project on health and health inequalities: A quasi-experimental study in Barcelona. *Journal of Epidemiology and Community Health*, *68*(9), 811–817. doi:10.1136/jech-2013-203434

Messing, J., Connor, L., King, A., Sheats, J., Winter, S., Buman, M., & Seguin, R. (2015). Novel assessment of built environment assets and barriers to healthy eating and active living in rural communities. *The FASEB Journal*, *29*(1 Supplement), 273.278.

Metcalf, B., Voss, L., Jeffery, A., Perkins, J., & Wilkin, T. (2004). Physical activity cost of the school run: Impact on schoolchildren of being driven to school (EarlyBird 22). *BMJ, 329*(7470), 832–833. doi:10.1136/bmj.38169.688102.F71 bmj.38169.688102.F71 [pii]

Molnar, B. E., Gortmaker, S. L., Bull, F. C., & Buka, S. L. (2004). Unsafe to play? Neighborhood disorder and lack of safety predict reduced physical activity among urban children and adolescents. *American Journal of Health Promotion, 18*(5), 378–386.

Mooney, S. J., DiMaggio, C. J., Lovasi, G. S., Neckerman, K. M., Bader, M. D., Teitler, J. O., . . . Rundle, A. G. (2016). Use of Google Street View to assess environmental contributions to pedestrian injury. *American Journal of Public Health, 106*(3), 462–469. doi:10.2105/AJPH.2015.302978

Moudon, A. V., & Lee, C. (2003). Walking and bicycling: An evaluation of environmental audit instruments. *American Journal of Health Promotion, 18*(1), 21–37.

Moudon, A. V., Lee, C., Cheadle, A. D., Garvin, C., Johnson, D., Schmid, T. L, . . . Lin, L. (2006). Operational definitions of walkable neighborhood: Theoretical and empirical insights. *Journal of Physical Activity and Health, 3*(1 Suppl), S99–S117.

Mozaffarian, D., Afshin, A., Benowitz, N. L., Bittner, V., Daniels, S. R., Franch, H. A., . . . Metabolism, Council on Clinical Cardiology Council on Cardiovascular Disease in the Young Council on the Kidney in Cardiovasc. (2012). Population approaches to improve diet, physical activity, and smoking habits: A scientific statement from the American Heart Association. *Circulation, 126*(12), 1514–1563. doi:10.1161/CIR.0b013e318260a20b

Mujahid, M. S., Diez Roux, A. V., Morenoff, J. D., & Raghunathan, T. (2007). Assessing the measurement properties of neighborhood scales: From psychometrics to ecometrics. *American Journal of Epidemiology, 165*(8), 858–867. doi:10.1093/aje/kwm040

Northridge, M. E., Sclar, E. D., & Biswas, P. (2003a). Sorting out the connections between the built environment and health: A conceptual framework for navigating pathways and planning healthy cities. *Journal of Urban Health, 80*(4), 556–568. doi:10.1093/jurban/jtg064

Northridge, M. E., Sclar, E. D., & Biswas, P. (2003b). Sorting out the connections between the built environment and health: A conceptual framework for navigating pathways and planning healthy cities. *Journal of Urban Health, 80*(4), 556–568.

Ottoson, J. M., Green, L. W., Beery, W. L., Senter, S. K., Cahill, C. L., Pearson, D. C., . . . Leviton, L. (2009). Policy-contribution assessment and field-building analysis of the Robert Wood Johnson Foundation's Active Living Research Program. *American Journal of Preventive Medicine, 36*(2 Suppl), S34–S43. doi:S0749-3797(08)00901-X [pii] 10.1016/j.amepre.2008.10.010

Papas, M. A., Alberg, A. J., Ewing, R., Helzlsouer, K. J., Gary, T. L., & Klassen, A. C. (2007). The built environment and obesity. *Epidemiology Review, 29*, 129–143.

Perdue, W. C., Stone, L. A., & Gostin, L. O. (2003). The built environment and its relationship to the public's health: The legal framework. *American Journal of Public Health, 93*(9), 1390–1394.

Perusse, L., Tremblay, A., Leblanc, C., & Bouchard, C. (1989). Genetic and environmental influences on level of habitual physical activity and exercise participation. *American Journal of Epidemiology, 129*(5), 1012–1022.

Pikora, T., Giles-Corti, B., Bull, F., Jamrozik, K., & Donovan, R. (2003). Developing a framework for assessment of the environmental determinants of walking and cycling. *Social Science & Medicine, 56*(8), 1693–1703.

Prasad, A., Gray, C. B., Ross, A., & Kano, M. (2016). Metrics in Urban Health: Current Developments and Future Prospects. *Annual Review of Public Health, 37*, 113–133. doi:10.1146/annurev-publhealth-032315-021749

Razum, O., & Gerhardus, A. (1999). Editorial: Methodological triangulation in public health research–advancement or mirage? *Tropical Medicine & International Health, 4*(4), 243–244.

Richardson, A. S., Troxel, W. M., Ghosh-Dastidar, M. B., Beckman, R., Hunter, G. P., DeSantis, A. S., . . . Dubowitz, T. (2017). One size doesn't fit all: Cross-sectional associations between neighborhood walkability, crime and physical activity depends on age and sex of residents. *BMC Public Health, 17*, 97. doi:10.1186/s12889-016-3959-z

Ritchie, L. D., Welk, G., Styne, D., Gerstein, D. E., & Crawford, P. B. (2005). Family environment and pediatric overweight: What is a parent to do? *Journal of American Dietetic Association, 105*(5 Suppl 1), S70–S79. doi:S0002822305001562 [pii] 10.1016/j.jada.2005.02.017

Rose, G. (1985). Sick individuals and sick populations. *International Journal of Epidemiology, 14*(1), 32–38.

Rundle, A. G., Bader, M. D., Richards, C. A., Neckerman, K. M., & Teitler, J. O. (2011). Using Google Street View to audit neighborhood environments. *American Journal of Preventive Medicine, 40*(1), 94–100. doi:10.1016/j.amepre.2010.09.034

Rundle, A., Goldstein, I. F., Mellins, R. B., Ashby-Thompson, M., Hoepner, L., & Jacobson, J. S. (2009). Physical activity and asthma symptoms among New York City Head Start Children. *Journal of Asthma, 46*(8), 803–809. doi:10.1080/02770900903114564 [pii]

Rydin, Y., Bleahu, A., Davies, M., Davila, J. D., Friel, S., De Grandis, G., . . . Wilson, J. (2012). Shaping cities for health: Complexity and the planning of urban environments in the 21st century. *Lancet, 379*(9831), 2079–2108. doi:10.1016/S0140-6736(12)60435-8

Sacher, P. M., Kolotourou, M., Chadwick, P. M., Cole, T. J., Lawson, M. S., Lucas, A., & Singhal, A. (2010). Randomized controlled trial of the MEND program: A family-based community intervention for childhood obesity. *Obesity (Silver Spring), 18*(Suppl 1), S62–S68. doi:oby2009433 [pii] 10.1038/oby.2009.433

Saelens, B. E., & Glanz, K. (2009). Work group I: Measures of the food and physical activity environment: Instruments. *American Journal of Preventive Medicine, 36*(4 Suppl), S166–170. doi:S0749-3797(09)00014-2 [pii] 10.1016/j.amepre.2009.01.006

Sallis, J. F., Cerin, E., Conway, T. L., Adams, M. A., Frank, L. D., Pratt, M., . . . Owen, N. (2016). Physical activity in relation to urban environments in 14 cities worldwide: A cross-sectional study. *The Lancet, 387*(10034), 2207–2217. doi:10.1016/S0140-6736(15)01284-2

Sallis, J. F., Linton, L. S., Kraft, M. K., Cutter, C. L., Kerr, J., Weitzel, J., . . . Pratt, M. (2009). The active living research program: Six years of grantmaking. *American Journal of Preventive Medicine, 36*(2 Suppl), S10–S21. doi:S0749-3797(08)00895-7 [pii] 10.1016/j.amepre.2008.10.007

Sallis, J. F., Owen, N., & Fisher, E. B. (2008). Ecological models of health behavior. *Health behavior and health education: Theory, research, and practice, 4*, 465–486.

Sallis, J. F., Prochaska, J. J., & Taylor, W. C. (2000). A review of correlates of physical activity of children and adolescents. *Medicine & Science in Sports & Exercise, 32*(5), 963–975.

Sarkar, C., & Webster, C. (2017). Healthy cities of tomorrow: The case for large scale built environment-health studies. *Journal of Urban Health, 94*(1), 4–19. doi:10.1007/s11524-016-0122-1

Savitch, H. V. (2003). How suburban sprawl shapes human well-being. *Journal of Urban Health, 80*(4), 590–607. doi:10.1093/jurban/jtg066

Seto, Karen C, Güneralp, Burak, & Hutyra, Lucy R. (2012). Global forecasts of urban expansion to 2030 and direct impacts on biodiversity and carbon pools. *Proceedings of the National Academy of Sciences, 109*(40), 16083–16088.

Shenassa, E. D., Liebhaber, A., & Ezeamama, A. (2006). Perceived safety of area of residence and exercise: A pan-European study. *American Journal of Epidemiology, 163*(11), 1012–1017.

Shiffman, S., Stone, A. A., & Hufford, M. R. (2008). Ecological momentary assessment. *Annual Review of Clinical Psychology. 4*, 1–32.

Silver, Mitchell. (2012). Planners and public health professionals need to partner. . . again. *North Carolina Medical Journal, 73*(4), 290.

Song, Y., & Knaap, G. (2003). New urbanism and housing values: A disaggregate assessment. *Journal of Urban Economics, 54*, 218–238.

Stewart, M., Makwarimba, E., Barnfather, A., Letourneau, N., & Neufeld, A. (2008). Researching reducing health disparities: Mixed-methods approaches. *Social Science & Medicine, 66*(6), 1406–1417. doi:10.1016/j.socscimed.2007.11.021

Stewart, O. T., Carlos, H. A., Lee, C., Berke, E. M., Hurvitz, P. M., Li, L., . . . Doescher, M. P. (2015). Secondary GIS built environment data for health research. *Journal of Transport and Health, 3*(4), 529–539.

Stewart, O. T., Vernez Moudon, A., Saelens, B. E., Lee, C., Kang, B., & Doescher, M. P. (2016). Comparing associations between the built environment and walking in rural small towns and a large metropolitan area. *Environment and Behavior, 48*(1), 13–36.

Stokols, D. (1996). Translating social ecological theory into guidelines for community health promotion. *American Journal of Health Promotion, 10*(4), 282–298.

Sugiyama, T., Howard, N. J., Paquet, C., Coffee, N. T., Taylor, A. W., & Daniel, M. (2015). Do relationships between environmental attributes and recreational walking vary according to area-level socioeconomic status? *Journal of Urban Health*. doi:10.1007/s11524-014-9932-1

Tanner, M., & Harpham, T. (2014). *Urban health in developing countries: progress and prospects*. New York, NY: Routledge.

Teschke, K., Dennis, J., Reynolds, C. C., Winters, M., & Harris, M. A. (2016). Bicycling crashes on streetcar (tram) or train tracks: Mixed methods to identify prevention measures. *BMC Public Health, 16*, 617. doi:10.1186/s12889-016-3242-3

Thornton, L. E., Pearce, J. R., Macdonald, L., Lamb, K. E., & Ellaway, A. (2012). Does the choice of neighbourhood supermarket access measure influence associations with individual-level fruit and vegetable consumption? A case study from Glasgow. *International Journal of Health Geographics, 11*(1), 29.

Tranter, P. J. (2010). Speed kills: The complex links between transport, lack of time and urban health. *Journal of Urban Health, 87*(2), 155–166. doi:10.1007/s11524-009-9433-9

TRB. (2005). *TRB Special Report 282: Does the built environment influence physical activity? Examining the evidence*. Washington, DC: The National Academies, Transportation Research Board.

Van Dyck, D., Cardon, G., Deforche, B., & De Bourdeaudhuij, I. (2011). Do adults like living in high-walkable neighborhoods? Associations of walkability parameters with neighborhood satisfaction and possible mediators. *Health Place, 17*(4), 971–977. doi:10.1016/j.healthplace.2011.04.001

van Ham, M., Manley, D., Bailey, N., Simpson, L., & Maclennan, D. (2012). *Understanding neighbourhood dynamics: New insights for neighbourhood effects research*. Dordrecht: Springer.

Vine, M. F., Degnan, D., & Hanchette, C. (1997). Geographic information systems: Their use in environmental epidemiologic research. *Environmental Health Perspectives, 105*(6), 598–605.

Weiss, C. C., Purciel, M., Bader, M., Quinn, J. W., Lovasi, G., Neckerman, K. M., & Rundle, A. G. (2011). Reconsidering access: Park facilities and neighborhood disamenities in New York City. *Journal of Urban Health*, *88*(2), 297–310. doi:10.1007/s11524-011-9551-z

Wilcox, S., Bopp, M., Oberrecht, L., Kammermann, S. K., & McElmurray, C. T. (2003). Psychosocial and perceived environmental correlates of physical activity in rural and older African American and white women. *Journal of Gerontology B Psychological Sciences & Social Sciences, 58*(6), P329–P337.

Willenberg, L. J., Ashbolt, R., Holland, D., Gibbs, L., MacDougall, C., Garrard, J., . . . Waters, E. (2010). Increasing school playground physical activity: A mixed methods study combining environmental measures and children's perspectives. *Journal of Science & Medicine & Sport, 13*(2), 210–216. doi:10.1016/j.jsams.2009.02.011

Williamson, T. (2002). Sprawl, politics, and participation: A preliminary analysis. *National Civic Review, 91*(3), 235–244.

Winters, M., Teschke, K., Brauer, M., & Fuller, D. (2016). Bike Score®: Associations between urban bikeability and cycling behavior in 24 cities. *International Journal of Behavioral Nutrition and Physical Activity, 13*(1), 18.

Wizemann, T. (2014). *Applying a health lens to decision making in non-health sectors: Workshop summary*. Washington, DC: National Academies Press.

Zick, C. D., Smith, K. R., Fan, J. X., Brown, B. B., Yamada, I., & Kowaleski-Jones, L. (2009). Running to the store? The relationship between neighborhood environments and the risk of obesity. *Social Sciences & Medicine, 69*(10), 1493–1500. doi:10.1016/j.socscimed.2009.08.032

9

FOOD ENVIRONMENT AND HEALTH

Jason Block, Michael Seward, and Peter James

One particular aspect of the environment that has generated great interest has been the link between access and exposure to food establishments and health, specifically diet quality, obesity, and other metabolic diseases. Over the last decade, the growth in this area of research has been exponential, as demonstrated by a PubMed search using the term "food environment" (Figure 9-1). This literature is varied and covers three aspects of food access or exposure. "Availability" refers to the adequacy of the supply of certain food types, such as the presence of supermarkets with available vegetables close to one's residence. "Accessibility" refers to the location of the food supply and ease of getting to that location, where travel time and distance may play a role. The price and perceptions of value relative to cost may be indicators of "affordability" (Caspi, Sorensen, Subramanian, & Kawachi, 2012). These food environment factors are hypothesized to drive food purchases, consumption, and ultimately chronic disease resulting from diet. In this chapter, we primarily focus on studies of accessibility rather than availability and affordability.

Much of the research on the food environment has examined access to "unhealthy" food establishments, such as fast food restaurants (e.g., McDonald's or Burger King), or "healthy" food establishments, such as supermarkets. Areas with high access to unhealthy establishments are often referred to as "food swamps" and areas with low access to healthy establishments as "food deserts." Although there is no standard definition of a food swamp (Hager et al., 2016; Luan, Law, & Quick, 2015), the US Department of Agriculture (USDA) defines census tracts (see Chapter 2) as food deserts if they are low income and have low access to a supermarket, supercenter, or large grocery store ("Economic Research Service [ERS], U.S. Department of Agriculture [USDA]. Food Access Research Atlas," 2017). In urban areas, the USDA uses the measure of 500 people or one third of the census tract population living greater than one half of a mile from a large food store as one definition of a food desert or the same number of people living more than 1 mile from a large food store as a second definition. In rural areas, the distances used vary from more than 10

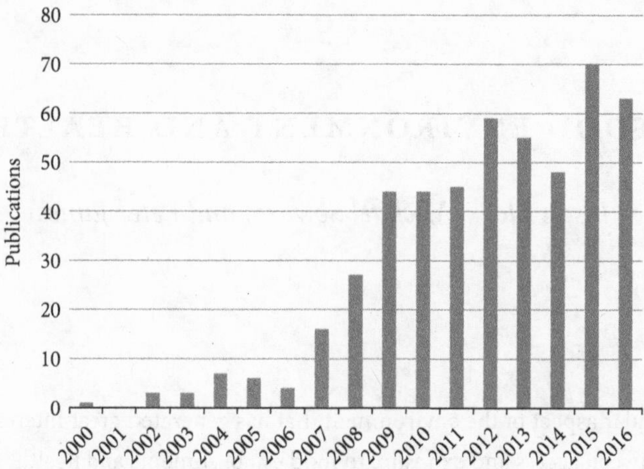

FIGURE 9-1 **Publications on the food environment, 2000 to 2016.**

or 20 miles from a large food store for the same number of people. Depending on how this measure is defined, 6% to 18% of the US population lives in a food desert. Another metric incorporates car ownership in the definition; approximately 2% of the US population does not own a car, lives in a low-income census tract, and has poor access to a large food store.

In this chapter, we examine multiple aspects of research on the food environment and health. First, we assess the methodology that has been used to conduct this research, including measures of food access and sources of information regarding food establishments. Second, we examine the literature on the relationship between food access and several important outcomes, including food consumption, obesity or body weight, hypertension, and other cardiometabolic outcomes. Third, we explore the move toward more comprehensive measures utilizing data outside residential environments and through wearable technologies and mobile devices.

MEASUREMENT OF FOOD ACCESS

Researchers have typically measured access to food establishments as the number and type of food outlets located near a person or population. In this section, we detail concepts and constructs that commonly drive development of these varied measures. We also cover commonly debated methodological questions and developing advancements in measurement.

Locus of Analysis

The majority of studies on the food environment focus on the home/residential environment. However, individuals have been shown to spend less than 50% of their time near their homes (Hurvitz & Moudon, 2012). Also, research conducted in Los Angeles found that fewer than 22% of respondents shop for groceries in their home census tract (Inagami, Cohen, Finch, & Asch, 2006). Therefore, other areas, including the workplace, school, or commuting environment, are relevant to understanding food access. To date, few studies have explored access outside the home/residential environment (see "Beyond Residential Access" later), though some initial work has found some correlation between access at home and work (K. Moore et al., 2013).

Food Establishment Types and Data Sources

Working around these loci of interest, researchers must identify specific types of food establishments that might be relevant to health. There is no standard for how to classify food establishments separately. In some cases, researchers use specific food establishment types to define access: fast food, convenience stores, small food stores, grocery stores, supermarkets, or full-service/sit-down restaurants (Block, Christakis, O'Malley, & Subramanian, 2011; Gamba, Schuchter, Rutt, & Seto, 2015). Others separately classify establishments based on perceptions of their healthfulness: grocery stores and supermarkets as "healthy" and fast food restaurants and convenience stores as "unhealthy" (Babey et al., 2008; Frankenfeld, Leslie, & Makara, 2015; Wilkins, Morris, Radley, & Griffiths, 2017). These broad healthy/unhealthy establishment definitions may not entirely match the characteristics of food sold in these locations, even if they align with public perception (Barnes, Freedman, Bell, Colabianchi, & Liese, 2016). For instance, while supermarkets may provide access to low-cost, nutritious foods, they simultaneously offer low-cost sugar-sweetened beverages, snack foods, and, increasingly, in-store fast food ("SupermarketGuru. Prepared Meals Will Outpace Foodservice, Packaged Foods Growth," 2014).

Data sources for geocoded food establishment data commonly include commercial databases, such as InfoUSA and Dun and Bradstreet (Lebel et al., 2017). These commercial databases, while developed for business purposes such as an assessment of a particular market area, often include detailed information including the business name, sales information, number of employees, and address, enabling researchers to identify and geocode food establishments. These databases also commonly include established industry classification codes which enable researchers to categorize food establishment types in a standardized manner. The standard coding system used is the North American Industry Classification System (NAICS), which precisely identifies a type of food establishment. For example, there are separate codes for fast food restaurants and full-service restaurants as well as for grocery stores and supermarkets. In addition to these commercial data sources, researchers also commonly use other secondary data sources for food establishments: government health records, such as governmental food inspection databases; other local directories such as Yellow Pages; internet searches; or a combination of sources (Block et al., 2011).

These secondary data sources provide an important shortcut for researchers examining food access; they forego the often costly and time-consuming endeavor of surveying geographic areas themselves to determine where food establishments are located. Further, the common use of standard industry classification codes, such as NAICS, enables comparison across studies. However, with shortcuts come limitations. Secondary databases of food establishments were created for purposes other than research and may have variable validity. According to one review (Fleischhacker, Evenson, Sharkey, Pitts, & Rodriguez, 2013), secondary data sources often failed validation attempts, such as verifying location and types of establishment through direct observation (sometimes referred to as "ground-truthing"). Sensitivity was reasonably high for commercial databases, such as Dun and Bradstreet and InfoUSA (correlation coefficients ranging from 0.60–0.96) and better than government sources (0.46–0.85), and local directories (0.52–0.74). But results are variable depending on the geographic area assessed. Studies have found that commercial databases undercount franchised fast food restaurants by 37%–59% compared to ground-truthed data (Liese et al., 2010, 2013; Powell et al., 2011); others have shown much greater accuracy (A. A. Gustafson, Lewis, Wilson, & Jilcott-Pitts, 2012). When uncertainty regarding establishment classification is present, using common business names (e.g., McDonald's) rather than industry codes (James, Arcaya, Parker, Tucker-Seeley, & Subramanian, 2014; Ohri-Vachaspati, Martinez, Yedidia, & Petlick, 2011; Simon, Kwan, Angelescu, Shih, & Fielding, 2008) may help to define establishment types properly.

Certain establishments may be harder to identify accurately in commercial databases. A review noted that convenience stores were one of the more challenging categories to match and were more often omitted by secondary data sources compared to other retail categories (Fleischhacker et al., 2013). Alternatively, commercial databases' capture of grocery stores had a broad range of sensitivity (0.46 to 0.99) and positive predictive value (0.59 to 0.98), perhaps because grocery stores can be part of chains or independent food stores that are difficult to assess without examining firsthand. Neighborhood characteristics affect the validity of secondary data sources; urban areas had more accurate data compared to rural areas. Conversely, neighborhood racial/ethnic makeup or socioeconomic status did not appear to play a major role in validity of these secondary data sources.

A recent review and meta-analysis of studies using commercially available business food establishment data found moderate- to high-quality studies (Lebel et al.,

2017). Authors reviewed 20 validation studies with sensitivity and positive predictive values ranging from 40% to 85% compared to ground-truthing as the gold standard. No major differences in quality were evident across different database types (e.g., Dun and Bradstreet v. InfoUSA) or by neighborhood racial or socioeconomic composition; however, the reviewers did observe some variability by country of origin (studies in the United States generally had lower validity) and by population density (lower validity in rural areas).

In general, the data sources for identifying food establishments are decent but not ideal. These data sources also have variable data quality depending on the geographic areas where they were utilized. Studies that use multiple data sources to identify or validate establishments are likely of a higher quality that those that rely on one data source.

Food Environment Metrics

While this book already discusses neighborhood boundaries and measures in previous chapters (see Chapters 2 and 3), there are a certain subset of metrics of the neighborhood food environment that are important to describe in this chapter. Researchers commonly use food environment metrics that can be categorized as density-based measures and proximity-based measures.

Density-based measures of the food environment are created by initially defining a neighborhood based around the locus of interest. Many studies use administrative boundaries, such as census tracts, to define neighborhoods and measures of food establishment access as a count per population or per land area within that area. Alternatively, researchers often create radial or circular buffers around a participant's geocoded home, work, or school address and then count the number of food establishments within that buffer. Network buffers, or polygons that follow the contours of the roads surrounding a participant's home (see Chapter 2), are also commonly used to define the area that would be considered easily accessible for a person. There is no standard size for buffers in the food environment literature. A recent review of food environment methodologies found that among 20 studies using buffers, 14 different buffer sizes were applied ranging from 0.1 to 10 miles. One mile (n = 9), 1/2 mile (n = 10), and 1/4 mile (n = 7) were the most commonly used buffer sizes (Gamba et al., 2015).

These density-based methods have shortcomings because they are subject to the modifiable areal unit problem. Different choices of administrative boundaries or buffers may yield different relationships between the food environment and health (Fotheringham & Wong, 1991). The radius or size of a buffer used for an urban area may not be appropriate for rural areas. Additionally, it is still unclear what spatial extent for measuring the food environment is most relevant to health behaviors (a concept known as the uncertain geographic context problem; Chen & Kwan, 2015). For instance, as stated earlier, some studies have shown that individuals are unlikely to shop for groceries within their home census tract (Inagami et al., 2006). Therefore, measuring the food environment within a census tract may have little bearing on food shopping behavior. Despite these shortcomings, density-based measures are the most commonly used metrics employed in food environment research, with radial buffers appearing most often (Charreire et al., 2010).

By measuring the distance to food establishments from a given locus, proximity-based methods circumvent some methodological concerns of density-based methods. Distance can be measured through straight-line, or Euclidean, distance or distance via the road network. Additionally, proximity-based measures can incorporate travel time, considering speed limits on roads. A common example of these types of measures includes the road distance from a home address to the closest supermarket or fast food restaurant. Other studies have measured the average driving distance to the five closest fast food establishments (Block et al., 2011; James et al., 2014), which may provide a more stable estimate of overall access. These proximity-based measures do not have the same assumptions as density-based measures in that access is not constrained within the borders of a buffer or administrative boundary. There is no assumption of maximal distance or travel time. Proximity studies appear less often in the literature, but among proximity studies, Euclidean distance is the most common approach (Charreire et al., 2010).

Additional metrics are less widespread. Gravity measures use a weighting algorithm such that more proximal food establishments are weighted more highly than those that are further away (Charreire et al., 2010). Kernel density estimation has been applied to create a smooth spatial surface of the density and proximity of food establishments over a given area (L. V. Moore, Diez Roux, Nettleton, & Jacobs, 2008). Studies also have developed ratio measures that compare the ratio of access to one destination compared to another. For example, one study created an index calculated with a numerator of fast food restaurants, convenience stores, and small food stores ("unhealthy" establishments) within a census tract and a denominator of fast food restaurants, convenience stores, small food stores, supermarkets, and produce vendors (all census tract establishments) (Truong, Fernandes, An, Shier, & Sturm, 2010). Finally, subjective perception-based measures query study participants regarding their beliefs about the food environment (Flint, Cummins, & Matthews, 2013; L. V. Moore, Diez Roux, & Brines, 2008). Participants are asked, as in one study, if they agree that "there is a good choice of different types of grocery stores in my neighbourhood" or if "the choice of fresh fruit and vegetables to purchase in my neighbourhood is good" (Flint et al., 2013). One study comparing these perception-based measures to objective density-based measures found that the two measures were associated but not completely identical, suggesting that they may be capturing different underlying constructs (L. V. Moore, Diez Roux, & Brines, 2008).

Table 9-1 summarizes the various components of food environment measurement. As we move forward with this chapter, we will review studies of the food environment and health. This table should provide a guide to the metrics that each study applied to measure the food environment.

Table 9-1 Measuring the Food Environment

Locus	Home
	School
	Worksite
	Commute
Food establishments	Fast food
	Convenience stores
	Small food stores
	Grocery stores
	Supermarkets
	Full service restaurants
Data sources	Commercial databases
	Government health departments
	Ground-truthed
Food environment metric	Density
	Administrative boundary
	Buffer
	Euclidean
	Network
	Proximity
	Euclidean
	Network
	Distance
	Travel time

NEIGHBORHOOD ENVIRONMENT, DIET, AND OBESITY

Observational Studies

The overwhelming majority of research on the food environment has focused on its potential effect on diet and body weight. This research is highly inconsistent and faces significant obstacles. Most studies are cross-sectional, although the use of more robust study designs methods, such as longitudinal cohorts, is increasing. As discussed earlier, measures of the food environment are highly variable, making comparisons across studies difficult. Density measures may be capturing something entirely different than proximity measures or measures defined by perceptions. The quality of the food environment data also can be limited, especially in nonurban areas. Even when longitudinal data on diet or weight is available, the acquisition of historic, high-quality data on the food environment might not be. Although some of the commercially available business data might be available historically, they cannot be ground-truthed or validated, making them somewhat less reliable.

Causal inference can also be difficult in this research. Although longitudinal data can overcome problems related to temporality of exposure and outcome that are inherent in cross-sectional studies, it cannot solve others. Restaurant chains and other retail food stores may choose to locate in neighborhoods whose populations have certain characteristics. Any findings connecting the food environment to diet or weight outcomes could be subject to confounding by those factors or reverse causality. Strong study designs, such as the use of natural and quasi-experiments, can account for this somewhat but not completely. Problems related to individual self-selection into neighborhoods might also create problems related to causal inference. People may choose to live (or work) in neighborhoods based on certain amenities, including access to food retail options; conversely, some individuals may avoid neighborhoods with an abundance of food retailers. These patterns might result in spurious associations, even with strong study designs. Interpretation of studies requires attention to all of these issues.

Several systematic reviews have examined the relationship between food access and dietary outcomes, most commonly fruit and vegetable intake or fast food consumption (Caspi et al., 2012; Cobb et al., 2015; A. Gustafson, Hankins, & Jilcott, 2012). These studies have been highly variable (Caspi et al., 2012). A review of the food environment and dietary outcomes, through 2011, included publications that assessed both the density of and proximity to food establishments. Of those studies that included objective, GIS measures of the food environment, 12 of 20 found some relationship between the food environment and dietary measures. In some of these "positive" studies, results demonstrated associations only for subgroups or for specific measures of food access. For example, in a study of over 10,000 cohort participants in the Atherosclerosis Risk in Communities Study (ARIC), the presence of supermarkets in residential neighborhoods, captured from government records, was associated with a greater odds of meeting guideline-recommended intake of fruits and vegetables, fat and saturated fat (Morland, Wing, & Diez Roux, 2002). When stratified by race, an association was present only for Black participants. When assessed among nearly 2,500 participants in the Multi-ethnic Study of Atherosclerosis (MESA) for whom GIS measures of food establishments were available, there was no association found between the density of fast food restaurants and most dietary outcomes, including fast food intake and overall ratings of diet quality (L. V. Moore, Diez Roux, Nettleton, Jacobs, & Franco, 2009). However, self-reported availability of fast food was associated with higher odds of consuming fast food near one's home. Only two longitudinal studies were included in the Caspi et al., review; both examined the dietary effect of a new supermarket opening. One study found improvements in diet quality after the opening of a supermarket in Leeds, England (Wrigley, 2003), but the other in Glasgow, Scotland, did not (S. Cummins, Petticrew, Higgins, Findlay, & Sparks, 2005).

The most up-to-date systematic review of the food environment and obesity covered 71 studies across 65 separate samples (Cobb et al., 2015); some of these studies also measured dietary outcomes. The overwhelming majority of studies were cross-sectional and found no significant relationship between food access and obesity. Among studies that did find an effect, closer proximity to supermarkets was associated with less obesity or lower weight, whereas closer proximity to fast food restaurants was associated with greater obesity or higher weight. Most studies were fairly low quality, as rated by the authors of this review using eight criteria regarding the capture of weight or food establishment data, the analysis, and study design. Among the most highly rated papers that were also longitudinal, results were highly divergent.

A few studies of adults were among those that were highly rated. Block and colleagues analyzed the Framingham Heart Study Offspring cohort, using data from 3,113 participants living in a geographically contiguous area from 1971 to 2000 (Block et al., 2011). They examined associations between longitudinal exposure to six different types of food establishments and measured body mass index (BMI) and found very limited relationships. The food establishment data were captured from several sources, including government food inspection records and commercial data. The only significant finding was between proximity to fast food establishments and BMI, such that BMI was 0.19 kg/m^2 higher for every kilometer closer that women lived to fast food establishments. For a woman of average height, this difference in BMI translated to a difference of 0.5 kg for every 1 kilometer closer to a fast food restaurant. A study by Powell and Han found similar small associations between food access and BMI for women only (Powell & Han, 2011). They used commercially available data on food establishments over time, linked to self-reported height/weight data for nearly 13,000 men and women followed from 1999 to 2005 in the Panel Study of Income Dynamics. Close proximity to fast food restaurants and convenience stores had a limited association with higher BMI for women, as did supermarket proximity with lower BMI among low-income women.

A series of studies conducted using the Coronary Artery Risk Development in Young Adults (CARDIA) cohort found some supporting evidence for how the food environment might influence health or consumption. Using commercially available business data to find food establishments, higher exposure to fast food establishments was associated with more fast food consumption for low-income men (Boone-Heinonen et al., 2011a). More diversity of food retail types and places for physical activity were associated with higher diet quality in low population density areas (Meyer et al., 2015). More specialty stores, places for physical activity, and fewer convenience stores were associated with higher diet quality in places with high population density. This finding on convenience stores was replicated in another study but found to be strongest for individuals with lower income (Rummo et al., 2015). Limited evidence linked the food environment to body weight except for one study showing that BMI was lower in residential neighborhoods with large increases in the number of supermarkets over time (Boone-Heinonen et al., 2013).

Results are similar among children, with no consistent evidence of a relationship between the food environment and weight. In a study of over 11,000 school-age children, followed from kindergarten to fifth grade, children living in lower income neighborhoods were more likely to be exposed to fast food; however, they were also more likely to live near retail food stores, such as large grocery stores (Lee, 2012). There was no association between food establishment proximity and weight outcomes. Another study using the same data set but extended through eighth grade examined BMI change among over 6,000 children who had weight measures in fifth and eighth grade (Shier, An, & Sturm, 2012). No consistent association was apparent between the food environment and body weight. In fact, there was some evidence that BMI measures were higher for those living closer to supermarkets and grocery stores. A longitudinal study of over 400 six- to seven-year-old girls in California found that living closer to convenience stores was associated with a small rise in weight over 3 years (Leung et al., 2011). All of these studies used commercially available business data.

Natural Experiments and Quasi-Experimental Studies

Some of the most innovative and methodologically rigorous studies have examined natural experiments (see Chapter 6) related to the food environment. Most of these studies have followed dietary or weight measures after the opening of a supermarket in a food desert. In general, building supermarkets has not been found to influence dietary patterns or body weight, but perceptions of the food environment invariably improve. These studies have typically had some limitations related to dropout of study participants and relatively short-term follow-up, and they have only focused on one neighborhood at a time.

Two of the natural experiments were conducted in Pennsylvania, in large part due to the development of the Pennsylvania Food Financing Initiative, a public-private effort to construct 88 supermarkets in food deserts across the state of Pennsylvania (Karpyn et al., 2010; "Reinvestment Fund"). In the first of these studies, Cummins and colleagues investigated a new supermarket in a food desert in Philadelphia (S. Cummins, Flint, & Matthews, 2014). In 2006, they enrolled a cohort of mostly female, Black, low-income residents of the neighborhood where the supermarket was built and a matched comparison neighborhood without a new supermarket. The supermarket opened in 2009. In 2010, 656 of 1,400 original cohort members completed telephone questionnaires regarding food consumption, healthy food access, and body weight. Just over one quarter in the intervention neighborhood adopted the new supermarket as their main food shopping store, with another 50% using it as a secondary store. No change in fruit and vegetable consumption or body weight was evident after the opening of the supermarket. However, perceptions of food access improved, with more positive assessments of the quality and choice of grocery stores and fruit and vegetables and the cost of fruit and vegetables. Surprisingly, these improvements in perceptions were concentrated among those who did not use the store as their primary food shopping location.

Dubowitz and colleagues conducted a quasi-experimental analysis after the 2013 opening of a new supermarket in a food desert in Pittsburgh (Dubowitz, Ghosh-Dastidar, et al., 2015). The study design and demographics were similar to the aforementioned study with 831 of 1,372 cohort participants interviewed in 2014 after the supermarket opening; the initial cohort was enrolled in 2011. Overall, residents of the neighborhood with the new supermarket reported declines in calorie intake as well as improvements in diet quality and perceptions of food access compared to the control neighborhood; fruit and vegetable intake and body weight did not change relative to controls. Surprisingly, diet quality as well as fruit and vegetable consumption actually declined in both intervention and control neighborhoods after the store opened; diet quality just fell more in the control neighborhood. Over two thirds of the intervention neighborhood participants were considered to be regular users of the new supermarket; these users had no demonstrable change in calorie intake pre- versus post-intervention compared to people living in the neighborhood who were not regular users. Regular users had better perceptions of food access than nonusers.

A study by Elbel and colleagues examined the effect of a new supermarket in New York City on diet and BMI (Elbel et al., 2015). Using a street intercept, repeated cross-sectional method, researchers approached 2,230 parents/caregivers of young children in a neighborhood with a new supermarket, before and after opening, or a matched control neighborhood. Only 13% of residents surveyed in the intervention neighborhood shopped at the new supermarket at least sometimes. No change in fruit and vegetable intake or BMI was evident after the opening of the new supermarket; some reductions in salty snacks, pastries, and milk were evident in the intervention community relative to the control, but these results were not consistent across two postopening measures. As with the Pittsburgh study, there was a trend toward lower consumption of fruit and vegetables in both communities over time.

What about the flip side of the food access equation? Can restricting "bad food" improve diets? Only two studies have captured the effect of a strategy to restrict the availability of unhealthy foods. In 2008, Los Angeles passed a moratorium on new "stand-alone fast food restaurants" in South and Southeastern Los Angeles. The Los Angeles City Council enacted the moratorium as a means to both improve neighborhood aesthetics and the health of residents. Sturm and Cohen (2009) initially questioned the moratorium, upon discovering that the density of fast food restaurants was actually lower in South LA compared to some other neighborhoods in the city and county. Los Angeles County as a whole had 60% higher major chain fast food density per capita than South LA and also a higher overall density of restaurants.

Using data from food inspection records and ongoing surveys of the Los Angeles population regarding diet and obesity, Sturm and Hattori (2015) analyzed the effect of the moratorium in South LA compared to other parts of Los Angeles city and county. After the moratorium, more new permits were issued for small food stores in South LA compared to other neighborhoods; fewer permits for large independent restaurants were issued in South LA. However, the number of permits issued for fast food restaurants was similar between South LA and other LA county neighborhoods. While all of the new permits for fast food restaurants in South LA met the standards outlined in the moratorium (i.e., not "stand alone"), there were enough permits for fast food restaurants connected to other retail buildings to offset the moratorium. Fast food consumption increased and sugary beverage consumption decreased after the moratorium, but these changes were not different between South LA and other neighborhoods. Overweight/obesity prevalence actually increased more in South LA than in other neighborhoods, indicating worsening disparities. In other words, the fast food moratorium did not have the intended effects.

The use of methods such as instrumental variables (see Chapter 6) is akin to a quasi-experimental design, even if data available are only cross-sectional. A few studies have used this approach to assess links between the food environment and health. In a study of over 1,000 residents of a rural area of Texas, Dunn and colleagues used cross-sectional data, with an instrumental variable that accounted for selection of restaurants into areas that were close to interstate highways (Dunn, Sharkey, & Horel, 2012). They found no association between fast food availability with consumption or self-reported obesity; however, once stratified by race, they found significant and strong relationships for non-White study participants, such that living closer to fast food restaurants was associated with both higher fast food consumption and obesity rates. Another study in 11 states, focused on rural areas, similarly used interstate highway proximity as an instrumental variable when evaluating the association between restaurant proximity (fast food or full service) and BMI. No association was found (Anderson & Matsa, 2011).

THE FOOD ENVIRONMENT AND OTHER HEALTH OUTCOMES

Although diet and weight dominate the literature in food environment research, several clinical conditions or diseases have been considered as potentially linked to elements of the food environment. Here we review those conditions with the most robust research, including hypertension, diabetes, prediabetes, and gestational diabetes. In general, findings are similar to those for diet and weight, with mixed results and mostly cross-sectional studies. However, because of the relative dearth of this research, much more work has to be done on these areas to develop firm conclusions.

Hypertension

Mujahid et al. (2008) completed the first study of food availability and hypertension. The cross-sectional study included 2,612 adults enrolled in the Multi-Ethnic Study of Atherosclerosis (MESA) study. In addition to surveying and measuring participants, MESA also included community surveys, in which individuals living in the same census tracts as MESA participants (but not enrolled in the study) were asked to rate the availability of healthy food within 1 mile of their homes. Those living in tracts that were perceived by residents to have high availability of healthy food had a 28% lower risk of hypertension than those living in areas with the least healthy food availability; race/ethnicity attenuated this association to some degree. Kaiser et al. (2016) conducted a longitudinal study in the same cohort, with over 3,000 MESA participants followed for over 10 years. In that study, the healthy food availability summary score, calculated through a combination of participant surveys, GIS measures of food availability, and community surveys, was inversely associated with hypertension such that each standard deviation increase in the score was associated with a 6% lower risk of hypertension. The perceptions of the food environment seemed to drive the association more than GIS-based measures.

Another cross-sectional study examined the association between blood pressure and residential food establishment densities using data from 60,775 postmenopausal women in the Women's Health Initiative clinical trial (Dubowitz et al., 2012). The authors found a very small negative association between diastolic blood pressure and closer access to grocery stores and supermarkets; diastolic blood pressure decreased by 0.31 mmHg as grocery store availability increased from the lowest to highest strata (10th to 90th percentile). No association was present for access to establishments and systolic blood pressure, and fast food access was not associated with diastolic or systolic blood pressure.

Diabetes

A cross-sectional study examined health data from almost 40,000 California Health Interview Survey participants to investigate the relationship between the food environment and diabetes (Babey et al., 2008). Using commercially available business data, the authors calculated a Retail Food Environment Index (RFEI) for each survey participant that was a ratio of fast food restaurants and convenience stores to grocery stores, supermarkets, and produce vendors around a participant's home. Adults living in areas with an RFEI ≥ 5.0 (≥ 5 times more fast food and convenience store options to grocery, supermarkets, and produce vendors) had a 23% higher prevalence of diabetes compared to those living in areas with an RFEI < 3.0 (absolute prevalence difference of 1.5%). Those living in low-income communities with high RFEIs had the highest prevalence of diabetes. Another similar study using data from metropolitan DC counties found a limited association between diabetes and the RFEI ratio. When counties were stratified by their RFEI level, among counties with a "healthy" food environment ratio, those with higher density of grocery stores had higher prevalence of diabetes, which ran counter to the hypothesized direction of association (Frankenfeld et al., 2015).

A longitudinal study among millions of Swedish adults found that access to individual food establishment types was not associated with incident or prevalent diabetes (Mezuk et al., 2016). However, the ratio of "health-harming food outlets" (fast food restaurants and convenience stores) to all outlets was associated with both incident and prevalent diabetes. The absolute differences were rather small despite large odds ratios; the range of obesity prevalence across quintiles of the "health-harming food outlet" ratio was 7.2% to 8.4%. This contrasts with the range across neighborhood deprivation measures, which was 5.5% to 10.5%. When accounting for changing food access over time, participants who moved to areas with a greater "health-harming" food outlet ratio as well as those who stayed in neighborhoods that had a rising ratio over time had a higher risk of diabetes. The risk was more than double for the "movers" than "stayers," suggesting some residential self-selection.

Gestational Diabetes

Janevic et al. were the first to analyze the relationship between the food environment and gestational diabetes (Janevic, Borrell, Savitz, Herring, & Rundle, 2010). The study linked hospital birth data from 210,926 births in New York City to food environment data from a retail food database. The authors summed the number of "healthy" (defined as supermarkets, fruit and vegetable stores, and natural food stores) and "unhealthy" (defined as fast food, pizza, convenience stores, bodegas, bakeries, candy and nut stores, and meat stores) establishments within each residential census tract. The authors did not observe an association between the number of healthy or unhealthy food establishments and gestational diabetes. However, a more recent study of a low-income, primarily Hispanic population in Texas found a higher risk of developing gestational diabetes for those living in neighborhoods with the highest density (fourth vs. first quartile) of either fast food restaurants (63% higher risk) or supermarkets (56% higher risk) (Kahr et al., 2016).

SUSCEPTIBLE POPULATIONS/SUBGROUPS

Studies on the food environment are notable for their mixed results, with many of the studies, as discussed earlier, showing no relationship with diet, obesity, or health outcomes. However, where associations exist, these often are present only (or are stronger) for particular subgroups. Some studies have demonstrated that minority race and lower socioeconomic status populations are exposed to less healthy food environments (Block, Scribner, & DeSalvo, 2004; S. C. Cummins, McKay, & MacIntyre, 2005; Fraser, Edwards, Cade, & Clarke, 2010; Hilmers, Hilmers, & Dave, 2012; James et al., 2014; Kwate, Yau, Loh, & Williams, 2009; Powell, Slater, Mirtcheva, Bao, & Chaloupka, 2007; Richardson et al., 2014; Walker, Keane, & Burke, 2010). Among studies cited earlier, some studies show links between the food environment and health for non-White (Dunn et al., 2012; Morland et al., 2002), low-income (Babey et al., 2008; Boone-Heinonen et al., 2011b; Rummo et al., 2015), or female participants (Block et al., 2011; Powell & Han, 2011). One study of children had a similar finding, in which census tract median household income was an effect modifier between the association of proximity to food establishments and weight; proximity to convenience stores and full-service restaurants were associated with higher weight only among children living in low-income census tracts (Fiechtner et al., 2015). Many studies of the food environment involved lower income or lower resource communities, and as discussed earlier, studies are very mixed with many showing no relationship with diet or health outcomes. However, it is notable that most studies that do find an effect involve these populations.

One potential mechanism to explain the stronger associations in these populations is that the local food environment may be more relevant to health among individuals with no access to an automobile. Illustrating this concept, a study in Los Angeles demonstrated stronger associations between the food environment and BMI among individuals who did not own cars (Inagami, Cohen, Brown, & Asch, 2009). Among participants without cars, those living in areas with a high concentration of fast food outlets weighed approximately 12 pounds more on average compared to those living in areas without fast food outlets. Alternatively, among participants who did own cars, there was a 1 pound difference between those who lived in areas with high concentrations of fast food versus no fast food.

The relationship between the food environment and health is little studied among rural populations, where the burden of diet-associated comorbidities is high. Studies of the food environment in rural communities have shown limited availability of healthy foods in addition to specific individual factors that might drive poor diet quality and obesity, such as inhospitable climate, regional and cultural preferences, poor transportation access, and remoteness (Lenardson, Hansen, & Hartley, 2015). Coupled with lower income, substandard housing, and less educational attainment compared to their urban counterparts, rural communities are particularly vulnerable to poor health outcomes. And research on rural food environments has unique challenges. Commercially available business data are less reliable and estimating the exact location of food establishments can be challenging, leading to a greater need for labor-intensive ground-truthing to identify establishments (Sharkey, 2009). As discussed previously, measuring only the residential food environment does not account for the dynamic exposures that people have throughout a day. This may be more important in rural communities where people travel greater distances to access resources. Researchers must develop metrics of accessibility that incorporate multipurpose trips and trip chaining (combining multiple errands into one trip). In addition, studies have shown that factors such as federal programs, civic engagement, informal transportation networks, long travel distances, bulk items, community gardens, and supplementing of harvested, hunted, and bartered food may be relevant to the diet of rural communities (Smith & Morton, 2009; Yousefian, Leighton, Fox, & Hartley, 2011). Studies on rural areas should account for unique features to these environments rather than assuming that urban and rural settings have similar attributes.

WHY MIGHT FOOD ACCESS NOT BE LINKED TO IMPROVEMENTS IN CONSUMPTION OR OBESITY?

Even in neighborhoods that are food deserts, residents tend to shop at supermarkets. In the Pittsburgh study referenced earlier, 75% of residents of the intervention and control communities shopped at a supermarket, even though they traveled long distances to do so (Dubowitz, Zenk, et al., 2015). In New York City, with compressed distances due to the dense urban environment, more than 90% of residents in two food deserts reported shopping at supermarkets or discount stores (Elbel et al., 2015). In a study of more than 1,300 residents of King County, Washington, less than 20% of participants chose the supermarket closest to their home as their primary shopping location (Drewnowski, Aggarwal, Hurvitz, Monsivais, & Moudon, 2012). On average, individuals traveled a median of 2.5 miles to their primary shopping location, more than double the distance to the closest supermarket from their home. Price was a deterministic factor regarding supermarket choice. Lower income participants were much more likely to shop at low-price supermarkets compared to higher income participants. Similar findings were evident in Pittsburgh (Dubowitz, Zenk, et al., 2015).

Even when new supermarkets open, the change in distance to a supermarket might not change enough to alter patterns. For example, in 2009 and 2010, 12 supermarkets opened in eight separate Northern California neighborhoods. Researchers studied the effect of these openings on weight outcomes and distances travelled (Zhang et al., 2016). Among over 3,000 patients with diabetes receiving care in the Kaiser Permanent Northern California network, approximately one third experienced a reduction in distance to the nearest supermarket after these supermarkets opened. The mean reduction was 0.7 miles, and the greatest reduction in mean distance for a single neighborhood was 1.4 miles. When comparing patients who experienced a reduction in distance versus those who did not, there was no differential change in BMI overall or when stratified by neighborhood.

Even beyond access, there has been a blurring of lines between food establishment types. While supermarkets and grocery stores have traditionally been viewed as "healthy" food retailers and fast food restaurants and convenience stores as "unhealthy," these dichotomous distinctions no longer exist. Most supermarkets now have embedded fast food restaurants in them (Zenk et al., 2015). Prepared food sold in supermarkets has become a $26 billion market ("SupermarketGuru," 2014). In coming years, sales in this food sector are projected to grow at a faster rate than retail food or restaurant sales (Food Business News, 2013; Kearney, 2013). Also, supermarkets have extensive offerings of calorie-dense, packaged foods (Farley et al., 2009). They might offer more healthy foods, such as fresh produce, than restaurants or convenience stores, but unhealthy snacks still outnumber fruits and vegetables, especially in supermarkets located in low-income neighborhoods (Cameron, Thornton, McNaughton, & Crawford).

Despite these findings, provocative evidence regarding neighborhood effects on weight still exist. One of the most convincing studies of this comes from the Moving to Opportunity study, a randomized trial of housing vouchers conducted in the 1990s in five US cities (see Chapter 6). Families living in public housing located in high-poverty neighborhoods were randomized to receive a housing voucher to move to any new neighborhood or a voucher to move to a low-poverty neighborhood, or they were part of a control group. Ultimately, only about 50% of those receiving the low-poverty voucher used it to move. In 2008 to 2010, approximately 4,500 women participated in a 10- to 15-year, follow-up health study, in which weight and glycosylated hemoglobin were measured (Ludwig et al., 2011). By 10 years, those randomized to the low-poverty voucher were living in slightly lower poverty neighborhoods compared to those in the control group. After 10 to 15 years, compared to the control group, those in the low-poverty voucher group had 3% absolute lower rates of extreme obesity, defined as BMI ≥ 40 kg/m^2, and 4% absolute lower rates of diabetes. No differences were evident between the control group and the group that received the traditional voucher. There were no data on why these outcomes might have been realized over time and no measurement of the food environment. Although other factors might have driven these health benefits from moving, it is provocative that moving neighborhoods led to a reduction in diet-related conditions.

PERCEPTIONS OF THE FOOD ENVIRONMENT AND INTERACTION OF THE FOOD ENVIRONMENT WITH INTERVENTIONS

Although the overall food environment and health literature, especially the most robust studies, has shown limited effects, studies of perceptions of participants appear to differ from those on diet or health outcomes. Studies routinely find that perceptions of the food environment improve in neighborhoods after a supermarket opens. Both studies of new supermarkets in food deserts in Pennsylvania found improvements in perceptions of neighborhood access to healthy foods. This was present for the entire participant sample in the study in Philadelphia (S. Cummins et al., 2014) and for regular users of the new supermarket in Pittsburgh (Dubowitz, Ghosh-Dastidar, et al., 2015). When the measure of the food environment is participant perception, a relationship with diet or health outcomes may emerge, even when objective measures of food establishments are not associated. For example, while there was no relationship with objective measures of the food environment in a study among participants enrolled in the MESA cohort, self-reported availability of fast food was associated with higher odds of consuming fast food near one's home (L. V. Moore et al., 2009). Perception measures could indicate important unmeasured confounding in studies. A person who is more prone to believe that the food environment is healthier (or less healthy) may be more or less likely to eat healthfully and participate in other health-promoting behaviors. These findings regarding improvements in perception after supermarket openings associated with diet and health should be more thoroughly explored. There might be opportunities to target perceptions as a means of improving diet and health.

The food environment also might work in concert with health interventions. Very few studies cover this possibility but what has emerged is intriguing. A study of several community dietary interventions in Colorado, mostly focused on educating consumers or working with local restaurants to offer more healthy options, found that baseline positive perceptions of the food environment were linked to greater response to the interventions (Caldwell, Miller Kobayashi, DuBow, & Wytinck, 2009). These interventions were in 24 communities and lasted from 4 to 16 weeks. Among those relatively few study participants with access to data at baseline and 1-year post intervention (260 out of 1,075), reporting greater baseline ease at obtaining fruits and vegetables was associated with a greater increase in fruit and vegetable consumption over the course of the community interventions. This association was attenuated 1 year after the completion of the program.

A study of 500 children with obesity participating in an obesity treatment randomized controlled trial found similar effect modification, this time measured by objective access to food establishments (Fiechtner et al., 2016). Living close to a supermarket was associated with a larger effect of obesity treatment. For every 1 mile closer a child lived to a supermarket, the intervention led to 0.3 larger increase in intake of fruits and vegetables and a small decrease in weight, compared to children in the study's control arm. These findings on effect modification might portend an important future direction for food environment research.

THE ALCOHOL ENVIRONMENT

A subset of the food environment literature has examined the potential role of access to alcohol establishments in driving alcohol purchases and alcohol consumption. For example, a set of studies in Finland have shown consistent associations between alcohol access and alcohol use. Among almost 79,000 individuals in Finland, the cross-sectional likelihood of heavy alcohol use was higher among those who lived less than 1 km from a bar (Halonen et al., 2013). In longitudinal analyses, those people who moved closer to a bar were more likely to become heavy users of alcohol.

Another analysis of these data showed that living close to any outlet that sold beer was associated with an increase in incident alcohol use in women, but not in men. In an analysis of 34,000 Finnish adults, living within 0.5 km of a wine outlet was associated with a higher odds of consuming wine over time (Halonen et al., 2014).

More recently, one study demonstrated that over 22 years of follow-up in young adults in Australia, increasing density of liquor stores or club licenses was related to higher alcohol consumption (adding one liquor store in 1600 m network buffers around the home was related to increased alcohol consumption of 1.22 g/day or 8%) (Foster et al., 2017). In another study in Australia, lower access to alcohol outlets was related to healthy alcohol consumption, defined by guidelines (Lamb et al., 2017).

Alcohol outlets also may be associated with other health issues. Tabb, Ballester, and Grubesic (2016) capitalized on a policy change in Seattle that privatized liquor sales and distribution to examine the effect of this natural experiment on assaults. For each additional alcohol outlet in a given census block group, there was a 5%–8% increase in aggravated assaults and a 5%–6% increase in nonaggravated assaults. Researchers in New York City analyzed pedestrian/bicyclist injury data over 10 years and found that the presence of one or more alcohol outlets in a census tract increased the risk of a pedestrian or bicyclist being struck by a car by 47% (DiMaggio, Mooney, Frangos, & Wall, 2016).

A systematic review of studies on the alcohol environment found that overall alcohol consumption, drinking patterns, and alcohol-related damage (e.g., fatal motor vehicle accidents, crime, suicide, sexually transmitted diseases) were consistently related to the availability of alcohol in terms of hours and days of sale and density of alcohol outlets (Popova, Giesbrecht, Bekmuradov, & Patra, 2009). Another recent systematic review of spatial and temporal availability of alcohol added information from 79 studies through 2014 (Holmes et al., 2014). Of the 136 spatial measures included in the reviewed studies, the majority measured outlet density (N = 118), while some measured proximity (N = 16), and one study examined alcohol outlet clustering. Most studies focused on acute consumption or harms, including violence and drunk driving, while a minority of studies addressed long-term consumption and other health conditions or factors. The authors identified a number of limitations in the literature, including little information about outlet-level temporal availability; empirical analyses focused on acute over chronic outcomes; outlets generally classified into broad categories (e.g., bars) with little empirical analysis of variation within outlet categories; studies mainly set in the United States, Australia, and Europe; and sparse information on availability of alcohol away from home or online and interactions between availability, price, and place. Further studies on the alcohol environment and health should consider and address these concerns.

BEYOND RESIDENTIAL FOOD ACCESS

The overwhelming majority of studies on the food environment have relied on residential exposures, rather than accounting for the dynamic daily exposure to food establishments that we know exists. A series of studies in the United Kingdom explored these relationships beyond residential exposures. Among over 2,500 adults living in Cambridgeshire, residential exposure to food establishments accounted for only 30% of total exposure (Burgoine & Monsivais, 2013). The density of food establishments was 125% greater at work than home, and participants passed about one food establishment every 100 meters on their commutes. The greatest difference in exposure between work and home was for restaurants, but exposure to convenience stores, supermarkets, and take-away restaurants also was higher at work. In their assessment of the link between the food environment, body weight, and food consumption, associations were fairly similar across all domains, with evidence for more food consumption and body weight with closest proximity to take-away restaurants at home, work, and along commuter routes (Burgoine, Forouhi, Griffin, Wareham, & Monsivais, 2014). When all exposures were combined, obesity levels were about 80% higher in the highest exposure quartile compared to the lowest, and take-away food consumption was nearly 6 grams higher per day. This study was cross-sectional and unable to untangle some contextual factors that might confound these relationships.

What is particularly needed in future research on the food environment and health is robust data that properly account for the complex dynamic of food environment exposures. In light of the uncertain geographic context problem (Chen & Kwan, 2015), we need to identify the specific geographic area most germane to health behaviors. The use of mobile technologies and increasingly sophisticated geographic information should allow for this (see Chapter 2). The increasing ubiquity of global positioning systems (GPS) technology to assess high-resolution spatial and temporal data provides a new data stream for researchers to better understand where exactly participants obtain their food and can directly address the uncertain geographic context problem. A recent review of six GPS-based studies of the food environment showed that findings were inconsistent across studies (Cetateanu & Jones, 2016). Some studies showed that GPS-based measures of exposure to food establishments were related to diet, while others did not. The reviewed literature suggested that exposure to unhealthy food environments was inversely related to whole grain intake and positively associated with saturated fat intake. Results were equivocal for fruit and vegetable consumption. Higher access to calorically dense, ready-to-eat foods was associated with higher weight status. One analysis demonstrated that the average time a child spent within 50 m of a fast food restaurant or convenience store was directly related to the likelihood of junk food purchasing (Sadler, Clark, Wilk, O'Connor, & Gilliland, 2016).

Importantly, one study estimated differences between GPS-measured food environment exposure and neighborhood-based exposure and found that neighborhood-based measures overestimated the relationship between the food environment and diet (Shearer et al., 2015). This suggests that the uncertain geographic context problem may plague the residential food environment literature. Similar to GPS-based studies, smartphones provide a novel data stream to gather location data but also allow for real-time survey administration. One study has used smartphones to log GPS data in coordination with videos of meals, physical activity from the phone's accelerometer, and mood through periodic questionnaires (Seto et al., 2016). In concert with high-resolution data on location, novel spatial datasets may enable new understandings of food environments. For instance, studies have increasingly shown that Google Street View images are a reliable and valid way to identify food establishments and to assess the objective food environment (Bethlehem et al., 2014; Clarke, Ailshire, Melendez, Bader, & Morenoff, 2010). In turn, researchers have used Google Street View images to test associations between perceived and objective measures of the food environment (Roda et al., 2016).

Although very few studies have been published in this area, as research on the food environment evolves, more studies capitalizing on high-resolution location data will add to our understanding of how the food environment influences health.

CONCLUSIONS

Is the food environment associated with health? The verdict is messy and unclear. These studies are inherently difficult to conduct and compare. Data sources on food establishments are of variable quality and differ greatly from study to study, and measures of the food environment are inconsistent. These factors limit comparisons in the food environment literature. Most studies are cross-sectional with no ability to make causal inferences, and nearly all rely on the home food environment only. Furthermore, sorting through complex factors such as self-selection into neighborhoods and food companies targeting specific neighborhoods can be challenging, if not impossible. Overall, there appears to be limited connection between the food environment and diet or health outcomes. The most robust studies, including quasi-experimental studies and those evaluating natural experiments, have shown limited to no effect. More studies of this type are needed to make definitive conclusions, especially studies using more advanced technologies that can account for the complex food environment exposures that people experience. Studies on cardiometabolic conditions such as hypertension and diabetes have found stronger effects, perhaps because this is an area of investigation still in its infancy.

Studies on low-income populations and those focused on people of a minority race or ethnicity are more likely to find associations between the food environment and diet or health outcomes than other studies. This may be because low-income individuals are uniquely vulnerable to the characteristics of their neighborhoods, especially if they do not own a car. Perceptions of the food environment are more reliably associated with diet, and perceptions appear to improve when new supermarkets are built within food deserts. More research on how to change perceptions and how changing perceptions of the food environment may be associated with health are needed. Lastly, the literature on the link between access to alcohol outlets and alcohol consumption and other negative outcomes, such as assaults, is more robust than the food environment literature.

Despite the lack of evidence, policy makers have responded to concerns about poor access to healthy foods or high exposure to unhealthy foods. Among others, the White House Task Force on Childhood Obesity and the World Health Organization have called for action to improve geographic access to healthy foods as a means of addressing the obesity epidemic (Nishtar, Gluckman, & Armstrong, 2016; White House Task Force on Childhood Obesity, 2010). In 2010, the US federal government initiated a public-private program, the Healthy Food Financing Initiative, to encourage the placement of supermarkets and grocery stores in low-income communities without access (Lytle & Sokol, 2017). The program built on successful state-based programs in Pennsylvania, Louisiana, and New York that led to the construction of supermarkets in food deserts (Karpyn et al., 2010). Less policy action has directly addressed the proliferation of food swamps. However, one notable policy was the 2008 moratorium on new fast food restaurants in South Los Angeles (Sturm & Cohen, 2009). Until we better understand how and if the food environment is really associated with health, policy makers should consider how best to frame these policies, especially when implemented in isolation without additional assistance to help guide individuals toward better food choices once they enter retail establishments. There are goals that can be achieved with these policies, such as neighborhood economic development or social justice, even without improvements in health. For now, these are the outcomes that may be more achievable, until we learn more about how the food environment may drive health.

REFERENCES

Anderson, M. L., & Matsa, D. A. (2011). Are restaurants really supersizing America? *American Economic Journal: Applied Economics*, *3*(1), 152–188.

Babey, S. H., Diamant, A., Hastert, T. A., Harvey, S., Goldstein, H., Flournoy, R., Banthia, R., Rubin, V., & Treuhaft, S. (2008). Designed for disease: The link between local food environments and obesity and diabetes. California Center for Public Health Advocacy, PolicyLink, and the UCLA Center for Health Policy Research.

Barnes, T. L., Freedman, D. A., Bell, B. A., Colabianchi, N., & Liese, A. D. (2016). Geographic measures of retail food outlets and perceived availability of healthy foods in neighbourhoods. *Public Health & Nutrition, 19*(8), 1368–1374.

Bethlehem, J. R., Mackenbach, J. D., Ben-Rebah, M., Compernolle, S., Glonti, K., Bardos, H., . . . Lakerveld, J. (2014). The SPOTLIGHT virtual audit tool: A valid and reliable tool to assess obesogenic characteristics of the built environment. *International Journal of Health Geography, 13*, 52. doi:10.1186/1476-072X-13-52

Block, J. P., Christakis, N. A., O'Malley, A. J., & Subramanian, S. V. (2011). Proximity to food establishments and body mass index in the Framingham Heart Study offspring cohort over 30 years. *American Journal of Epidemiology, 174*(10), 1108–1114.

Block, J. P., Scribner, R. A., & DeSalvo, K. B. (2004). Fast food, race/ethnicity, and income: A geographic analysis. *American Journal of Preventive Medicine, 27*(3), 211–217. doi:10.1016/j.amepre.2004.06.007

Boone-Heinonen, J., Diez-Roux, A. V., Goff, D. C., Loria, C. M., Kiefe, C. I., Popkin, B. M., & Gordon-Larsen, P. (2013). The neighborhood energy balance equation: Does neighborhood food retail environment + physical activity environment = obesity? The CARDIA study. *PLoS One, 8*(12), e85141.

Boone-Heinonen, J., Gordon-Larsen, P., Kiefe, C. I., Shikany, J. M., Lewis, C. E., & Popkin, B. M. (2011a). Fast food restaurants and food stores: longitudinal associations with diet in young and middle-aged adults: The Cardia Study. *Archives in Internal Medicine, 171*(13), 1162–1170. Retrieved from https://www.ncbi.nlm.nih.gov/pmc/articles/PMC3178268/pdf/nihms321590.pdf

Boone-Heinonen, J., Gordon-Larsen, P., Kiefe, C. I., Shikany, J. M., Lewis, C. E., & Popkin, B. M. (2011b). Fast food restaurants and food stores: Longitudinal associations with diet in young to middle-aged adults: The CARDIA study. *Archives in Internal Medicine, 171*(13), 1162–1170. doi:10.1001/archinternmed.2011.283

Burgoine, T., Forouhi, N. G., Griffin, S. J., Wareham, N. J., & Monsivais, P. (2014). Associations between exposure to takeaway food outlets, takeaway food consumption, and body weight in Cambridgeshire, UK: Population based, cross sectional study. *British Medical Journal, 348*(348), g1464.

Burgoine, T., & Monsivais, P. (2013). Characterising food environment exposure at home, at work, and along commuting journeys using data on adults in the UK. *International Journal of Behavioral Nutrition and Physical Activity, 10*(85), 85.

Caldwell, E. M., Miller Kobayashi, M., DuBow, W. M., & Wytinck, S. M. (2009). Perceived access to fruits and vegetables associated with increased consumption. *Public Health & Nutrition, 12*(10), 1743–1750.

Cameron, A. J., Thornton, L. E., McNaughton, S. A., & Crawford, D. Variation in supermarket exposure to energy-dense snack foods by socio-economic position. *Public Health & Nutrition*, 1–8. doi:S1368980012002649 [pii] 10.1017/S1368980012002649 [doi]

Caspi, C. E., Sorensen, G., Subramanian, S. V., & Kawachi, I. (2012). The local food environment and diet: A systematic review. *Health & Place, 18*(5), 1172–1187. Retrieved from https://www.ncbi.nlm.nih.gov/pmc/articles/PMC3684395/pdf/nihms381700.pdf

Cetateanu, A., & Jones, A. (2016). How can GPS technology help us better understand exposure to the food environment? A systematic review. *SSM Population Health, 2*, 196–205. doi:10.1016/j.ssmph.2016.04.001

Charreire, H., Casey, R., Salze, P., Simon, C., Chaix, B., Banos, A., . . . Oppert, J. M. (2010). Measuring the food environment using geographical information systems: A methodological review. *Public Health & Nutrition, 13*(11), 1773–1785. doi:10.1017/S1368980010000753

Chen, X., & Kwan, M. P. (2015). Contextual uncertainties, human mobility, and perceived food environment: The uncertain geographic context problem in food access research. *American Journal of Public Health, 105*(9), 1734–1737. doi:10.2105/AJPH.2015.302792

Clarke, P., Ailshire, J., Melendez, R., Bader, M., & Morenoff, J. (2010). Using Google Earth to conduct a neighborhood audit: Reliability of a virtual audit instrument. *Health & Place, 16*(6), 1224–1229. doi:10.1016/j.healthplace.2010.08.007

Cobb, L. K., Appel, L. J., Franco, M., Jones-Smith, J. C., Nur, A., & Anderson, C. A. (2015). The relationship of the local food environment with obesity: A systematic review of methods, study quality, and results. *Obesity (Silver Spring), 23*(7), 1331–1344.

Cummins, S., Flint, E., & Matthews, S. A. (2014). New neighborhood grocery store increased awareness of food access but did not alter dietary habits or obesity. *Health Affairs (Millwood), 33*(2), 283–291. doi:33/2/283 [pii] 10.1377/hlthaff.2013.0512 [doi]

Cummins, S., Petticrew, M., Higgins, C., Findlay, A., & Sparks, L. (2005). Large scale food retailing as an intervention for diet and health: Quasi-experimental evaluation of a natural experiment. *Journal of Epidemiology and Community Health, 59*(12), 1035–1040.

Cummins, S. C., McKay, L., & MacIntyre, S. (2005). McDonald's restaurants and neighborhood deprivation in Scotland and England. *American Journal of Preventive Medicine, 29*(4), 308–310. doi:10.1016/j.amepre.2005.06.011

DiMaggio, C., Mooney, S., Frangos, S., & Wall, S. (2016). Spatial analysis of the association of alcohol outlets and alcohol-related pedestrian/bicyclist injuries in New York City. *Injury Epidemiology, 3*, 11. doi:10.1186/s40621-016-0076-5

Drewnowski, A., Aggarwal, A., Hurvitz, P. M., Monsivais, P., & Moudon, A. V. (2012). Obesity and supermarket access: Proximity or price? *American Journal of Public Health, 102*(8), e74–e80. doi:10.2105/AJPH.2012.300660 [doi]

Dubowitz, T., Ghosh-Dastidar, M., Cohen, D. A., Beckman, R., Steiner, E. D., Hunter, G. P., . . . Collins, R. L. (2015). Diet and perceptions change with supermarket introduction in a food desert, but not because of supermarket use. *Health Affairs (Millwood), 34*(11), 1858–1868. Retrieved from http://content.healthaffairs.org/content/34/11/1858.long https://www.ncbi.nlm.nih.gov/pmc/articles/PMC4977027/pdf/nihms801755.pdf

Dubowitz, T., Ghosh-Dastidar, M., Eibner, C., Slaughter, M. E., Fernandes, M., Whitsel, E. A., . . . Escarce, J. J. (2012). The Women's Health Initiative: The food environment, neighborhood socioeconomic status, BMI, and blood pressure. *Obesity (Silver Spring), 20*(4), 862–871. doi:10.1038/oby.2011.141

Dubowitz, T., Zenk, S. N., Ghosh-Dastidar, B., Cohen, D. A., Beckman, R., Hunter, G., . . . Collins, R. L. (2015). Healthy food access for urban food desert residents: Examination of the food environment, food purchasing practices, diet and BMI. *Public Health and Nutrition, 18*(12), 2220–2230. Retrieved from http://www.ncbi.nlm.nih.gov/pmc/articles/PMC4457716/pdf/nihms654087.pdf

Dunn, R. A., Sharkey, J. R., & Horel, S. (2012). The effect of fast-food availability on fast-food consumption and obesity among rural residents: An analysis by race/ethnicity. *Economics and Human Biology, 10*(1), 1–13.

Economic Research Service (ERS), U.S. Department of Agriculture (USDA). Food Access Research Atlas. (2017). Retrieved from https://www.ers.usda.gov/data-products/food-access-research-atlas/

Elbel, B., Moran, A., Dixon, L. B., Kiszko, K., Cantor, J., Abrams, C., & Mijanovich, T. (2015). Assessment of a government-subsidized supermarket in a high-need area on household food availability and children's dietary intakes. *Public Health & Nutrition*, 1–10. doi:S1368980015000282 [pii] 10.1017/S1368980015000282 [doi]

Farley, T. A., Rice, J., Bodor, J. N., Cohen, D. A., Bluthenthal, R. N., & Rose, D. (2009). Measuring the food environment: Shelf space of fruits, vegetables, and snack foods in stores. *Journal of Urban Health*, *86*(5), 672–682. doi:10.1007/s11524-009-9390-3 [doi]

Fiechtner, L., Kleinman, K., Melly, S. J., Sharifi, M., Marshall, R., Block, J., . . . Taveras, E. M. (2016). Effects of proximity to supermarkets on a randomized trial studying interventions for obesity. *American Journal of Public Health*, *106*(3), 557–562.

Fiechtner, L., Sharifi, M., Sequist, T., Block, J., Duncan, D. T., Melly, S. J., . . . Taveras, E. M. (2015). Food environments and childhood weight status: effects of neighborhood median income. *Childhood Obesity*, *11*(3), 260–268.

Fleischhacker, S. E., Evenson, K. R., Sharkey, J., Pitts, S. B., & Rodriguez, D. A. (2013). Validity of secondary retail food outlet data: A systematic review. *American Journal of Preventive Medicine*, *45*(4), 462–473. doi:10.1016/j.amepre.2013.06.009

Flint, E., Cummins, S., & Matthews, S. (2013). Do perceptions of the neighbourhood food environment predict fruit and vegetable intake in low-income neighbourhoods? *Health & Place*, *24*, 11–15. doi:10.1016/j.healthplace.2013.07.005

Food Business News. Prepared foods threaten restaurant industry. (2013). Retrieved from http://www.foodbusinessnews.net/articles/news_home/Food-Service-Retail/2013/07/Prepared_foods_threaten_restau.aspx?ID={71818C36-BC1D-4C87-93EA-6D05E414C456}&cck=1

Foster, S., Trapp, G., Hooper, P., Oddy, W. H., Wood, L., & Knuiman, M. (2017). Liquor landscapes: Does access to alcohol outlets influence alcohol consumption in young adults? *Health & Place*, *45*, 17–23. doi:10.1016/j.healthplace.2017.02.008

Fotheringham, A. S., & Wong, D. W. S. (1991). The modifiable areal unit problem in multivariate statistical analysis. *Environment and Planning A*, *23*(7), 1025–1044.

Frankenfeld, C. L., Leslie, T. F., & Makara, M. A. (2015). Diabetes, obesity, and recommended fruit and vegetable consumption in relation to food environment sub-types: A cross-sectional analysis of Behavioral Risk Factor Surveillance System, United States Census, and food establishment data. *BMC Public Health*, *15*, 491. doi:10.1186/s12889-015-1819-x

Fraser, L. K., Edwards, K. L., Cade, J., & Clarke, G. P. (2010). The geography of fast food outlets: A review. *International Journal of Environmental Research and Public Health*, *7*(5), 2290–2308. doi:10.3390/ijerph7052290

Gamba, R. J., Schuchter, J., Rutt, C., & Seto, E. Y. (2015). Measuring the food environment and its effects on obesity in the United States: A systematic review of methods and results. *Journal of Community Health*, *40*(3), 464–475. doi:10.1007/s10900-014-9958-z

Gustafson, A., Hankins, S., & Jilcott, S. (2012). Measures of the consumer food store environment: A systematic review of the evidence 2000–2011. *Journal of Community Health*, *37*(4), 897–911.

Gustafson, A. A., Lewis, S., Wilson, C., & Jilcott-Pitts, S. (2012). Validation of food store environment secondary data source and the role of neighborhood deprivation in Appalachia, Kentucky. *BMC Public Health*, *12*, 688. doi:10.1186/1471-2458-12-688

Hager, E. R., Cockerham, A., O'Reilly, N., Harrington, D., Harding, J., Hurley, K. M., & Black, M. M. (2016). Food swamps and food deserts in Baltimore City, MD, USA: Associations with dietary behaviours among urban adolescent girls. *Public Health and Nutrition, 22*, 1–10.

Halonen, J. I., Kivimaki, M., Pentti, J., Virtanen, M., Subramanian, S. V., Kawachi, I., & Vahtera, J. (2014). Association of the availability of beer, wine, and liquor outlets with beverage-specific alcohol consumption: A cohort study. *Alcoholism Clinical and Experimental Research, 38*(4), 1086–1093. doi:10.1111/acer.12350

Halonen, J. I., Kivimaki, M., Virtanen, M., Pentti, J., Subramanian, S. V., Kawachi, I., & Vahtera, J. (2013). Living in proximity of a bar and risky alcohol behaviours: A longitudinal study. *Addiction, 108*(2), 320–328. doi:10.1111/j.1360-0443.2012.04053.x

Hilmers, A., Hilmers, D. C., & Dave, J. (2012). Neighborhood disparities in access to healthy foods and their effects on environmental justice. *American Journal of Public Health, 102*(9), 1644–1654. doi:10.2105/AJPH.2012.300865

Holmes, J., Guo, Y., Maheswaran, R., Nicholls, J., Meier, P. S., & Brennan, A. (2014). The impact of spatial and temporal availability of alcohol on its consumption and related harms: A critical review in the context of UK licensing policies. *Drug Alcohol Review, 33*(5), 515–525. doi:10.1111/dar.12191

Hurvitz, P. M., & Moudon, A. V. (2012). Home versus nonhome neighborhood: Quantifying differences in exposure to the built environment. *American Journal of Preventive Medicine, 42*(4), 411–417. doi:10.1016/j.amepre.2011.11.015

Inagami, S., Cohen, D. A., Brown, A. F., & Asch, S. M. (2009). Body mass index, neighborhood fast food and restaurant concentration, and car ownership. *Journal of Urban Health, 86*(5), 683–695. doi:10.1007/s11524-009-9379-y

Inagami, S., Cohen, D. A., Finch, B. K., & Asch, S. M. (2006). You are where you shop: Grocery store locations, weight, and neighborhoods. *American Journal of Preventive Medicine, 31*(1), 10–17. doi:10.1016/j.amepre.2006.03.019

James, P., Arcaya, M. C., Parker, D. M., Tucker-Seeley, R. D., & Subramanian, S. V. (2014). Do minority and poor neighborhoods have higher access to fast-food restaurants in the United States? *Health & Place, 29*, 10–17. Retrieved from http://www.sciencedirect.com/science/article/pii/S1353829214000690;https://www.ncbi.nlm.nih.gov/pmc/articles/PMC4783380/pdf/nihms744161.pdf

Janevic, T., Borrell, L. N., Savitz, D. A., Herring, A. H., & Rundle, A. (2010). Neighbourhood food environment and gestational diabetes in New York City. *Paediatric Perinatal Epidemiology, 24*(3), 249–254. doi:10.1111/j.1365-3016.2010.01107.x

Kahr, M. K., Suter, M. A., Ballas, J., Ramin, S. M., Monga, M., Lee, W., . . . Aagaard, K. M. (2016). Geospatial analysis of food environment demonstrates associations with gestational diabetes. *American Journal of Obstetrics and Gynecology, 214*(1), 110 e111–e119. doi:10.1016/j.ajog.2015.08.048

Kaiser, P., Diez Roux, A. V., Mujahid, M., Carnethon, M., Bertoni, A., Adar, S. D., . . . Lisabeth, L. (2016). Neighborhood environments and incident hypertension in the multi-ethnic study of atherosclerosis. *American Journal of Epidemiology, 183*(11), 988–997. doi:10.1093/aje/kwv296

Karpyn, A., Manon, M., Treuhaft, S., Giang, T., Harries, C., & McCoubrey, K. (2010). Policy solutions to the "grocery gap." *Health Affairs, 29*(3), 473–480.

Kearney, A. T. (2013). Fresh prepared foods—A growth driver for your company. Retrieved from http://www.middle-east.atkearney.com/consumer-products-retail/ideas-insights/

-/asset_publisher/3wUhKxoRuuW6/content/fresh-prepared-foods-a-growth-driver-for-your-company/10192

Kwate, N. O., Yau, C. Y., Loh, J. M., & Williams, D. (2009). Inequality in obesigenic environments: Fast food density in New York City. *Health & Place, 15*(1), 364–373. doi:10.1016/j.healthplace.2008.07.003

Lamb, K. E., Thornton, L. E., Teychenne, M., Milte, C., Cerin, E., & Ball, K. (2017). Associations between access to alcohol outlets and alcohol intake and depressive symptoms in women from socioeconomically disadvantaged neighbourhoods in Australia. *BMC Public Health, 17*(1), 83. doi:10.1186/s12889-017-4022-4

Lebel, A., Daepp, M. I., Block, J. P., Walker, R., Lalonde, B., Kestens, Y., & Subramanian, S. V. (2017). Quantifying the foodscape: A systematic review and meta-analysis of the validity of commercially available business data. *PLoS One, 12*(3), e0174417.

Lee, H. (2012). The role of local food availability in explaining obesity risk among young school-aged children. *Social Science Medicine, 74*(8), 1193–1203.

Lenardson, J. D., Hansen, A. Y., & Hartley, D. (2015). Rural and remote food environments and obesity. *Current Obesity Report, 4*(1), 46–53. doi:10.1007/s13679-014-0136-5

Leung, C. W., Laraia, B. A., Kelly, M., Nickleach, D., Adler, N. E., Kushi, L. H., & Yen, I. H. (2011). The influence of neighborhood food stores on change in young girls' body mass index. *American Journal of Preventive Medicine, 41*(1), 43–51.

Liese, A. D., Barnes, T. L., Lamichhane, A. P., Hibbert, J. D., Colabianchi, N., & Lawson, A. B. (2013). Characterizing the food retail environment: Impact of count, type, and geospatial error in two secondary data sources. *Journal of Nutrition Education and Behavior, 45*(5), 435–442. doi:10.1016/j.jneb.2013.01.021

Liese, A. D., Colabianchi, N., Lamichhane, A. P., Barnes, T. L., Hibbert, J. D., Porter, D. E., . . . Lawson, A. B. (2010). Validation of 3 food outlet databases: Completeness and geospatial accuracy in rural and urban food environments. *American Journal of Epidemiology, 172*(11), 1324–1333. doi:10.1093/aje/kwq292

Luan, H., Law, J., & Quick, M. (2015). Identifying food deserts and swamps based on relative healthy food access: A spatio-temporal Bayesian approach. *International Journal of Health Geography, 14*(37), 37.

Ludwig, J., Sanbonmatsu, L., Gennetian, L., Adam, E., Duncan, G. J., Katz, L. F., . . . McDade, T. W. (2011). Neighborhoods, obesity, and diabetes—a randomized social experiment. *New England Journal of Medicine, 365*(16), 1509–1519. Retrieved from http://www.nejm.org/doi/pdf/10.1056/NEJMsa1103216

Lytle, L. A., & Sokol, R. L. (2017). Measures of the food environment: A systematic review of the field, 2007-2015. *Health & Place, 44*, 18–34.

Meyer, K. A., Boone-Heinonen, J., Duffey, K. J., Rodriguez, D. A., Kiefe, C. I., Lewis, C. E., & Gordon-Larsen, P. (2015). Combined measure of neighborhood food and physical activity environments and weight-related outcomes: The CARDIA study. *Health Place, 33*, 9–18.

Mezuk, B., Li, X., Cederin, K., Rice, K., Sundquist, J., & Sundquist, K. (2016). Beyond access: Characteristics of the food environment and risk of diabetes. *American Journal of Epidemiology, 183*(12), 1129–1137. doi:10.1093/aje/kwv318

Moore, K., Diez Roux, A. V., Auchincloss, A., Evenson, K. R., Kaufman, J., Mujahid, M., & Williams, K. (2013). Home and work neighbourhood environments in relation to body mass index: The multi-ethnic study of atherosclerosis (MESA). *Journal of Epidemiology and Community Health, 67*(10), 846–853. doi:10.1136/jech-2013-202682

Moore, L. V., Diez Roux, A. V., & Brines, S. (2008). Comparing perception-based and geographic information system (GIS)-based characterizations of the local food environment. *Journal of Urban Health, 85*(2), 206–216. doi:10.1007/s11524-008-9259-x

Moore, L. V., Diez Roux, A. V., Nettleton, J. A., Jacobs, D. R., & Franco, M. (2009). Fast-food consumption, diet quality, and neighborhood exposure to fast food: The multi-ethnic study of atherosclerosis. *American Journal of Epidemiology, 170*(1), 29–36.

Moore, L. V., Diez Roux, A. V., Nettleton, J. A., & Jacobs, D. R., Jr. (2008). Associations of the local food environment with diet quality—a comparison of assessments based on surveys and geographic information systems: The multi-ethnic study of atherosclerosis. *American Journal of Epidemiology, 167*(8), 917–924. doi:10.1093/aje/kwm394

Morland, K., Wing, S., & Diez Roux, A. (2002). The contextual effect of the local food environment on residents' diets: The atherosclerosis risk in communities study. *American Journal of Public Health, 92*(11), 1761–1767.

Mujahid, M. S., Diez Roux, A. V., Morenoff, J. D., Raghunathan, T. E., Cooper, R. S., Ni, H., & Shea, S. (2008). Neighborhood characteristics and hypertension. *Epidemiology, 19*(4), 590–598. doi:10.1097/EDE.0b013e3181772cb2

Nishtar, S., Gluckman, P., & Armstrong, T. (2016). Ending childhood obesity: A time for action. *Lancet, 387*(10021), 825–827.

Ohri-Vachaspati, P., Martinez, D., Yedidia, M. J., & Petlick, N. (2011). Improving data accuracy of commercial food outlet databases. *American Journal of Health Promotion, 26*(2), 116–122. doi:10.4278/ajhp.100120-QUAN-21

Popova, S., Giesbrecht, N., Bekmuradov, D., & Patra, J. (2009). Hours and days of sale and density of alcohol outlets: Impacts on alcohol consumption and damage: A systematic review. *Alcohol and Alcoholism, 44*(5), 500–516. doi:10.1093/alcalc/agp054

Powell, L. M., & Han, E. (2011). Adult obesity and the price and availability of food in the United States. *American Journal of Agricultural Economics, 93*(2), 378–384.

Powell, L. M., Han, E., Zenk, S. N., Khan, T., Quinn, C. M., Gibbs, K. P., . . . Chaloupka, F. J. (2011). Field validation of secondary commercial data sources on the retail food outlet environment in the U.S. *Health & Place, 17*(5), 1122–1131. doi:10.1016/j.healthplace.2011.05.010

Powell, L. M., Slater, S., Mirtcheva, D., Bao, Y., & Chaloupka, F. J. (2007). Food store availability and neighborhood characteristics in the United States. *Preventive Medicine, 44*(3), 189–195. doi:10.1016/j.ypmed.2006.08.008

Reinvestment Fund. Success story: Pennsylvania Fresh Food Financing Initiative. Retrieved from https://www.reinvestment.com/success-story/pennsylvania-fresh-food-financing-initiative/

Richardson, A. S., Meyer, K. A., Howard, A. G., Boone-Heinonen, J., Popkin, B. M., Evenson, K. R., . . . Gordon-Larsen, P. (2014). Neighborhood socioeconomic status and food environment: A 20-year longitudinal latent class analysis among CARDIA participants. *Health & Place, 30*, 145–153. doi:10.1016/j.healthplace.2014.08.011

Roda, C., Charreire, H., Feuillet, T., Mackenbach, J. D., Compernolle, S., Glonti, K., . . . Oppert, J. M. (2016). Mismatch between perceived and objectively measured environmental obesogenic features in European neighbourhoods. *Obesity Review, 17* (Suppl 1), 31–41. doi:10.1111/obr.12376

Rummo, P. E., Meyer, K. A., Boone-Heinonen, J., Jacobs, D. R., Jr., Kiefe, C. I., Lewis, C. E., . . . Gordon-Larsen, P. (2015). Neighborhood availability of convenience stores and diet quality: Findings from 20 years of follow-up in the coronary artery risk development in young adults study. *American Journal of Public Health, 105*(5), e65–73.

Sadler, R. C., Clark, A. F., Wilk, P., O'Connor, C., & Gilliland, J. A. (2016). Using GPS and activity tracking to reveal the influence of adolescents' food environment exposure on junk food purchasing. *Canadian Journal of Public Health, 107*(Suppl 1), 5346. doi:10.17269/cjph.107.5346

Seto, E., Hua, J., Wu, L., Shia, V., Eom, S., Wang, M., & Li, Y. (2016). Models of individual dietary behavior based on smartphone data: The influence of routine, physical activity, emotion, and food environment. *PLoS One, 11*(4), e0153085. doi:10.1371/journal.pone.0153085

Sharkey, J. R. (2009). Measuring potential access to food stores and food-service places in rural areas in the U.S. *American Journal of Preventive Medicine, 36*(4 Suppl), S151–S155. doi:10.1016/j.amepre.2009.01.004

Shearer, C., Rainham, D., Blanchard, C., Dummer, T., Lyons, R., & Kirk, S. (2015). Measuring food availability and accessibility among adolescents: Moving beyond the neighbourhood boundary. *Social Sciences & Medicine, 133*, 322–330. doi:10.1016/j.socscimed.2014.11.019

Shier, V., An, R., & Sturm, R. (2012). Is there a robust relationship between neighbourhood food environment and childhood obesity in the USA? *Public Health, 126*(9), 723–730.

Simon, P. A., Kwan, D., Angelescu, A., Shih, M., & Fielding, J. E. (2008). Proximity of fast food restaurants to schools: Do neighborhood income and type of school matter? *Preventive Medicine, 47*(3), 284–288. doi:10.1016/j.ypmed.2008.02.021

Smith, C., & Morton, L. W. (2009). Rural food deserts: Low-income perspectives on food access in Minnesota and Iowa. *Journal of Nutrition Education and Behavior, 41*(3), 176–187. doi:10.1016/j.jneb.2008.06.008

Sturm, R., & Cohen, D. A. (2009). Zoning for health? The year-old ban on new fast-food restaurants in South LA. *Health Affairs, 28*(6), w1088–w1097.

Sturm, R., & Hattori, A. (2015). Diet and obesity in Los Angeles County 2007–2012: Is there a measurable effect of the 2008 "Fast-Food Ban"? *Social Sciences & Medicine, 133*, 205–211. Retrieved from http://www.sciencedirect.com/science/article/pii/S0277953615001409 https://www.ncbi.nlm.nih.gov/pmc/articles/PMC4410074/pdf/nihms669718.pdf

SupermarketGuru. Prepared meals will outpace foodservice, packaged foods growth. (2014). Retrieved from http://www.supermarketguru.com/articles/prepared-meals-will-outpace-foodservice,-packaged-foods-growth.html

Tabb, L. P., Ballester, L., & Grubesic, T. H. (2016). The spatio-temporal relationship between alcohol outlets and violence before and after privatization: A natural experiment, Seattle, WA 2010–2013. *Spatial and Spatiotemporal Epidemiology, 19*, 115–124. doi:10.1016/j.sste.2016.08.003

Truong, K., Fernandes, M., An, R., Shier, V., & Sturm, R. (2010). Measuring the physical food environment and its relationship with obesity: Evidence from California. *Public Health, 124*(2), 115–118. doi:10.1016/j.puhe.2009.12.004

Walker, R. E., Keane, C. R., & Burke, J. G. (2010). Disparities and access to healthy food in the United States: A review of food deserts literature. *Health & Place, 16*(5), 876–884. doi:10.1016/j.healthplace.2010.04.013

White House Task Force on Childhood Obesity. *Solving the problem of childhood obesity within a generation.* (2010). Retrieved from Washington, DC: http://www.letsmove.gov/sites/letsmove.gov/files/TaskForce_on_Childhood_Obesity_May2010_FullReport.pdf

Wilkins, E. L., Morris, M. A., Radley, D., & Griffiths, C. (2017). Using Geographic Information Systems to measure retail food environments: Discussion of methodological considerations and a proposed reporting checklist (Geo-FERN). *Health & Place*, *44*, 110–117. doi:10.1016/j.healthplace.2017.01.008

Wrigley, N., Warm, D., Margetts, B. (2003). Deprivation, diet, and food-retail access: Findings from the Leeds "food deserts" study. *Environment and Planning*, *A35*(1), 151–188.

Yousefian, A., Leighton, A., Fox, K., & Hartley, D. (2011). Understanding the rural food environment—perspectives of low-income parents. *Rural and Remote Health*, *11*(2), 1631. Retrieved from https://www.ncbi.nlm.nih.gov/pubmed/21513422

Zenk, S. N., Powell, L. M., Isgor, Z., Rimkus, L., Barker, D. C., & Chaloupka, F. J. (2015). Prepared food availability in U.S. food stores: A national study. *American Journal of Preventive Medicine*, *23*(15), 00100–00102.

Zhang, Y. T., Laraia, B. A., Mujahid, M. S., Blanchard, S. D., Warton, E. M., Moffet, H. H., & Karter, A. J. (2016). Is a reduction in distance to nearest supermarket associated with BMI change among type 2 diabetes patients? *Health & Place*, *40*, 15–20.

10

NEIGHBORHOODS, SPATIAL STIGMA, AND HEALTH

Danya E. Keene and Mark B. Padilla

A large literature has considered the way that places contribute to the health of their residents. The bulk of this literature has considered these place effects to operate through the risks and resources that are contained within a particular geographic area. However, places also carry symbolic meanings that are produced and reproduced both within and beyond the boundaries of neighborhood and communities (Bourdieu, 1999; Gieryn, 2000; Wacquant, 2007). These representations of places may have implications for the health and well-being of their residents. In particular, recent research has examined how negative representations of place, or *spatial stigmas*, adversely affect the health of those who reside in or relocate from stigmatized locales (Duncan et al., 2016; Keene & Padilla, 2014; Kelaher, Warr, Feldman, & Tacticos, 2010). This research finds that spatial stigma can affect residents' sense of self, their experiences of stress, their behaviors, and their social interactions (Keene & Padilla, 2014). It also suggests that the negative representation of structurally disadvantaged neighborhoods may be an understudied pathway that contributes to the disproportionate burden of poor health that residents of these areas experience.

In this chapter, we review the literature on spatial stigma, as it relates to neighborhood health inequality. We first describe how spatial stigma is conceptualized in the literature, both in relation to neighborhoods—which we describe here as *neighborhood stigma*—as well as other geographic areas. We then describe the pathways and processes that connect spatial or neighborhood stigma to health. We describe how stigma related to neighborhoods and place can affect access to resources, stress exposure, and identity. We also describe the agency that individuals employ to navigate, manage, and resist spatial stigma and the implications of these strategies for their health and well-being. Finally, we review the existing empirical literature that connects measures of spatial stigma to health outcomes.

SPATIAL STIGMA AND SOCIAL INEQUALITY

The concept of spatial stigma posits that those who reside in or relocate from vilified and degraded locales may become marked by a stigma of place that influences their sense of self, their access to resources, their daily experiences, and their mobility beyond their communities (Keene & Padilla, 2014). In this sense, spatial stigma can act as a degrading mark of "spoiled identity" (Goffman, 1963) that is associated with an individual's current or former home and "reduces them from a whole and usual person to a tainted and discounted one" (Goffman, 1963, p. 3).

The concept of spatial stigma is part of a growing literature on structural stigma, which describes the societal conditions, cultural norms, and institutional policies that constrain the opportunities, resources, and well-being of stigmatized groups (Hatzenbuehler & Link, 2014). Recent studies find that geographic variation in expressions of structural stigma predict geographic variations in health outcomes (Chae et al., 2015; Hatzenbuehler et al., 2014). This research introduces a spatial dimension to the existing stigma literature, examining stigma as a feature of a particular setting. The concept of spatial stigma extends this geographic focus by considering place itself as a source of stigma.

The larger structural stigma literature shows how the construction and maintenance of stigma are dependent on social, economic, and political power (Hatzenbuehler, Phelan, & Link, 2013; Parker & Aggleton, 2003). Likewise, the concept of spatial stigma is related to structural forces that produce and maintain inequality. For example, in his seminal work on "territorial stigmatization," Loic Wacquant (2007, 2008) argues that in the late 20th century, racialized urban poverty became highly spatialized in the form of geographically isolated and symbolically degraded urban ghettos. He describes "discourses of vilification" (2007, p. 67) that proliferate around and within these areas, creating a "blemish of place" (2007, p. 67) that is superimposed on existing stigmas of poverty, race, and ethnic origin. Sampson and Raudenbush (2004) empirically examine the racialization of neighborhood reputation in a study of Chicago neighborhoods. They find that the racial composition of an area significantly moderated the relationship between objective and subjective measures of neighborhood disorder such that predominantly Black neighborhoods were perceived to be more disordered than White neighborhoods, independent of objective characteristics. Their study shows how places can "inherit the stigma" of those who occupy them (Pearce, 2012). Here racial stereotypes are assigned, not only to bodies, but to neighborhoods, furthering both symbolic as well as material ghettoization (Wacquant, 2008). Similarly, these findings show how racial stigma can function through places to affect their residents. Looking beyond the boundaries of stigmatized neighborhoods, Anderson (2015) shows how the symbolic icon of the "ghetto" can act as a source of stigma that affects African Americans more broadly, regardless of their actual association with these urban spaces.

Research has also documented how racialized spatial stigma can intersect with the stigma of illness. For example, Smith-Morris (2017) illustrates how the Ebola epidemic contributed to place-based stigma for African immigrants living in the United States. Here, stigma associated with Ebola mapped onto a broad and imprecise geographic identifier of Africa. Smith-Morris explains, "While Africa and Africanness had some level of epidemiological justification for Ebola blame, the non-specificity of this prejudice merged placism with racism, allowing one to camouflage the other" (p. 112). In a similar and classic example of this process from more than four decades earlier, Haitian Americans bore the stigma of the global HIV/AIDS epidemic. Haiti was falsely accused of bringing the epidemic to the United States, when in fact the epidemiological evidence suggested the opposite was true (Farmer, 1992). Farmer argues that US anti-Haitianism was symbolically expressed in scientific theories positing the "endemic" nature of HIV/AIDS in Haiti—origin stories of AIDS that included unsubstantiated notions of blood exchange in voodoo rituals, for example, and neglected colonial and postcolonial relations of dependency and poverty that contributed to the vulnerability of Haitians to HIV infection on the island.

The concept of spatial stigma has also been applied to places that are blemished by litter, pollution, and industrial waste (Atari, Luginaah, & Baxter, 2011; Bush, Moffatt, & Dunn, 2001; Murphy, 2012; Wakefield & McMullan, 2005), or physical disorder (Draus, Roddy, & Greenwald, 2010; Graham et al., 2016). For example, in their study of spatial stigma in Detroit, Graham and colleagues (2016) describe how structural abandonment, deindustrialization the global outsourcing of labor markets, and resultant conditions of urban decay contributed to a symbolic marginalization that Detroit residents experienced, and in some cases resisted. Such examples demonstrate that as political-economic conditions evolve, such as the collapse of industrial zones in Detroit, the contours and expression of spatial stigma can similarly transform. Thus historicization is required to fully grasp spatial stigma as it operates in specific settings and populations.

SPATIAL STIGMA PATHWAYS AND PROCESSES

The existing literature provides a framework for thinking about the multiple processes through which spatial or neighborhood stigma can operate to affect health outcomes and health behaviors. We summarize these processes in the next section, focusing on the following questions: (1) How does spatial stigma limit access to resources that promote health and protect against illness? (2) How does spatial stigma contribute to psychosocial stress and its negative health sequelae? (3) How does spatial stigma contribute to a sense of self and identity formation? (4) How do those who reside in or relocate from stigmatized locales manage and resist spatial stigma, with implications for their health and well-being?

Access to Resources

A central function of stigma is the exclusion of individuals from resources that they need to support their life chances and well-being (Link & Phelan, 2001). Both qualitative and quantitative studies have documented the role that neighborhood reputation can play in limiting access to health-promoting resources for residents of socially marginalized neighborhoods. For example, research finds that neighborhood stigma serves as a barrier to employment among residents of disadvantaged neighborhoods (Moss, Kirschenman, & Kennelly, 2001). Extending this research on spatial stigma and economic opportunity, Besbris and colleagues (2015) used an experimental audit study design to compare responses to classified advertisements (posted to Craigslist) based on the neighborhood of the seller. They found that advertisements from disadvantaged neighborhoods received significantly fewer responses than advertisements from more advantaged neighborhoods, suggesting that negative conceptions of neighborhoods influence the prospects for economic exchange among those who reside in them. By limiting employment options and other economic opportunities, neighborhood stigma can serve to limit both economic and neighborhood mobility. As Kelaher et al. (2010, p. 386) note, neighborhood stigma may be quite literally a way of keeping people "in their place."

Additionally, research finds that spatial stigma can shape access to health-promoting, or even health-essential services within stigmatized neighborhoods. A Glasgow-based study finds that residents of disadvantaged neighborhoods experienced more denial of emergency medical services than residents of more advantaged neighborhoods, likely in part due to stigma (Macintyre & Ellaway, 2003). Similarly, in their Harlem-based ethnography (see Chapter 7), Mullings and Wali (1999) describe delays in ambulance service that residents attributed to the reputation of their neighborhoods. Relatedly, in qualitative interviews, former Chicago public housing residents describe, how stigmatization of their housing complexes reduced their access to healthcare resources. For example, one participant noted, "Therapists would come to the home, you know to do therapy on their children, but with me, they wouldn't even come you know, people shut down on us because of where we lived" (McCormick, Joseph, & Chaskin, 2012, p. 293).

Some research also suggests that spatial stigma can be carried to new destinations, where it can contribute to ongoing marginalization, and reduced access to resources and opportunities. For example, in our qualitative study of low-income African American Chicago residents who had moved to eastern Iowa in search of safer communities and affordable housing, participants described how racialized stereotypes of Chicago's urban neighborhoods constrained their opportunities in multiple ways. As one participant stated, "Well, it's like when you say you're from Chicago around certain people and I ain't just going to say the police, I'm saying other people like, if you're trying to get housing or some kind of low income for your family, it's like they discriminate on you because you say where you're from, Chicago" (Keene & Padilla, 2010, p. 1219).

These examples illustrate how spatial stigma that is enacted by outsiders and attributed to residents of stigmatized areas may function to limit access to resources. Alternatively, when stigma is anticipated by those who reside in a stigmatized area, it may prevent them from seeking health supporting resources. For example, Collins and colleagues (2016) show how the placement of HIV services in a stigmatized neighborhood, Toronto's Downtown Eastside, reduced their utilization by those residents who had moved out of this neighborhood and wanted to distance themselves from it. For these relocated residents, the stigma associated with their former neighborhood also created challenges as they attempted to access services outside of the Downtown Eastside.

On a structural level, the meanings that places hold may also reinforce their existing material conditions and further limit access to health-promoting resources for their residents. Grocery stores, businesses, and regional investments that can contribute to the health of neighborhood residents may avoid stigmatized places (Eisenhauer, 2001). Likewise, real-estate values may be strongly affected by spatial stigma, thereby reducing wealth acquisition for residents of these areas, (Musterd & Andersson, 2006). Thus, the effects of stigma can be multilayered, exerting themselves on both individuals and the places in which they reside.

When spatial stigma undermines property values in disadvantaged areas, it can also pave the way for gentrification, community dispossession, and displacement. It can also be employed by those in power for the purpose of appropriating places that are occupied by economically and racially marginalized populations (Bennett & Reed, 1999; Gans, 1990). For example, Kallin and Slater (2014) show how spatial stigma was employed by the state to justify gentrification of industrial neighborhoods outside of Edinburgh, and the resulting economic displacement of their residents. Though such gentrification may lead to neighborhood improvements, associated increases in housing costs, and displacement can contribute to poor health among economically marginalized residents of gentrifying areas.

Interpersonal Discrimination and Psychosocial Stress

To the extent that spatial stigma excludes individuals from resources, it can act as a source of chronic stress that has detrimental consequences for mental and physical health (Keene & Padilla, 2014). Furthermore, spatial stigma may lead to interpersonal discrimination that can create stress responses. For example, qualitative interviews with residents in an impoverished Australian neighborhood find experiences of social rejection following disclosure of their residence. As one participant says about revealing the name of her neighborhood, "You've lost them there. They don't want to know you" (Warr, 2005, p. 298). Similarly, research conducted in a disadvantaged neighborhood in Scotland finds that experiences of spatial stigma contributed to psychosocial distress, anger, and shame among neighborhood residents (Airey, 2003).

For participants in our Iowa research, negative perceptions of Chicago seemed to be a source of stress even after they had moved away. For example, one participant described the way Chicago migrants were repeatedly vilified in local media and often blamed for crime and drug activity. She explained, "It's just Chicago, Chicago, Chicago, everywhere you go. It makes me mad when they say Chicago, Chicago, Chicago, when this is happening all over the United States. There was drugs in Iowa long before anyone from Chicago ever came" (Keene & Padilla, 2010, p. 1218).

Similarly, a study of former Chicago public housing residents who had relocated to newly constructed, mixed-income developments in that city described ongoing experiences of stress that were associated with the stigmatization of "the projects." As one respondent explained when describing a community meeting in her new mixed-income housing complex, "And the lady [homeowner] was sitting up there saying, 'I'm telling everything. The people from the projects, they ain't no good.' I'm from the projects but I didn't say nothing. I'm getting heated and my blood getting heated" (McCormick, Joseph, & Chaskins, 2012, p. 302). Here, the respondent's experience of getting "heated" upon hearing negative comments about her former home and its residents points to the potential physical effects of exposure to stigma-related stress. Some research suggests that discrimination and related psychosocial stress may also contribute to unhealthy coping behaviors in stigmatized neighborhoods (Stead, MacAskill, MacKintosh, Reece, & Eadie, 2001).

Research also suggests that one way residents of stigmatized areas avoid discrimination and stress associated with spatial stigma is by concealing their neighborhood of residence or neighborhood of origin (Keene & Padilla, 2010; Palmer, Ziersch, Arthurson, & Baum, 2004; Wacquant, 2007; Warr, 2005). While this may help individuals to avoid the negative interactions described earlier, stigma research suggests that the process of concealment itself can be stressful and health demoting

(Chaudoir, Earnshaw, & Andel, 2013; Pachankis, 2007). For example, research on minority stress among populations vulnerable to HIV/AIDS demonstrates that the felt need to conceal aspects of the self can lead to chronic stress, contributing to HIV risk and undermining prevention and treatment outcomes (Meyer, Schwartz, & Frost, 2008). Concealment related to spatial stigma may operate in a similar way.

Identity Formation and Management

Negative perceptions of place that are held by others affect the health and well-being of those who reside in stigmatized areas. However, these spatial stigmas can also be internalized in ways that affect health. A significant amount of literature has examined the relationships between place and identity (Dixon & Durrheim, 2000) and has also described the threats to self-esteem that are associated with living in discredited places (Bolam, Murphy, & Gleeson, 2006). This literature raises important questions about the connection between spatial stigma and identity formation, about the ways that individuals manage the spatial stigma that they experience, and whether and how they attribute these qualities to themselves.

Several studies have described how individuals who reside in a stigmatized locale manage this stigma in order to construct positive identities (Castro & Lindbladh, 2004; Fast, Shoveller, Shannon, & Kerr, 2010; Garbin & Millington, 2011; Keene & Padilla, 2010; Popay et al., 2003; Thomas, 2016). For example, some studies find that residents of stigmatized neighborhoods attempt to create symbolic distance between themselves and neighborhood stigma by differentiating their specific area from other parts of the neighborhood (Popay, 2003; Thomas, 2016). They create what Popay (2003) refers to as "subtle cartographies of difference" to positively define their own homes, while denigrating other portions of the neighborhood.

Residents of stigmatized areas may also manage this stigma by symbolically or physically distancing themselves from their neighbors. For example, research finds that some residents of stigmatized areas engage in a discursive strategy of lateral denigration that accepts the stigmatizing discourse, but applies it to neighbors, rather than themselves (Thomas, 2016; Wacquant, 2007). Other research finds that residents of stigmatized places may mange these negative representations by withdrawing to the private sphere of their homes (Castro & Lindbladh, 2004; Wacquant, 2007). These forms of discursive and physical distancing may be effective personal strategies for negotiating stigmatized identities and stigmatized landscapes. However, these strategies may also have consequences for individual and collective well-being by weakening the social fabric of marginalized communities and limiting residents' access to health-promoting, community-based, social support resources. Additionally, the withdrawal from collective life that participants describe may reduce the ability of neighborhood residents to advocate for their collective well-being (Keene & Padilla, 2014).

In contrast, other research describes the way that residents of stigmatized neighborhoods manage to create strong social ties within their communities despite stigma (August, 2014; Thomas, 2016; Wutich, Ruth, Brewis, & Boone, 2014). For example, August (2014) describes how residents of Toronto's Regent Park housing estate valued this stigmatized community as an anchor for the deep webs of friendship and collective life that it held. Similarly, Thomas (2016) finds that residents of one stigmatized neighborhood in the United Kingdom describe social relationships as a positive feature of their community that is often ignored in primarily negative media portrayals.

Research also shows how residents of stigmatized communities have come together to actively reject spatial stigma, by speaking out against it, by emphasizing the positive features of their neighborhoods, and by advocating for more balanced media representation (Kirkness, 2014; Slater, 2015; Thomas, 2016). In his account of resistance to spatial stigma among residents of defamed housing estates in France, Kirkness (2014) shows that "territorial stigmatization can lead to the strengthening of networks of solidarity and a deepening attachment to place" (p. 1285), as residents come together in solidarity against those who stigmatize them. Though this resistance may be beneficial to stigmatized communities and their residents, this active fight against stigma may also consume time, energy, and resources, and produce stress that is health demoting.

OPERATIONALIZING SPATIAL STIGMA AND MEASURING ASSOCIATIONS WITH HEALTH

Although the majority of existing research on spatial stigma has been qualitative in nature, documenting experiences and processes associated with the stigmatization of place, emerging research has operationalized this concept and empirically measured its association with health outcomes. For example, Kelaher (2010) and colleagues operationalize spatial stigma as an assessment of reputation, asking survey participants to report their agreement with the following statement: "Generally, this neighborhood has a good reputation with people living in the surrounding area." They find that residents who live in more disadvantaged "renewal areas" of Victoria, Australia, report less agreement with this statement that those who reside outside of renewal areas. They also find that perceptions of more positive neighborhood reputations are associated with better self-rated health, independent of other measured individual and neighborhood characteristics.

Going beyond self-reported health, Duncan and colleagues (2016) examine how perceptions of spatial stigma are associated with obesity and high blood pressure among a sample of low-income subsidized housing residents in New York City. They operationalize spatial stigma as a function of neighborhood reputation, representation in the media, and discrimination. Specifically, they ask survey respondents the following four questions: What is the reputation of this neighborhood? What is the image of the neighborhood in the media? Are people who live in your neighborhood seen negatively? Do you feel that people judge you because you live in low-income subsidized housing? Controlling for a range of neighborhood characteristics, they find that participants who report living in a neighborhood with a bad reputation have higher body mass index (BMI) as well as higher systolic blood pressure and diastolic blood pressure. A related study, conducted with the same sample, finds that perceived negative media representation of one's neighborhood is negatively associated with both poor sleep quality and shorter sleep duration (Ruff et al., 2016). These findings speak to the potential role of stress, manifesting here as sleep disruption, in mediating relationships between spatial stigma and health outcomes.

Whereas the aforementioned studies focus on the reputational aspects of spatial stigma, Tabuchi and colleagues (2012) focus specifically on discrimination associated with place of residence, a concept they refer to as "geographically based discrimination." They consider discrimination associated with two types of geography. First, they consider the Buraku district, a neighborhood that was historically home to a marginalized class of workers. Although the ancestry of this marginalized group is not documented in the Japanese census, place of residence has become a marker of this stigmatized identity. Second, they examine stigma associated with Nishinari ward, an area marked by poverty and poor housing, and held in almost universal poor esteem by the media and residents of surrounding areas. They ask residents of one Buraku district in the Nishinari ward of Osaka, Japan, whether they are "treated with a lack of courtesy, threatened or harassed by any kind of discrimination." The survey then asks about reasons for reported discrimination, including living in their district, living in their ward, and a range of other demographic characteristics. They find that geographically based discrimination associated with both ward and district is significantly and positively associated with depressive symptoms and mental illness diagnosis, independent of socioeconomic status, social relationship, and lifestyle factors.

The surveys described earlier employ different measures to capture various dimensions of spatial stigma. Future research may be able to develop a more comprehensive instrument that assesses residents' experiences of spatial stigma across geographies and their associations with health outcomes. Future research may also be able to assess spatial stigma as a neighborhood-level variable by aggregating survey responses across neighborhood residents (Duncan et al., 2016). In constructing neighborhood-level measures of spatial stigma, it may also be useful for future research to move beyond the perceptions of disadvantaged neighborhood residents themselves (the stigmatized) to consider the perspectives and actions of those who produce and enact spatial stigma (the stigmatizers). Content analyses of newspaper reports, analyses of Google search terms, and data on taxi cab or food delivery refusals may all be useful in constructing neighborhood-level variables that capture forms of enacted spatial stigma. Neighborhood measures of both perceived and enacted spatial stigma can be used to examine the contributions of spatial stigma to health variation across neighborhoods.

CONCLUSION

The literature described herein considers the various pathways through which spatial stigma may operate and also begins to operationalize this concept and relate it to health outcomes. Our discussion points to spatial stigma as an important understudied mechanism by which spatialized social inequalities contribute to health disparities, particularly in predominantly minority urban areas that are often marked by stigmas of race, class, and underresourced physical environments.

Although the growing literature on spatial stigma represents a new concept for the study of neighborhood effects, it also represents a fundamental departure from this literature. Rather than focusing on the conditions that exist within disadvantaged neighborhoods, and are considered to be the cause of poor health for their residents, spatial stigma turns our attention to a "gaze that is trained on the neighborhood" (Slater & Hannigan, 2015, p. 12). Though spatial stigma may be reproduced, or contested within neighborhoods, it is predominantly produced by neighborhood outsiders; in the media; and in public, political, or even academic discourse. Indeed, it is possible that by locating the problems that disadvantaged neighborhoods face within their boundaries, academic research on neighborhood effects may unintentionally contribute to spatial stigma. Well-intentioned research that makes presumptions about the conditions of stigmatized neighborhoods may be unwittingly replicating the denigrating discourses associated with them in the first place.

The concept of spatial stigma turns our attention away from causes of poor health that are inherent to the neighborhood to focus attention on the ways that broader societal meanings and cultural logics are manifested and expressed in specific local settings (Keene & Padilla, 2014). From this perspective, the expression of spatial stigma in many predominantly minority and high-poverty urban areas cannot be separated from the global, structural, and symbolic systems that shape the conditions of these spaces and the (often racialized) tropes that circulate widely about their "failings." In order to move beyond a framing of spatial stigma that confines itself to conditions within spaces, the conceptual frameworks that inform research and policy initiatives need to be expanded to include region, national, and global contexts within which knowledge about place is produced. Research and policy analysis that can trace pathways connecting global discourses to the production and maintenance of spatial stigma may ultimately be able to develop strategies for disrupting or reversing them.

Theoretical frameworks emerging from Foucauldian critiques of knowledge and power can foreground the contingent nature of the knowledge produced about places, and can provoke the kind of critical reflection about representation that is necessary for researchers working on the social construction of space (Parker & Aggleton, 2003). Additionally, community collaboration and dissemination of research on spatial stigma can help ensure that scientific knowledge is grounded in the realities and cognizant of the stakes of these symbolic representations, and foster means of constructively responding to spatial stigma in innovative ways. Finally, taking spatial stigma seriously requires an awareness of the fact that, scientific research on the health implications of spatial stigma is necessary but not sufficient to address the marginalization of denigrated areas or prevent their resulting health effects. Research must be paired with reflexive attention to the historical context of spatial stigma and to the inevitable participation of science in the shape and boundaries of the discourses that produce it.

REFERENCES

Airey, L. (2003). "Nae as nice a scheme as it used to be": Lay accounts of neighbourhood incivilities and well-being. *Health & place*, *9*(2), 129–137.

Anderson, E. (2015). The white space. *Sociology of Race and Ethnicity*, *1*(1), 10–21.

Atari, D. O., Luginaah, I., & Baxter, J. (2011). "This is the mess that we are living in": Residents everyday life experiences of living in a stigmatized community. *GeoJournal*, *76*(5), 483–500.

August, M. (2014). Challenging the rhetoric of stigmatization: The benefits of concentrated poverty in Toronto' s Regent Park. *Environment and Planning A*, *46*, 1317–1333.

Bennett, L., & Reed, A. (1999). The new face of urban renewal: The Near North Redevelopment Initiative and the Cabrini-Green neighborhood. In A. Reed (Ed.), *Without justice for all: The New Liberalism and our retreat from racial equality* (pp. 176–192). Boulder, CO: Westview Press.

Besbris, M., Faber, J. W., Rich, P., & Sharkey, P. (2015). Effect of neighborhood stigma on economic transactions. *Proceedings of the National Academy of Sciences*, *112*(16), 4994–4998.

Bolam, B., Murphy, S., & Gleeson, K. (2006). Place-identity and geographical inequalities in health: A qualitative study. *Psychology & Health*, *21*(3), 399–420. http://doi.org/10.1080/14768320500286526

Bourdieu, P. (1999). Site effects. In P. Bourdieu (Ed.), *The weight of the world* (pp. 123–130). Stanford, CA: Stanford University Press.

Bush, J., Moffatt, S., & Dunn, C. (2001). "Even the birds round here cough": Stigma, air pollution and health in Teesside. *Health & Place, 7*, 47–56.

Castro, P. B., & Lindbladh, E. (2004). Place, discourse and vulnerability—a qualitative study of young adults living in a Swedish urban poverty zone. *Health & Place, 10*(3), 259–272.

Chae, D. H., Clouston, S., Hatzenbuehler, M. L., Kramer, M. R., Cooper, H. L. F., Wilson, S. M., . . . Link, B. G. (2015). Association between an internet-based measure of area racism and black mortality. *PLoS ONE, 10*(4), 1–12.

Chaudoir, S. R., Earnshaw, V. A., & Andel, S. (2013). "Discredited" versus "discreditable": Understanding how shared and unique stigma mechanisms affect psychological and physical health disparities. *Basic and Applied Social Psychology, 35*(1), 75–87.

Collins, A. B., Parashar, S., Closson, K., Turje, R. B., Strike, C., & McNeil, R. (2016). Navigating identity, territorial stigma, and HIV care services in Vancouver, Canada: A qualitative study. *Health and Place, 40*, 169–177. http://doi.org/10.1016/j.healthplace.2016.06.005

Dixon, J., & Durrheim, K. (2000). Displacing place-identity: A discursive approach to locating self and other. *British Journal of Social Psychology, 39*(1), 27–44.

Draus, P. J., Roddy, J. K., & Greenwald, M. (2010). A hell of a life: Addiction and marginality in post-industrial Detroit. *Social & Cultural Geography, 11*(7), 663–680.

Duncan, D. T., Ruff, R. R., Chaix, B., Regan, S. D., Williams, J. H., Ravenell, J., . . . York, N. (2016). Perceived spatial stigma, body mass index and blood pressure: A global positioning system study among low-income housing residents in New York City. *Geospatial Health, 11*, 1–4.

Eisenhauer, E. (2001). In poor health: Supermarket redlining and urban nutrition. *GeoJournal, 53*(2), 125–133.

Farmer, P. (1992). *AIDS and accusation: Haiti and the geography of blame*. Berkeley: University of California Press.

Fast, D., Shoveller, J., Shannon, K., & Kerr, T. (2010). Safety and danger in downtown Vancouver: Understandings of place among young people entrenched in an urban drug scene. *Health & Place, 16*(1), 51–60.

Gans, H. (1990). Deconstructing the underclass: The term's dangers as a planning voncept. *Journal of the American Planning Association, 56*(3), 271–277.

Garbin, D., & Millington, G. (2011). Territorial stigma and the politics of resistance in a Parisian banlieue: La Courneuve and beyond. *Urban Studies, 49*(10), 2067–2083.

Gieryn, T. F. (2000). A space for place in sociology. *Annual Review of Sociology, 26*, 463–496.

Goffman, E. (1963). *Stigma: Notes on the management of a spoiled identity*. New York, NY: Simon and Shuster.

Graham, L. F., Padilla, M. B., Lopez, W. D., Stern, A. M., Peterson, J., & Keene, D. E. (2016). Spatial stigma and health in postindustrial Detroit. *International Quarterly of Community Health Education, 36*(2), 105–113.

Hatzenbuehler, M. L., Bellatorre, A., Lee, Y., Finch, B. K., Muennig, P., & Fiscella, K. (2014). Structural stigma and all-cause mortality in sexual minority populations. *Social Science and Medicine, 103*, 33–41.

Hatzenbuehler, M. L., & Link, B. G. (2014). Introduction to the special issue on structural stigma and health. *Social Science & Medicine (1982), 103*, 1–6.

Hatzenbuehler, M. L., Phelan, J. C., & Link, B. G. (2013). Stigma as a fundamental cause of population health inequalities. *American Journal of Public Health, 103*(5), 813–821.

Kallin, H., & Slater, T. (2014). Activating territorial stigma: Gentrifying marginality on Edinburgh's periphery. *Environment and Planning A*, *46*(6), 1351–1368.

Keene, D., & Padilla, M. (2010). Race, class and the stigma of place: Moving to "opportunity" in Eastern Iowa. *Health & Place*, *16*(6), 1216–1223.

Keene, D., & Padilla, M. (2014). Spatial stigma and health inequality. *Critical Public Health*, March, 1–13.

Kelaher, M., Warr, D. J., Feldman, P., & Tacticos, T. (2010). Living in "Birdsville": Exploring the impact of neighbourhood stigma on health. *Health & Place*, *16*(2), 381–8.

Kirkness, P. (2014). The cités strike back: Restive responses to territorial taint in the French banlieues. *Environment and Planning A*, *46*(6), 1281–1296.

Link, B. G., & Phelan, J. C. (2001). Conceptualizing stigma. *Annual Review of Sociology*, *27*, 363–385.

Macintyre, S., & Ellaway, A. (2003). An overview. In I. Kawachi & L. F. Berkman (Eds.), *Neighborhoods and health*. Cambridge, UK: Oxford University Press.

McCormick, N. J., Joseph, M. L., & Chaskin, R. J. (2012). The new stigma of relocated public housing residents: Challenges to social Identity in mixed-income developments. *City & Community*, *11*(3), 285–308.

Meyer, I. H., Schwartz, S., & Frost, D. M. (2008). Social patterning of stress and coping: Does disadvantaged social statuses confer more stress and fewer coping resources? *Social Science and Medicine*, *67*(3), 368–379.

Mullings, L., & Wali, A. (1999). *Stress and resilience: The social context of reproduction in Central Harlem*. New York, NY: Kluwer Academic/Plenum.

Murphy, A. K. (2012). Litterers. *The ANNALS of the American Academy of Political and Social Science*, *642*(1), 210–227.

Musterd, S., & Andersson, R. (2006). Employment, social ,mobility and neighbourhood effects: The case of Sweden. *International Journal of Urban and Regional Research*, *30*(1), 120–140.

Pachankis, J. E. (2007). The psychological implications of concealing a stigma: A cognitive-affective-behavioral model. *Psychological Bulletin*, *133*(2), 328–345.

Palmer, C., Ziersch, A., Arthurson, K., & Baum, F. (2004). Challenging the stigma of public housing: Preliminary findings from a qualitative study in South Australia. *Urban Policy & Research*, *22*(4), 411–426.

Parker, R., & Aggleton, P. (2003). HIV and AIDS-related stigma and discrimination: A conceptual framework and implications for action. *Social Science & Medicine*, *57*(1), 13–24.

Pearce, J. (2012). The "blemish of place": Stigma, geography and health inequalities. A commentary on Tabuchi, Fukuhara, & Iso. *Social Science and Medicine*, *75*(11), 1921–1924.

Popay, J., Thomas, C., Williams, G., Bennett, S., Gatrell, A., & Bostock, L. (2003). A proper place to live: Health inequalities, agency and the normative dimensions of space. *Social Science and Medicine*, *57*(1), 55–69.

Ruff, R., Ng, J., Jean-Louis, G., Elbel, B., Chaix, B., & Duncan, D. (2016). Neighborhood stigma and sleep: Findings from a pilot study of low-income housing residents in New York City. *Behavioral Medicine*, 1–6.

Sampson, R. J., & Raudenbush, S. W. (2004). Seeing disorder: Neighborhood stigma and the social construction of "broken windows." *Social Psychology Quarterly*, *67*(4), 319–342.

Slater, T. (2015). Territorial stigmatization: Symbolic defamation and the contemporany metropolis. In J. Hannigan & G. Richards (Eds.), *The Handbook of New Urban Studies* (pp. 111–125). Sage Publications.

Smith-Morris, C. (2017). Epidemiological placism in public health emergencies: Ebola in two Dallas neighborhoods. *Social Science & Medicine, 179*, 106–114.

Stead, M., MacAskill, S., MacKintosh, A.-M., Reece, J., & Eadie, D. (2001). "It's as if you're locked in": Qualitative explanations for area effects on smoking in disadvantaged communities. *Health & Place, 7*(4), 333–343.

Tabuchi, T., Fukuhara, H., & Iso, H. (2012). Geographically-based discrimination is a social determinant of mental health in a deprived or stigmatized area in Japan: A cross-sectional study. *Social Science & Medicine, 75*(6), 1015–1021.

Thomas, G. M. (2016). "It"s not that bad': Stigma, health, and place in a post-industrial community. *Health and Place, 38*, 1–7.

Tilly, C., Moss, P., Kirschenman, J., & Kennelly, I. C. (2001). Space as a signal: How employers perceive neighborhoods in four metropolitan labor markets. In C. T. and L. B. Alice O'Connor (Eds.), *Urban inequality: Evidence from four cities* (pp. 304–338). New York, NY: Russell Sage.

Wacquant, L. (2007). Territorial stigmatization in the age of advanced marginality. *Thesis Eleven, 91*(1), 66–77.

Wacquant, L. (2008). *Urban outcasts.* Cambridge, UK: Polity Press.

Wakefield, S., & McMullan, C. (2005). Healing in places of decline: (Re)imagining everyday landscapes in Hamilton, Ontario. *Health & Place, 11*(4), 299–312.

Warr, D. (2005). There goes the neighborhood. *Social City, 19*, 1–10.

Wutich, A., Ruth, A., Brewis, A., & Boone, C. (2014). Stigmatized neighborhoods, social bonding, and health. *Medical Anthropology Quarterly, 28*(4), 556–577.

11

NEIGHBORHOOD FORECLOSURES AND HEALTH

Mariana C. Arcaya

The year 2007 marked the beginning of an international financial and housing crisis, which, in the United States, was characterized by a drop in residential construction, steep declines in home prices, widespread mortgage delinquency, and a "foreclosure epidemic" (Bennett, Scharoun-Lee, & Tucker-Seeley, 2009; Joint Center for Housing Studies, 2010). In 2010 at the peak of the US crisis, roughly 2.8 million mortgages were subject to foreclosure notices, which, in just over 1 million cases, resulted in bank repossession of the home (RealtyTrac, 2011a). Expressed as a share of the nation's housing stock, these 2.8 million mortgages were held on about 2.2% of the country's housing units (RealtyTrac, 2011a). All told, over 9.4 million US homes have been lost to foreclosure and related mechanisms, such as "short sales" that can allow borrowers to avoid foreclosure when a home is worth less than is owed on the mortgage, since 2007 (Joint Center for Housing Studies, 2016).

These statistics caught the interest of public health researchers and practitioners in the midst of the crisis, prompting warnings that housing distress and many of its sequelae are well-documented health risk factors for individuals undergoing foreclosure, and that the community-level effects of foreclosure activity could also harm residents regardless of their personal housing exposures (Alameda County Public Health Department & Causa Justa, 2010; Bennett et al., 2009; Pollard, 2008; Raitt & Arcaya, 2010). Since the start of the crisis, over 40 empirical papers have been published examining foreclosure as a health risk factor. This chapter describes and interprets the current state of the evidence in four parts. First, I introduce the foreclosure process itself, which is critical to conceptualizing the mechanisms by which neighborhood-level foreclosure activity could exert a contextual influence on health. Second, I review the direct effects foreclosure activity has on neighborhood environments, as well as the evidence that these neighborhood conditions affect health. Third, I describe findings from empirical research on the health effects of neighborhood-level foreclosure activity. Finally, I close by interpreting the current evidence base and recommending future research directions.

THE FORECLOSURE PROCESS

Taking out a mortgage to purchase a home is, in many ways, no different than taking on any other sort of debt. In most cases, a lender and borrower enter into a legal agreement under which the lender advances the borrower a sum of money with specified repayment conditions. The borrower uses this money to purchase a home with the understanding that a newly purchased property secures the lender's investment. Just as failure to make car payments results in the repossession of a car, and falling short on student loans may lead to garnished wages, borrowers can lose their homes if they violate their mortgage contracts. When a borrower fails to make regular, in-full payments, the lender has a legal right to recover the full outstanding balance of the loan by seizing the collateral that secures the loan—in this case, the borrower's home. The events that occur from the time a lender begins to go about recovering an outstanding balance until the time the balance is paid off or made current is called the "foreclosure process" (Figure 11-1).

In other ways, a home mortgage is a unique form of debt. Policy makers have provided more protection for borrowers who fail to make payments on a home than is provided to those who fail to make others sorts of payments. US foreclosure laws, though they vary from state to state, generally require, as protection for homeowners, that lenders give advance warning before they seize a home, and that there be

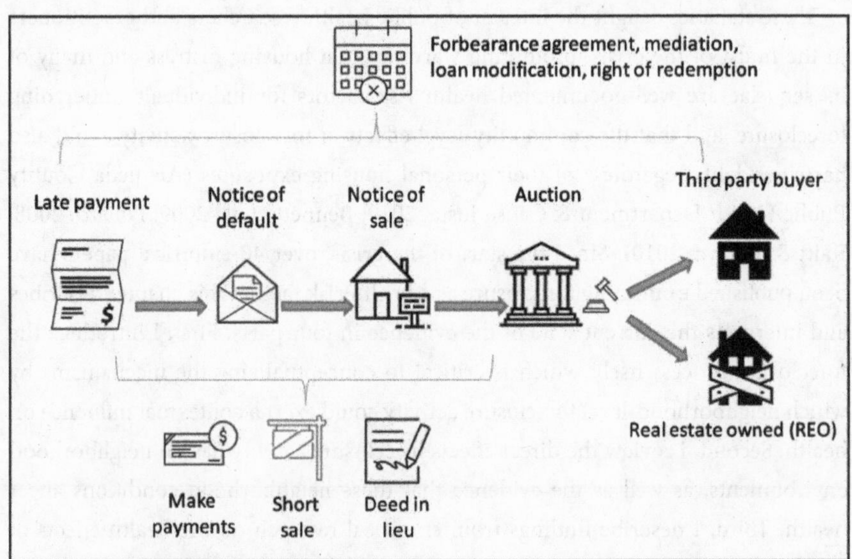

FIGURE 11-1 The foreclosure process.

opportunities for borrowers to catch up on payments. As the first step in the foreclosure process, a lender must send official notice to the borrower that the loan is in default and that the lender intends to seize the securing property. This notice is generally sent when a borrower has not made any mortgage payments in the past 60–90 days; this is called a "notice of default" (NOD) or "*lis pendens*" (LP), meaning "notice of pending lawsuit." NOD and LP filings indicate that a mortgage is in the preforeclosure stage, during which borrowers can make up late payments. If, after receiving one of these preforeclosure filings, borrowers do not become current on their payments, the bank moves to scheduling an auction, at which the home will be sold if a bid is made for the amount of the outstanding balance or higher. At this stage, the lender is required to post a notice announcing the public auction date, called a "Notice of Foreclosure Sale" (NFS), "Notice of Trustee Sale" (NTS), or simply a "Notice of Sale" (NOS). Lenders are usually required to list such notices in local newspapers, in a letter to the borrower, and often on signs at the property. Generally, a notice of sale must be filed 3–4 weeks prior to the auction date to give the borrower time to reinstate a loan by making payments, though the exact timeline varies by state. If the home is purchased at auction, the foreclosure is complete and a new owner becomes responsible for the property. In many cases, however, the home does not sell and the property is designated real estate owned (REO). At this point, the home often sits vacant as the bank tries to resell it on the regular market (RealtyTrac, 2011c).

Generically, the official notices described earlier, including LP, NOD, NTS, NFS, NOS, and REO, are called "foreclosure filings" or "foreclosure notices." "Foreclosure starts" include NOD and LP filings, while "completed foreclosures" comprise all foreclosure starts that ended in repossession. When the popular news media uses the term *foreclosure* to describe a specific property, as in "she lives next door to a foreclosure," this is usually shorthand for bank-owned, or REO, property. The "foreclosure inventory" refers to the total number of properties in foreclosure in a given place at a given time.

Home Mortgage Delinquencies

Foreclosure is only one manifestation of housing market distress; tracking delinquencies, which precede foreclosures, is important for several reasons. First, official foreclosure statistics may underestimate the true extent of housing distress. Borrowers who fall behind on mortgage payments and know they will not be able to catch up often prefer to sell their homes in "preforeclosure short sales" to avoid having foreclosures recorded on their credit histories. A preforeclosure short sale is one in which the borrower sells his or her home for less than the outstanding balance on the loan during the preforeclosure period, and uses the money to pay off the mortgage. Banks may also prefer to acquire homes through preforeclosure sales even if it means they must accept less than the outstanding balance of the loan. Such sales circumvent the lengthy, expensive, and often controversial foreclosure process. With each foreclosure costing lenders an estimated $50,000 and many months to complete (Apgar, Duda, Gorey, & Council, 2005), it is often in the bank's interest to seek an alternative to the foreclosure process. In practice, preforeclosure short sales function much like completed foreclosures; borrowers keep no profit from selling their homes and are forced to move. Because the lender is the new owner in some arrangements that serve as foreclosure alternatives, the property may also sit vacant just like an REO that failed to sell at auction. Foreclosure filings do not capture such transactions, but the mortgage distress that precedes them is documented in delinquency records.

Delinquencies may also give early warning of upcoming foreclosure activity, and they are usually reported along with foreclosure statistics in order to give a sense of how many loans are vulnerable to the official foreclosure process (Duke, 2010).

Heterogeneity in the Foreclosure Process

Although the foreclosure process is structured similarly across the United States, state and local conditions that help shape the foreclosure experience, and therefore its effects on communities and individuals, are highly variable. The prevalence of foreclosure activity also varies greatly.

State-level policy is critical in determining how long the foreclosure process takes and how much protection a borrower has along the way. For example, the required redemption period from the first notice of default to the auction, during which borrowers have the chance to catch up on payments, varies greatly by state. State location also matters for how borrowers subject to foreclosure are treated after an auction. Some US states offer a "right of redemption," meaning that for a certain number of weeks after an auction, the original borrower can make past-due payments and legally reclaim the home. States also determine if separate eviction proceedings are required apart from the foreclosure process, meaning that the original borrower may have the right to stay in the home even after it has been sold to a new buyer at auction, or while it is REO. In all, state-level factors cause the foreclosure timeline to range from less than 2 months in Texas, to over a year in New York (RealtyTrac, 2011b), and they can determine how likely it is that foreclosure will result in eviction. State-level factors also drive whether lenders must make their case before a judge, proving ownership of the mortgage debt, in order to foreclose. Local policy is the main driver of how REO and vacant properties are handled, including whether sidewalks are shoveled and how properties are otherwise maintained when not occupied. These sorts of local decisions influence what type of neighborhood-level impact the foreclosure process may have. Finally, local housing market conditions and neighborhood-level factors, which may include the existing density of REOs, determine how easily homes sell at auction and for how long they are vacant if they do not sell.

Heterogeneity in both the individual and community impact of foreclosure is also caused by—and reflected in—the varying prevalence of mortgage distress by state, city, and neighborhood. Five states, Arizona, California, Florida, Michigan, and Illinois, accounted for half the foreclosure activity in the nation at the peak of the recent 2007—2011 crisis despite the fact that they comprised much less than half of the housing. In Nevada, 9.4% of properties were subject to foreclosure in 2010, which was over four times the estimated national rate of 2.2% (RealtyTrac, 2011a). The degree of foreclosure activity is an important source of heterogeneity both because the sheer number of properties in foreclosure varies, and because the marginal impact of each REO may change in relation to how many other REOs are nearby (Harding, Rosenblatt, & Yao, 2009; Rogers & Winter, 2009; Schuetz, Been, & Ellen, 2008).

LOCALIZED FORECLOSURE ACTIVITY AND EFFECTS ON NEIGHBORHOOD ENVIRONMENTS

Neighborhood-level foreclosure activity has strong theoretical relevance as a contextual health risk factor. Many of the neighborhood outcomes that have shown to be sensitive to foreclosure activity are also upstream contextual determinants of health. Figure 11-2 summarizes some of the salient pathways by which neighborhood foreclosure rates may influence health, and the evidence for these pathways is described briefly next.

Lower Property Values and Financial Uncertainty for Neighbors

It is estimated that a completed foreclosure carries an economic cost of nearly $80,000. While about $57,000 of this is thought to be borne jointly by the lender and borrower who originally entered into the failed mortgage contract, over $20,000 is externalized to the local community (Kingsley, 2009). Housing researchers have argued over the past 10 years that REOs lower the value of nearby homes—even those with mortgages in good standing. One proposed mechanism for this discounting effect is that deferred maintenance on the foreclosed property leads to vandalism, neglect, and unsightliness, making the neighborhood less desirable (Harding et al.,

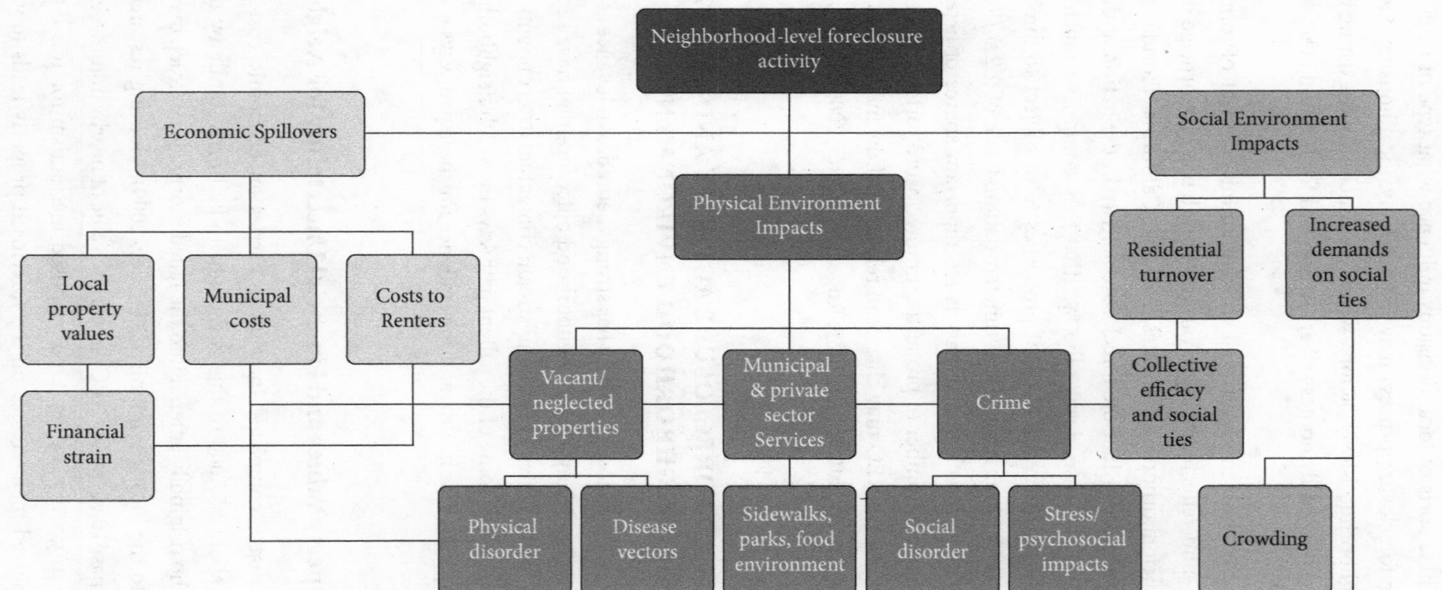

FIGURE 11-2 **Pathways from neighborhood-level foreclosure activity to health determinants.**

2009). Another proposed mechanism is the simple addition of low-cost properties into a localized housing market, whereby increased supply drives down price. The result is reduced home sales prices that persist up to .9 kilometers from the foreclosed property and up to 5 years from the date of foreclosure (Lin, Rosenblatt, & Yao, 2009). Although researchers disagree about how much temporal and spatial distance must separate for-sale and foreclosed properties before impacts of the foreclosed property decay to zero, the existence of an impact is broadly accepted. In fact, some estimate that for every 1 million additional foreclosures, at least 3–5 million homes will be negatively affected (Harding et al., 2009). The exact penalty associated with a nearby foreclosure is also a point of contention among researchers, with estimates ranging from drops of roughly 1% to 9% of the sales value of the nearby home (Harding et al., 2009; Lin et al., 2009). Conservative estimates place the total cost to neighbors of each foreclosure at around $3,000 (Immergluck & Smith, 2006; Kingsley, 2009). In addition to lower sales prices, neighbors may also realize economic losses in the form of higher barriers to accessing equity in their homes, missed employment opportunities contingent on relocation because their homes would not sell (Dietz & Haurin, 2003), or through a perceived loss of wealth that triggered different financial behavior.

While some home owners trying to sell or take out home equity will experience actual monetary losses due to proximate REOs, a much higher proportion are vulnerable to concerns that they have less home equity than they thought, or that they would not be able to sell if they needed to. Renters may also be financially strained if they are forced to move from foreclosed properties. The literature on financial strain, which captures whether respondents perceive that they can afford essential costs in their lives, might therefore be particularly relevant to understanding how neighborhood-level foreclosure exposures affect health. Early work on financial strain was conducted by Pearlin and colleagues (Pearlin, Lieberman, Menaghan, & Mullan, 1981), who acknowledged and measured it as a type of stressor, and by Krause (1987), who contributed methods for measuring the construct early on. A host of literature finds that financial strain is associated with worse health consistently across diverse populations and various stages of the life course, where health outcomes include cardiovascular disease, blood pressure, cortisol levels, psychological distress and depression, obesity, smoking, self-rated health, early disability, and mortality, though much of this research is cross-sectional or poorly controls for confounders (Angel, Frisco, Angel, & Chiriboga, 2003; de Castro, Gee, & Takeuchi, 2010; Duncan et al., 2017; Ferrie, Martikainen, Shipley, & Marmot, 2005; Ford et al., 2010; Garasky, Stewart, Gundersen, Lohman, & Eisenmann, 2009; Grossi, Perski, Lundberg, & Soares, 2001; Martica Hall et al., 2008; Jang, Chiriboga, Herrera, & Branch, 2009; J. R Kahn & Pearlin, 2006; Joan R Kahn & Fazio, 2005; Kendzor et al., 2010; Krause, 1987; Lincoln,

2007; Lynch, Kaplan, & Shema, 1997; Mattsson, Topor, Cullberg, & Forsell, 2008; Pyle, Haddock, Poston, Bray, & Williams, 2007; Rüger et al., 2010; Schulz et al., 2006; Steptoe, Brydon, & Kunz-Ebrecht, 2005; Szanton, Thorpe, & Whitfield, 2010; Tucker-Seeley, Harley, Stoddard, & Sorensen, 2013; Zimmerman & Katon, 2005).

Other potentially relevant financial exposures include debt and unaffordable or insecure housing. Homeowners' level of debt and monthly housing costs are tied to local levels of foreclosure activity because (1) lenders may be less likely to extend refinance loans to borrowers in distressed areas than they are to make refinance loans in more stable areas (Avery, Bhutta, Brevoort, & Canner, 2010); and (2) the loan-to-value ratio of a home goes up as home values decline in response to nearby REOs. In these ways, the economic spillover of neighborhood foreclosure activity makes mortgage debt both objectively and subjectively harder to manage. For all owners in general, barriers to refinancing mean that total mortgage debt and monthly housing are costs higher than they otherwise would be. For the subset owners on the brink of foreclosure themselves, the inability to refinance and higher debt-to-asset ratios may actually, or may be perceived to, threaten their housing security. Renters evicted from foreclosed properties may have to move to less affordable housing and could experience the stress associated with housing insecurity.

Other Economic Costs

The cost of foreclosure is also externalized to local governments that are often left footing the bill for clean-up or maintenance of vacant properties, housing court costs if needed, and even extra police and fire department visits to vacant and blighted structures (Apgar et al., 2005). All told, research from Chicago found that these costs totaled roughly $5,000–$19,000 per REO under most circumstances, but they could reach $35,000 per REO in extreme cases of property destruction (Apgar et al., 2005). In addition to direct costs, municipal governments also lose money through unpaid property taxes and sewer and water bills (Apgar et al., 2005). Perhaps more important, reductions in home values translate into lower property taxes overall. Cuyahoga County Ohio, for example, estimated during the crisis that it would lose $1 million annually if Cleveland area home values dropped just 1 percentage point (Axel-Lute, 2009). Renters living in foreclosed properties also face costs, including those associated with moving and unreturned security deposits (Kingsley, 2009).

Neighborhood Physical Environment Impacts

On top of economic costs to nearby homeowners, local governments, and renters, REOs have been shown to degrade the neighborhood environment, acting as a particularly detrimental form of local foreclosure exposure from a community perspective. More so than other types of properties in foreclosure, REOs uniquely impose hazardous spillovers that elicit complaints from neighbors, ranging from burst pipes that cause mold and sewage backups in basements, to squatters moving into unsecured properties (Lambie-Hanson, 2015). Abandoned properties can become havens for crime, and unkempt, blighted structures produce signs of "physical disorder." The Charlotte-Mecklenburg Police Department documented the impact of the housing crisis on its neighborhoods, noting that beginning in 2005, many recently built neighborhoods began to fill with "houses that were boarded up, broken streetlights, and junk and trash accumulating on the sidewalks (Bess, 2008)." Prompted by these observations, the department analyzed its blight, crime, and disorder statistics vis-à-vis foreclosure information and found that concentrated foreclosures were temporally and spatially associated with higher property and violent crime, noting in particular that foreclosed properties were frequently victim to appliance and building material theft. More rigorous research from Chicago found that for each additional foreclosure per 100 properties in a census tract, violent crime rates spiked by 2.3% in that tract (Immergluck & Smith, 2005). Since these studies were published at the beginning of the housing crisis, new papers have been published showing associations between foreclosure activity and burglary (Baumer et al., 2012), larceny, and aggravated assault (Goodstein & Lee, 2010), and violent (Ellen, Lacoe, & Sharygin, 2013; Lacoe & Ellen, 2015; Stucky, Ottensmann, & Payton, 2012), drug, and property crimes (Katz, Wallace, & Hedberg, 2013). At least one paper finds no association between annual violent crime rate and foreclosure rates (Kirk & Hyra, 2010).

Other sources of neighborhood degradation include reductions in municipal and private sector services. Municipal governments are particularly vulnerable to housing crises, as their budgets are triply penalized: first through costs introduced by REOs, secondly through lower revenue as property values decline and taxes go unpaid on abandoned properties, and finally in the form of increased needs for human and social services (Apgar et al., 2005; Hoene & Pagano, 2010; Kingsley, 2009). The best source of data on impacts to municipal services comes from surveys of elected and appointed local officials nationwide, conducted by the nonprofit organization the National League of Cities. A 2008 poll showed that even early in the market crash, about a fifth of cities represented reported cutting back on services and projects due to budget shortfalls, and that over half reported increased demand from residents for public assistance (McFarland & McCahan, 2008). In 2010, 87% of responding cities' finance officers said they were less able than in the previous year to meet their needs, demonstrating the impact of four straight years of city revenue decline (Hoene & Pagano, 2010). To deal with budget shortfalls, about 80% of cities were cutting municipal staff, nearly 70% were canceling or delaying capital improvements, and a quarter were making public safety cuts.

Blight and disorder are increasingly well-recognized upstream health risk factors. Directly related to foreclosures are vacant and abandoned lots. Vacant and abandoned lot area has been positively associated with neighborhood volume of outdoor advertising (e.g., billboards) after accounting for area-level racial and economic composition (Kwate & Lee, 2007). Longitudinal studies of advertising exposure and substance use in adolescents and young adults suggest that this is a potentially relevant health exposure (Biener & Siegel, 2000; West et al., 2010). Because racial/ethnic minority neighborhoods, which were disproportionately impacted by the most recent housing crisis, already have higher outdoor advertising volumes and that these ads are more likely to feature alcohol and tobacco (Stoddard & Boley-Cruz, 1998), REOs have the potential to worsen an existing source of health inequity. Vacant and abandoned properties have also been linked to higher body mass index, lower self-rated health, and worse mental health via their inclusion on neighborhood disorder indices. Data from Chicago show that an index of physical disorder comprising the presence of vacant properties, litter, glass, or trash on the sidewalk or street, and graffiti was associated with worse self-rated health (Chang, Hillier, & Mehta, 2009). This study controlled for a range of possible confounders, including individual-level sociodemographic factors and health behaviors, as well as neighborhood-level measures of socioeconomic status, heathcare facilities, and social resources. The magnitude of a one point difference on the nine-point neighborhood-level physical disorder index was greater than the impact of reporting high blood pressure (dichotomous) at the individual level. A Philadelphia-based study also used vacant lots and abandoned and vacant properties as components of a neighborhood physical disorder index that also included city code violations, fires, Philadelphia Housing Authority properties, and home sales prices (Chang et al., 2009). Results showed that after accounting for individual sociodemographic factors and neighborhood-level poverty, social resource, advertising, park and recreational facilities, and food environment factors, physical disorder was still a strong and significant predictor of obesity in women. Women living in the highest quartile of disorder compared to the lowest had 1.78 times the odds of obesity after full adjustment. A study of New Haven, Connecticut, that used a "loop analysis of causal feedback" approach to account for the self-perpetuating cycle of neighborhood decline, disinvestment, and resident exit concluded that vacant lots and vacant/abandoned properties exert a negative causal effect on residents' mental health after accounting for prior neighborhood-level conditions (Dinno, 2007).

Neighborhood disorder and perceived neighborhood problems that exclude explicit measurement of vacancy or blight are also relevant because the health effects of neighborhood-level foreclosure activity could be mediated through cuts to municipal services, private sector disinvestment, crime, and a degraded neighborhood environment. For example, a sample of nearly 8,000 diabetic adults from seven US states found that the perception of neighborhood problems, including litter, trash, graffiti, crime, and a lack of grocery stores, was associated with current smoking behavior after adjustment for individual sociodemographic and health factors and neighborhood-level poverty (Gary et al., 2008). In a sample of nearly 700 London adults, researchers found that after controlling for potential individual- and neighborhood-level confounders, neighborhood disorder, operationalized as vandalism, litter in the streets, and a lack of retail and entertainment outlets, among other items, was associated with 2.7 times the odds of mental health problems and 2.0 times the odds of worse self-rated health when comparing the worst to best quartiles of neighborhoods (Steptoe & Feldman, 2001). A large body of research links crime and exposure to violence with mental health problems, particularly depressive symptoms, though the crime measure used matters (Aisenberg & Herrenkohl, 2008; Curry, Latkin, & Davey-Rothwell, 2008; Schulz et al., 2006).

Mortgage distress, as indicated by foreclosure and delinquency, also impacts the social environment. In this sense, a community impacted by foreclosure can be conceptualized as geographic, social, or both. Geographic communities may be disrupted by foreclosure via residential turnover. Homeowners lose their homes in pre-foreclosure short sales or repossession, and renters are evicted after landlords default on loans. In a study of the Oakland area by the Alameda County Public Health Department and a community partner organization at the peak of the crisis, 33% of residents who reported recently or currently undergoing foreclosure had lived in the neighborhood 10 or more years, and another 49% had been there between 5 and 10 years (Alameda County Public Health Department & Causa Justa, 2010). Oakland data also show that the stress of foreclosure may seep into social networks, with those who report worrying about their contacts' vulnerability to foreclosure also reporting worse health. Finally, residents displaced by foreclosure report coping by moving in with family or friends and are therefore more likely to report living in crowded housing (Alameda County Public Health Department & Causa Justa, 2010). Nationally, between 2005 and 2009, foreclosure activity is estimated to have increased Black–White segregation by 1.1 dissimilarity points, and Latino–White segregation by 2.2 points (Matthew Hall, Crowder, & Spring, 2015).

In sum, neighborhood-level foreclosure activity has been shown to adversely impact the finances of nearby homeowners through lowered property values and higher barriers to refinancing, potentially translating to real and perceived increases in financial strain, debt burden, and housing insecurity. Renters living in seized properties may also experience financial strain associated with moving and the stress of housing insecurity. Neighborhood-level foreclosure activity may also create health risks by increasing levels of disorder, crime, and blight in neighborhoods, and by disrupting local social relationships. The epidemiologic literature suggests that these exposures are causally related to health behaviors, stress-related biomarkers, physical and mental health clinical end points, and self-rated health. In line with the theoretical model summarized in Figure 11-2, which views neighborhood-level foreclosure activity as a contextual health risk factor, empirical studies examining direct links between foreclosure and health have largely supported the idea that foreclosures are bad for both homeowners going through the process and for the surrounding local community.

EMPIRICAL EVIDENCE ON FORECLOSURE AND HEALTH

As of 2016, two systematic reviews had identified roughly 40 relevant epidemiologic studies on foreclosure and health, and both reported that the weight of the evidence links the personal experience of foreclosure, as well as exposure to neighborhood foreclosures, to worse health at the individual and population levels. Specific evidence from these studies is detailed next, but the weight of the evidence is also summarized by the authors of these two reviews. For example, across studies of both personal and contextual exposures, Tsai found that 91% of studies published to date showed associations between foreclosure and worse health, but noted that many were vulnerable to bias, for example, due to confounding where associations were cross-sectional (Tsai, 2015).

Downing reported that 80% of studies on the contextual effects of foreclosure showed a link to worse health (Downing, 2016). Since these reviews were conducted, five additional relevant empirical papers have been published and, between them, present a mix of null and positive results (Berger et al., 2015; Calo, Vernon, Lairson, & Linder, 2015; Christine et al., 2017; Downing, Karter, et al., 2016; Vásquez-Vera, Rodríguez-Sanz, Palència, & Borrell, 2016). Although the focus of this chapter is on foreclosure as a neighborhood-level health risk factor, I first review the health consequences of individual foreclosure experiences for two reasons. First, foreclosed homeowners contribute to overall burdens of disease in a community, and, second, many of the documented consequences are behavioral or psychological outcomes that have suspected contagious effects within communities (Christakis & Fowler, 2009).

Individual-Level Studies

The evidence base on the health effects of personal foreclosure experiences comprises roughly two dozen papers, most of which find associations with poor health outcomes using cross-sectional data, largely from the United States and Europe. Despite some examples of null findings (e.g., Lindblad & Riley, 2015), much of the evidence points to the potential psychological impacts of undergoing foreclosure. For example, a cross-sectional survey divided nearly 800 participants from states hard hit by the foreclosure crisis into four categories: renters, homeowners with no housing strain, homeowners with some housing strain, and homeowners who had defaulted on loans and/or had received foreclosure notices. After controlling for socioeconomic and demographic factors, homeowners who were delinquent or in foreclosure had higher rates of psychological stress, lower self-rated health, more physical health impairments, and more symptoms of physical health problems than did the other groups (Cannuscio et al., 2012). Similarly, a separate US study found that being behind on mortgage payments or in the foreclosure process, or recently going through foreclosure was cross-sectionally associated with fair/poor self-rated health and anxiety and depression outcomes, but not with a problematic drinking screening questions (Burgard, Seefeldt, & Zelner, 2012). Finally, Pollack and Lynch surveyed a convenience sample of 250 adults engaged in home mortgage foreclosure counseling in Philadelphia in 2008 and found that, compared to a community sample (n = 10,007), those enmeshed in the foreclosure process were more likely to report major depression, cost-related medication nonadherence, hypertension, and smoking behavior (Pollack & Lynch, 2009). About a third of the foreclosure sample was depressed, roughly 50% forwent prescription drugs because of cost, 40% were hypertensive, and 32% smoked.

Consequences for maternal child health have also been studied. Experiencing foreclosure in the 2 years before giving birth was associated with severe depression symptoms in a cohort of 662 new mothers in Detroit, Michigan, even after adjustments for a range of potential confounders and prepregnancy health status (Osypuk, Caldwell, Platt, & Misra, 2012), and data on over 60,000 Wisconsin households uncovered a link between receiving a foreclosure filing and Child Protective Services investigation or substantiation of child maltreatment leading up to the filing and immediately afterward (Berger et al., 2015).

Personal foreclosure experience has been implicated in suicide deaths as well. A case-control study of suicide deaths in one Ohio county found that compared to nonsuicide deaths, including unintentional injury deaths, suicide victims had roughly three times the odds of undergoing foreclosure in the year before death (Cook, 2012). Using data from 16 US states, different authors found that suicide-related foreclosures increased by over 250%, from 30 to 106 cases, between 2005 and 2010 (Fowler, Gladden, Vagi, Barnes, & Frazier, 2015). In addition to these studies on foreclosure specifically, mortgage delinquency has been associated with depressive symptoms and medication nonadherence (Alley, Pagán, & Lipman, 2010).

International cross-sectional data also support links between individual foreclosure experience and poorer health. Data on thousands of medical visits in Spain also showed cross-sectional associations between major depressive disorder and foreclosure (Gili, Roca, Basu, McKee, & Stuckler, 2013), while a cross-sectional survey of people struggling with their mortgages in Catalonia found that mental health was worse among people in the nonpayment stage of foreclosure compared to those who were still paying their mortgages, and that later stages in the foreclosure process were associated with worse self-reported health (Vásquez-Vera et al., 2016).

Longitudinal studies have also been conducted. Undergoing foreclosure was associated with subsequently developing major depression and with subsequently developing generalized anxiety disorder, controlling for prior mental health, in a sample of over 1,500, majority African American adults in Detroit, Michigan (McLaughlin et al., 2011). Using 17 waves of a longitudinal UK panel dataset established in 1991 (n = 12,390) to understand if home repossession was a risk factor for common mental illness, Pevalin found that homeowners whose homes were repossessed had 1.6 times the odds of developing common mental illness just after the repossession compared to those who did not undergo foreclosure (Pevalin, 2009), controlling for individual fixed-effects, social class, employment, marital status, and age. Using the same data set to examine mortgage debt and arrears, however, has shown no relationship with psychological distress in one study (Brown, Taylor, & Wheatley Price, 2005), and associations with poor self-reported health (Nettleton & Burrows, 1998) and psychological distress (Taylor, Pevalin, & Todd, 2007) in others. Examining Panel Study of Income Dynamics (PSID) data from 2007–2011 with fixed effects and time-varying controls, Yilmazer and colleagues showed that foreclosure was associated with both psychological distress and depression (Yilmazer, Babiarz, & Liu, 2015).

One challenge to isolating the causal effects of individual foreclosure experience on health is mounting evidence that health problems contribute to foreclosure. At least three studies find that health problems and changes in healthcare utilization precede and predict personal foreclosure experiences. To ascertain the extent to which medical problems contributed to the current wave of foreclosures, Robertson et al. surveyed home owners subject to foreclosure filings in California, Florida, Illinois, and New Jersey about a variety of experiences in the two before they received their foreclosure notices. Within each state, a random sample of 500 single family home or condominium owners who had received a preforeclosure filing (NOD or LP) within the past 30 days were mailed surveys, totaling 2,000 homeowners. Of the 128 owners that responded, 49% reported that medical factors had contributed to their mortgage distress. Add to this percentage the respondents who did not report a medical cause but had used home equity to pay medical bills, were unable to work due to medical issues, had high medical bills, or had missed more than 2 weeks of work due to a health problem, and nearly 70% had medical problems preceding their foreclosure filings (Robertson, Egelhof, & Hoke, 2008). Robertson et al. concluded that medical problems were common drivers of mortgage distress.

A case-control study of homeowners' health and healthcare utilization in the time leading up to foreclosure also suggests that changes in medical needs precede foreclosure. Matching patients undergoing foreclosure to geographically proximate controls, the authors found that emergency department utilization, outpatient visits, lacking a primary care provider, and failing to arrive for a scheduled appointment were associated with a subsequent foreclosure notice (Pollack, Kurd, Livshits, Weiner, & Lynch, 2011). Houle and Keene explored the medical causes of foreclosure using longitudinal data and found that worsening health increased the risk of foreclosure in a nationally representative sample (Houle & Keene, 2015).

Research on the health causes of foreclosure demonstrate methodological challenges associated with disentangling complex and likely bidirectional relationships between health and individual foreclosure risk, but also uncover potential areas of intervention to help mitigate the socioeconomic consequences of poor health. For example, Houle and Keene note loss of insurance and family income as partial mediators of the health–foreclosure relationship (Houle & Keene, 2015), while Robertson's findings highlight medical bills and inability to work as relevant pathways (Robertson et al., 2008). These results suggest that expanded access to affordable health insurance and paid sick leave may be worth debating as housing policy interventions.

Neighborhood-Level Studies

Since 2007, roughly 20 papers have examined associations between neighborhood-level foreclosure activity and health, and most have found that various measures of foreclosure intensity predict worse health outcomes (Downing, 2016). The first peer-reviewed study on this topic investigated why Bakersfield, California, saw a spike in West Nile virus cases during the summer of 2007 that could not be explained by weather patterns. Researchers discovered that neglected swimming pools, ornamental ponds, and hot tubs on foreclosed or abandoned property that had become mosquito breeding grounds were responsible for the sudden rise in cases (Reisen, Takahashi, Carroll, & Quiring, 2008). Since then, researchers have tested associations between a range of contextual foreclosure measures and psychological, physical, behavioral, and healthcare utilization outcomes across geographic locations.

Many of the positive findings from this literature are reported in studies that examined exposure to REOs as a health risk factor. For example, Cagney et al. found that in a nationally representative US sample observed between 2005 and 2011, living in a zip code that experienced large increases in the percent of housing units that became REO was linked to developing depressive symptoms, but increases in the overall completed foreclosure rate was not (Cagney, Browning, Iveniuk, & English, 2014). Houle also examined a range of foreclosure measures as predictors of mental health outcomes using nationally representative data; however, foreclosure rates were measured at the county level between 2006 and 2011. He found that both the overall foreclosure and REO rates were associated with worse mental health, although REO activity had a stronger effect than did foreclosure activity overall (Houle, 2014). Likewise, when Houle and Light examined suicide rates in relation to state-level foreclosure activity, they showed that while both overall foreclosure and REO foreclosure rates were associated with higher suicide rates, REO rates were more strongly predictive (Houle & Light, 2014). In terms of physical health outcomes, Arcaya and colleagues found that REO properties located within 100 meters of Framingham Heart Study participants' homes predicted higher measured body mass index (M. Arcaya et al., 2013) and systolic blood pressure, and that blood pressure increases were partially mediated by alcohol consumption and weight gain (M. Arcaya et al., 2014). In sum, across a range of geographic scales and health outcomes, contextual measures of REO activity have been linked to poor health.

A mix of null and positive associations have been found in studies that examine overall foreclosure rates. Three studies investigate foreclosure rates' relationship to child maltreatment outcomes at various geographies. State-level foreclosure rate was not associated with maternal spanking between 2007 and 2010 in a representative sample of families living in large US cities (Brooks-Gunn, Schneider, & Waldfogel, 2013). In contrast, the county-level foreclosure rate was positively associated with Child Protective Services investigations and substantiated child abuse allegations in Pennsylvania between 1990 and 2010 (Frioux et al., 2014). Changes in regional foreclosure rates were predictive of admissions to a sample of US children's hospitals for physical abuse among children under 6 years old, and for traumatic brain injuries not caused by car crashes or birth injuries among infants (Wood et al., 2012).

Overall foreclosure rates have also been used to examine healthcare demand and somatic morbidity. Curie and Tekin show that increases in the ZIP code–level foreclosure rate predicted increases in nonelective hospitalizations and emergency department visits in Arizona, California, Florida, and New Jersey during the recent housing crisis (Currie & Tekin, 2015), while Calo finds that census tract-level foreclosure starts were not associated with colorectal screening in Houston, Texas. Higher foreclosure filing rates have also been associated with increases in Google searches for information about psychological distress symptoms (Ayers et al., 2012).

Associations between foreclosure rates and somatic morbidity have been mixed. For example, Downing et al. examined whether census block-level foreclosure rates predicted glycemic control (Downing, Laraia, Rodriguez, Dow, & Adler, 2016) or body weight (Downing, Karter, et al., 2016) during the recent housing crisis (2007–2011) in a population of roughly 100,000 Kaiser Permanent Northern California patients with type 2 diabetes. Individual fixed effects models showed null associations between the completed foreclosure rate and a measure of glycemic control, annual average HbA1C, over time, as were associations with weight changes. A study with a similarly fine-grained view of localized foreclosure activity, measured by changes in the number of foreclosures within 1/4 mile of study participants' homes, assessed changes in health among Multi-Ethnic Study of Atherosclerosis participants between 2005 and 2012. Results show that each additional foreclosure was associated with an increase in fasting blood glucose, a decrease in systolic blood pressure, and no change in weight (Christine et al., 2017).

Other less direct measures of foreclosure have also been studied. The federal Housing and Urban Development (HUD) agency's foreclosure risk at the census tract level was associated with the odds of reporting fair or poor health among breast cancer survivors in Missouri, 2006–2008 (Schootman, Deshpande, Pruitt, & Jeffe, 2012). Results obtained using delinquency measures are mixed. Large increases in percent of housing units per ZIP code to receive a NOD filing were associated with the development of serious depressive symptoms in one nationally representative sample (Cagney et al., 2014), whereas county-level NOD rates were unrelated to mental health in another nationally representative sample (Houle, 2014). Regional delinquency rates were associated with hospital admissions among children under 6 years old for physical abuse, and among infants for traumatic brain injuries not caused by car crashes or birth injuries (Wood et al., 2012).

RECOMMENDATIONS FOR FUTURE RESEARCH IN THE FACE OF MIXED FINDINGS

Although the weight of the evidence suggests that foreclosures harm health both when individuals undergo foreclosure themselves and when they are exposed to foreclosure activity in their neighborhoods, mixed findings underscore the fact that relationships between foreclosure and health are not yet well understood, and they highlight opportunities for further research. A critical priority is to replicate studies that have found negative health effects associated with foreclosure in different populations and time periods in order to establish if previously published relationships are the product of statistical variability or if results are replicable. Publication bias introduces a substantial risk that positive findings are a result of chance but have become amplified above null results (M. C. Arcaya, 2017). In replication efforts, it will be important to use consistent measures of foreclosure and health outcomes, as differences in measuring foreclosure activity may help explain why results are inconsistent across the literature. Prior work suggests that the presence of REO foreclosures may matter more for residents than does the completed foreclosure rate, even though the completed foreclosure rate is the most commonly used measure of foreclosure activity in the literature.

Although overall foreclosure measures have been linked to worse health outcomes in many cases, the handful of papers that provided separate estimates of the effects of REO and of other foreclosure activity would urge a focus on REOs. There are two ways in which the foreclosure rate may not perform as well as measures of REO density or proximity. First, while many foreclosed properties will eventually become REO, completed foreclosure rates include foreclosure sales to third parties who may immediately move in and put the property back into productive use. Second, foreclosure rate only counts transaction filings that occurred during a specific time period, which is analogous to an incidence measure, rather than foreclosed properties themselves, which is analogous to prevalence. As a consequence, an REO that has been vacant for 1 year will not be counted toward neighbors' exposure measured by an annual foreclosure rate because the filing occurred in the previous year, despite the fact that neighbors have been coping with a proximate REO for at least 12 months. Understanding the implications of using different foreclosure measures in epidemiologic studies is not simply of methodological concern. Testing the health effects of different foreclosure measures is crucial for practice as well. Knowing if REOs are the driving force behind contextual effects on foreclosure on health is critical for intervention planning; equal effects of any foreclosure deed transfers might imply a focus on foreclosure prevention, while uniquely harmful effects of bank-owned properties could direct attention more toward property maintenance. Other explanations for mixed findings that should be controlled in deliberate replication efforts include the use of widely variable neighborhood definitions and spatial scales across which researchers look for effects.

In addition to further probing suspected relationships between neighborhood-level foreclosure and health, new research should also examine how the changing social meaning of foreclosure over time and place may generate health risks in some context but not others. Better understanding the circumstances under which neighborhood foreclosures matter for health, which likely changes over time, will require stronger investigations of neighborhood context. For example, high foreclosure rates could change the social meaning of extremely localized, marginal differences in foreclosure activity. Some work has assessed how community context modifies the effect of foreclosures on health (Houle, 2014), but more work spanning large geographic areas is needed. Similarly, we currently have a poor understanding of which health outcomes are sensitive to neighborhood-level foreclosure activity. Mixed results in the literature could reflect true etiologic differences in how blood glucose versus blood pressure problems develop and respond to neighborhood foreclosures, for example. Ultimately, public health and housing researchers and practitioners need to understand what health outcomes are at risk from what types of foreclosure activity, at what geographic scale (see Chapter 2 for a more detailed discussion), and under what social conditions. Creating a robust evidence base to answer these questions will require a mix of replication studies and new research questions be investigated in diverse populations and places.

Finally, evaluating the potential health effects of housing crisis-era interventions to stem the tide and impact of foreclosures, including neighborhood stabilization programs and policy differences that shorten or lengthen foreclosure timelines, will also be important. Understanding the potential of such interventions to protect health and health equity will be crucial in preparing for future downturns in the housing market. In perhaps the most convincing study on the causal effects of blight on crime, researchers used a quasi-experimental design to study the effects of blight remediation on violence in Philadelphia between 1999 and 2013. They found that remediating abandoned buildings and vacant lots reduced firearm violence but not nonfirearm violence, and created tax and social returns that outweighed the cost of remediation as a result (Branas et al., 2016). Foreclosure researchers should consider taking advantage of data on federal and local interventions implemented in response to the housing crisis (Immergluck, 2008; NSP: Neighborhood Stabilization Program—HUD Exchange, 2014), which may offer similarly rich opportunities to explore whether health improved when foreclosures were prevented or addressed.

The most recent US foreclosure crisis, which affected the neighborhood environments of tens of millions of people (Joint Center for Housing Studies, 2016), was not the first housing crisis to affect the United States, nor will it be the last. Continuing to study if, how, and when neighborhood-level foreclosure activity affects health is critical. Understanding how the underlying causes of the financial crisis, which include recklessness of profit-seeking financial firms, regulatory failures, and breaches in accountability and ethics at multiple levels (Commission, 2011), translated into population health risks, should help inform financial and housing regulatory policy going forward. Looking forward, evidence on mechanisms that link foreclosure and health, as well as interventions to protect neighborhoods, will help us prepare for future crises.

REFERENCES

Aisenberg, E., & Herrenkohl, T. (2008). Community violence in context: Risk and resilience in children and families. *Journal of Interpersonal Violence*, *23*(3), 296–315. https://doi.org/10.1177/0886260507312287

Alameda County Public Health Department, & Causa Justa. (2010, September). Rebuilding neighborhoods, restoring health: A report on the impact of foreclosure on public health. The California Endowment. Retrieved from http://www.acphd.org/media/53643/foreclose2.pdf

Alley, D. E., Pagán, J., & Lipman, T. (2010, December 1). *Economic strain and poor health: Associations between housing foreclosure and health*. Unpublished manuscript, University of Maryland School of Medicine.

Angel, R. J., Frisco, M., Angel, J. L., & Chiriboga, D. A. (2003). Financial strain and health among elderly Mexican-origin individuals. *Journal of Health and Social Behavior*, *44*(4), 536–551.

Apgar, W. C., Duda, M., Gorey, R. N., & Council, H. P. (2005). The municipal cost of foreclosures: A Chicago case study. Unpublished report, Homeownership Preservation Foundation, Minneapolis, MN.

Arcaya, M. C. (2017). Invited commentary: Foreclosures and health in a neighborhood context. *American Journal of Epidemiology*, *185*(6), 436–439. doi: 10.1093/aje/kww169.

Arcaya, M., Glymour, M. M., Chakrabarti, P., Christakis, N. A., Kawachi, I., & Subramanian, S. V. (2013). Effects of proximate foreclosed properties on individuals' weight gain in Massachusetts, 1987–2008. *American Journal of Public Health*, *103*(9), e50–e56.

Arcaya, M., Glymour, M. M., Chakrabarti, P., Christakis, N. A., Kawachi, I., & Subramanian, S. V. (2014). Effects of proximate foreclosed properties on individuals' systolic blood pressure in Massachusetts, 1987 to 2008. *Circulation*, *129*(22), 2262–2268. https://doi.org/10.1161/CIRCULATIONAHA.113.006205

Avery, R. B., Bhutta, N., Brevoort, K. P., & Canner, G. B. (2010). The 2009 HMDA data: The mortgage market during a time of low interest rates and economic distress. *Federal Reserve Bulletin*, December 2010. Retrieved from http:/papers.ssrn.com.ezp-prod1.hul.harvard.edu/sol3/papers.cfm?abstract_id=1682909

Axel-Lute, M. (2009). *Communities at risk: How the foreclosure crisis is damaging urban areas and what is being done about it*. New York, NY: Living Cities. Retrieved from http://backend.livingcities.org/_backend.livingcities.org/files/Living_Cities-communities-at-risk.pdf

Ayers, J. W., Althouse, B. M., Allem, J.-P., Childers, M. A., Zafar, W., Latkin, C., . . . Brownstein, J. S. (2012). Novel surveillance of psychological distress during the great recession. *Journal of Affective Disorders*, *142*(1–3), 323–330. https://doi.org/10.1016/j.jad.2012.05.005

Baumer, E. P., Wolff, K. T., & Arnio, A. N. (2012). A multicity neighborhood analysis of foreclosure and crime. *Social Science Quarterly*, *93*(3), 577–601. https://doi.org/10.1111/j.1540-6237.2012.00888.x

Bennett, G. G., Scharoun-Lee, M., & Tucker-Seeley, R. (2009). Will the public's health fall victim to the home foreclosure epidemic? *PLoS Medicine*, *6*(6), e1000087. https://doi.org/10.1371/journal.pmed.1000087

Berger, L. M., Collins, J. M., Font, S. A., Gjertson, L., Slack, K. S., & Smeeding, T. (2015). Home foreclosure and Child Protective Services involvement. *Pediatrics*, *136*(2), 299–307. https://doi.org/10.1542/peds.2014-2832

Bess, M. (2008). Assessing the impact of home foreclosures in Charlotte neighborhoods. *Geography and Public Safety*, *1*(3), 2–4.

Biener, L., & Siegel, M. (2000). Tobacco marketing and adolescent smoking: More support for a causal inference. *American Journal of Public Health*, *90*(3), 407–411. https://doi.org/10.2105/AJPH.90.3.407

Branas, C. C., Kondo, M. C., Murphy, S. M., South, E. C., Polsky, D., & MacDonald, J. M. (2016). Urban blight remediation as a cost-beneficial solution to firearm violence. *American Journal of Public Health*, *106*(12), 2158–2164. https://doi.org/10.2105/AJPH.2016.303434

Brooks-Gunn, J., Schneider, W., & Waldfogel, J. (2013). The Great Recession and the risk for child maltreatment. *Child Abuse & Neglect*, *37*(10), 721–729. https://doi.org/10.1016/j.chiabu.2013.08.004

Brown, S., Taylor, K., & Wheatley Price, S. (2005). Debt and distress: Evaluating the psychological cost of credit. *Journal of Economic Psychology*, *26*(5), 642–663. https://doi.org/10.1016/j.joep.2005.01.002

Burgard, S. A., Seefeldt, K. S., & Zelner, S. (2012). Housing instability and health: Findings from the Michigan recession and recovery study. *Social Science & Medicine*, *75*(12), 2215–2224. https://doi.org/10.1016/j.socscimed.2012.08.020

Cagney, K. A., Browning, C. R., Iveniuk, J., & English, N. (2014). The onset of depression during the Great Recession: Foreclosure and older adult mental health. *American Journal of Public Health*, *104*(3), 498–505. https://doi.org/10.2105/AJPH.2013.301566

Calo, W. A., Vernon, S. W., Lairson, D. R., & Linder, S. H. (2015). Associations between contextual factors and colorectal cancer screening in a racially and ethnically diverse population in Texas. *Cancer Epidemiology*, *39*(6), 798–804. https://doi.org/10.1016/j.canep.2015.09.012

Cannuscio, C. C., Alley, D. E., Pagán, J. A., Soldo, B., Krasny, S., Shardell, M., . . . Lipman, T. H. (2012). Housing strain, mortgage foreclosure, and health. *Nursing Outlook*, *60*(3), 134–142. https://doi.org/10.1016/j.outlook.2011.08.004

Chang, V. W., Hillier, A. E., & Mehta, N. K. (2009). Neighborhood racial isolation, disorder and obesity. *Social Forces; a Scientific Medium of Social Study and Interpretation*, *87*(4), 2063–2092. https://doi.org/10.1353/sof.0.0188

Christakis, N. A., & Fowler, J. H. (2009). *Connected: The surprising power of our social networks and how they shape our lives*. New York: Hachette Digital, Inc.

Christine, P. J., Moore, K., Crawford, N. D., Barrientos-Gutierrez, T., Sánchez, B. N., Seeman, T., & Diez Roux, A. V. (2017). Exposure to neighborhood foreclosures and changes in cardiometabolic health: Results from MESA. *American Journal of Epidemiology*, *185*(2), 106–114. https://doi.org/10.1093/aje/kww186

Cook, T. B. (2012). Assessing legal strains and risk of suicide using archived court data. *Suicide and Life-Threatening Behavior*, *42*(5), 495–506. https://doi.org/10.1111/j.1943-278X.2012.00107.x

Currie, J., & Tekin, E. (2015). Is there a link between foreclosure and health? *American Economic Journal: Economic Policy*, *7*(1), 63–94.

Curry, A., Latkin, C., & Davey-Rothwell, M. (2008). Pathways to depression: The impact of neighborhood violent crime on inner-city residents in Baltimore, Maryland, USA. *Social Science & Medicine (1982)*, *67*(1), 23–30. https://doi.org/10.1016/j.socscimed.2008.03.007

de Castro, A. B., Gee, G. C., & Takeuchi, D. T. (2010). Examining alternative measures of social disadvantage among Asian Americans: The relevance of economic opportunity, subjective social status, and financial strain for health. *Journal of Immigrant and Minority*

Health/Center for Minority Public Health, 12(5), 659–671. https://doi.org/10.1007/s10903-009-9258-3

Dietz, R. D., & Haurin, D. R. (2003). The social and private micro-level consequences of homeownership. *Journal of Urban Economics, 54*(3), 401–450.

Dinno, A. (2007). Loop analysis of causal feedback in epidemiology: An illustration relating to urban neighborhoods and resident depressive experiences. *Social Science & Medicine (1982), 65*(10), 2043–2057. https://doi.org/10.1016/j.socscimed.2007.06.018

Downing, J. (2016). The health effects of the foreclosure crisis and unaffordable housing: A systematic review and explanation of evidence. *Social Science & Medicine, 162*, 88–96. https://doi.org/10.1016/j.socscimed.2016.06.014

Downing, J., Karter, A., Rodriguez, H., Dow, W. H., Adler, N., Schillinger, D., . . . Laraia, B. (2016). No spillover effect of the foreclosure crisis on weight change: The Diabetes Study of Northern California (DISTANCE). *PloS One, 11*(3), e0151334. https://doi.org/10.1371/journal.pone.0151334

Downing, J., Laraia, Rodriguez, Dow, & Adler, N. (2016). Beyond the Great Recession: Was the foreclosure crisis harmful to the health of diabetics? *American Journal of Epidemiology, 185*(6), 429–435. doi: 10.1093/aje/kww171.

Duke, E. Foreclosure documentation issues. Financial Services Subcommittee on Housing and Community Opportunity, U.S. House of Representatives (2010). Washington DC. Retrieved from http://www.federalreserve.gov/newsevents/testimony/duke20101118a.htm

Duncan, D. T., Hyun Park, S., Al-Ajlouni, Y. A., Hale, L., Jean-Louis, G., Goedel, W. C., . . . Elbel, B. (2017). Association of financial hardship with poor sleep health outcomes among men who have sex with men. *SSM—Population Health, 3*, 594–599. https://doi.org/10.1016/j.ssmph.2017.07.006

Ellen, I. G., Lacoe, J., & Sharygin, C. A. (2013). Do foreclosures cause crime? *Journal of Urban Economics, 74*, 59–70. https://doi.org/10.1016/j.jue.2012.09.003

Ferrie, J. E., Martikainen, P., Shipley, M. J., & Marmot, M. G. (2005). Self-reported economic difficulties and coronary events in men: Evidence from the Whitehall II study. *International Journal of Epidemiology, 34*(3), 640–648.

Financial Crisis Inquiry Commission (2011). *The financial crisis inquiry report: Final report of the National Commission on the Causes of the Financial and Economic Crisis in the United States*. Public Affairs. Available at https://www.gpo.gov/fdsys/pkg/GPO-FCIC/pdf/GPO-FCIC.pdf

Ford, E., Clark, C., McManus, S., Harris, J., Jenkins, R., Bebbington, P., . . . Stansfeld, S. A. (2010). Common mental disorders, unemployment and welfare benefits in England. *Public Health, 124*(12), 675–681. https://doi.org/10.1016/j.puhe.2010.08.019

Fowler, K. A., Gladden, R. M., Vagi, K. J., Barnes, J., & Frazier, L. (2015). Increase in suicides associated with home eviction and foreclosure during the US housing crisis: Findings from 16 national violent death reporting system states, 2005–2010. *American Journal of Public Health, 105*(2), 311–316. https://doi.org/10.2105/AJPH.2014.301945

Frioux, S., Wood, J. N., Fakeye, O., Luan, X., Localio, R., & Rubin, D. M. (2014). Longitudinal association of county-level economic indicators and child maltreatment incidents. *Maternal and Child Health Journal, 18*(9), 2202–2208. https://doi.org/10.1007/s10995-014-1469-0

Garasky, S. a, Stewart, S. D., Gundersen, C., Lohman, B. J., & Eisenmann, J. C. (2009). Family stressors and child obesity. *Social Science Research, 38*(4), 755–766.

Gary, T. L., Safford, M. M., Gerzoff, R. B., Ettner, S. L., Karter, A. J., Beckles, G. L., & Brown, A. F. (2008). Perception of neighborhood problems, health behaviors, and diabetes outcomes among adults with diabetes in managed care: The Translating Research Into Action for Diabetes (TRIAD) study. *Diabetes Care*, *31*(2), 273–278. https://doi.org/10.2337/dc07-1111

Gili, M., Roca, M., Basu, S., McKee, M., & Stuckler, D. (2013). The mental health risks of economic crisis in Spain: Evidence from primary care centres, 2006 and 2010. *European Journal of Public Health*, *23*(1), 103–108. https://doi.org/10.1093/eurpub/cks035

Goodstein, R., & Lee, Y. Y. (2010). *Do foreclosures increase crime?* (SSRN Scholarly Paper No. ID 1670842). Rochester, NY: Social Science Research Network. Retrieved from https://papers.ssrn.com/abstract=1670842

Grossi, G., Perski, A., Lundberg, U., & Soares, J. (2001). Associations between financial strain and the diurnal salivary cortisol secretion of long-term unemployed individuals. *Integrative Physiological and Behavioral Science: The Official Journal of the Pavlovian Society*, *36*(3), 205–219.

Hall, M., Buysse, D. J., Nofzinger, E. A., Reynolds, C. F., Thompson, W., Mazumdar, S., & Monk, T. H. (2008). Financial strain is a significant correlate of sleep continuity disturbances in late-life. *Biological Psychology*, *77*(2), 217–222. https://doi.org/10.1016/j.biopsycho.2007.10.012

Hall, M., Crowder, K., & Spring, A. (2015). Neighborhood foreclosures, racial/ethnic transitions, and residential segregation. *American Sociological Review*. https://doi.org/10.1177/0003122415581334

Harding, J. P., Rosenblatt, E., & Yao, V. W. (2009). The contagion effect of foreclosed properties. *Journal of Urban Economics*, *66*(3), 164–178. https://doi.org/10.1016/j.jue.2009.07.003

Hoene, C., & Pagano, M. (2010). *City Fiscal Conditions in 2010*. Washington, DC: National League of Cities. Retrieved from http://www.nlc.org/ASSETS/AE26793318A645C795C9CD11DAB3B39B/RB_CityFiscalConditions2010.pdf

Houle, J. N. (2014). Mental health in the foreclosure crisis. *Social Science & Medicine*, *118*, 1–8. https://doi.org/10.1016/j.socscimed.2014.07.054

Houle, J. N., & Keene, D. E. (2015). Getting sick and falling behind: Health and the risk of mortgage default and home foreclosure. *Journal of Epidemiology and Community Health*, *69*(4), 382–387. https://doi.org/10.1136/jech-2014-204637

Houle, J. N., & Light, M. T. (2014). The home foreclosure crisis and rising suicide rates, 2005 to 2010. *American Journal of Public Health*, *104*(6), 1073–1079. https://doi.org/10.2105/AJPH.2013.301774

Immergluck, D. (2008). Community response to the foreclosure crisis: Thoughts on local interventions. *Institute of Urban & Regional Development*. Community Affairs Discussion Paper 01-08, Federal Reserve Bank of Atlanta: Community Affairs. Available at https://www.frbatlanta.org/-/media/documents/community-development/publications/discussion-papers/2008/01-community-response-to-foreclosure-crisis-2008-10-10.pdf

Immergluck, D., & Smith, G. (2005). *There goes the neighborhood: The effect of single-family mortgage foreclosures on property values*. Chicago IL: Woodstock Institute.

Immergluck, D., & Smith, G. (2006). The impact of single-family mortgage foreclosures on neighborhood crime. *Housing Studies*, *21*(6), 851–866.

Jang, Y., Chiriboga, D. A., Herrera, J. R., & Branch, L. G. (2009). Self-rating of poor health: A comparison of Cuban elders in Havana and Miami. *Journal of Cross-Cultural Gerontology*, *24*(2), 181–191. https://doi.org/10.1007/s10823-009-9094-x

Joint Center for Housing Studies. (2010). *The state of the nation's housing*. Cambridge, MA: Harvard University. Retrieved from http://www.jchs.harvard.edu/sites/jchs.harvard.edu/files/son2010.pdf

Joint Center for Housing Studies. (2016). *The state of the nation's housing*. Cambridge, MA: Harvard University. Retrieved from http://www.jchs.harvard.edu/research/state_nations_housing

Kahn, J. R., & Fazio, E. M. (2005). Economic status over the life course and racial disparities in health. *The Journals of Gerontology. Series B, Psychological Sciences and Social Sciences*, *60*(2), 76–84.

Kahn, J. R., & Pearlin, L. I. (2006). Financial strain over the life course and health among older adults. *Journal of Health and Social Behavior*, *47*(1), 17.

Katz, C. M., Wallace, D., & Hedberg, E. C. (2013). A longitudinal assessment of the impact of foreclosure on neighborhood crime. *Journal of Research in Crime and Delinquency*, *50*(3), 359–389. https://doi.org/10.1177/0022427811431155

Kendzor, D. E., Businelle, M. S., Costello, T. J., Castro, Y., Reitzel, L. R., Cofta-Woerpel, L. M., . . . Wetter, D. W. (2010). Financial strain and smoking cessation among racially/ethnically diverse smokers. *American Journal of Public Health*, *100*(4), 702–706. https://doi.org/10.2105/AJPH.2009.172676

Kingsley, G. T. (2009, June 22). The impacts of foreclosures on families and communities. Retrieved January 23, 2011, from http://www.urban.org/publications/411909.html

Kirk, D., & Hyra, D. (2010). Home foreclosures and community crime: Causal or spurious association? *SSRN ELibrary*. Retrieved from http://papers.ssrn.com.ezp-prod1.hul.harvard.edu/sol3/papers.cfm?abstract_id=1697871

Krause, N. (1987). Chronic financial strain, social support, and depressive symptoms among older adults. *Psychology and Aging*, *2*(2), 185–192.

Kwate, N. O. A., & Lee, T. H. (2007). Ghettoizing outdoor advertising: Disadvantage and ad panel density in black neighborhoods. *Journal of Urban Health: Bulletin of the New York Academy of Medicine*, *84*(1), 21–31. https://doi.org/10.1007/s11524-006-9127-5

Lacoe, J., & Ellen, I. G. (2015). Mortgage foreclosures and the changing mix of crime in microneighborhoods. *Journal of Research in Crime and Delinquency*, *52*(5), 717–746. https://doi.org/10.1177/0022427815572633

Lambie-Hanson, L. (2015). When does delinquency result in neglect? Mortgage distress and property maintenance. *Journal of Urban Economics*, *90*, 1–16. https://doi.org/10.1016/j.jue.2015.07.002

Lin, Z., Rosenblatt, E., & Yao, V. W. (2009). Spillover effects of foreclosures on neighborhood property values. *The Journal of Real Estate Finance and Economics*, *38*(4), 387–407.

Lincoln, K. D. (2007). Financial strain, negative interactions, and mastery: Pathways to mental health among older African Americans. *The Journal of Black Psychology*, *33*(4), 439–462. https://doi.org/10.1177/0095798407307045

Lindblad, M. R., & Riley, S. F. (2015). Loan modifications and foreclosure sales during the financial crisis: Consequences for health and stress. *Housing Studies*, *30*(7), 1092–1115. https://doi.org/10.1080/02673037.2015.1008425

Lynch, J. W., Kaplan, G. A., & Shema, S. J. (1997). Cumulative impact of sustained economic hardship on physical, cognitive, psychological, and social functioning. *The New England Journal of Medicine*, *337*(26), 1889–1895. https://doi.org/10.1056/NEJM199712253372606

Mattsson, M., Topor, A., Cullberg, J., & Forsell, Y. (2008). Association between financial strain, social network and five-year recovery from first episode psychosis. *Social Psychiatry and Psychiatric Epidemiology*, *43*(12), 947–952. https://doi.org/10.1007/s00127-008-0392-3

McFarland, C., & McCahan, W. (2008). *Housing finance and foreclosures crisis: Local impacts and responses* (No. 2008-1). Washington, DC: National League of Cities. Retrieved from http://www.nlc.org/ASSETS/580A9E2DD59E42809E3C4FBBD6AC1A99/PARHousingRB2008.pdf

McLaughlin, K. A., Nandi, A., Keyes, K. M., Uddin, M., Aiello, A. E., Galea, S., & Koenen, K. C. (2011). Home foreclosure and risk of psychiatric morbidity during the recent financial crisis. *Psychological Medicine*, 1–8. https://doi.org/10.1017/S0033291711002613

Nettleton, S., & Burrows, R. (1998). Mortgage debt, insecure home ownership and health: An exploratory analysis. *Sociology of Health & Illness*, *20*(5), 731–753. https://doi.org/10.1111/1467-9566.00127

NSP: Neighborhood Stabilization Program—HUD Exchange. (2014). Retrieved August 24, 2016, from https://www.hudexchange.info/programs/nsp/

Osypuk, T. L., Caldwell, C. H., Platt, R. W., & Misra, D. P. (2012). The consequences of foreclosure for depressive symptomatology. *Annals of Epidemiology*, *22*(6), 379–387. https://doi.org/10.1016/j.annepidem.2012.04.012

Pearlin, L. I., Lieberman, M. A., Menaghan, E. G., & Mullan, J. T. (1981). The stress process. *Journal of Health and Social Behavior*, *22*(4), 337–356.

Pevalin, D. J. (2009). Housing repossessions, evictions and common mental illness in the UK: Results from a household panel study. *Journal of Epidemiology and Community Health*, *63*(11), 949–951. https://doi.org/10.1136/jech.2008.083477

Pollack, C. E., Kurd, S. K., Livshits, A., Weiner, M., & Lynch, J. (2011). A case-control study of home foreclosure, health conditions, and health care utilization. *Journal of Urban Health: Bulletin of the New York Academy of Medicine*, *88*(3), 469–478. https://doi.org/10.1007/s11524-011-9564-7

Pollack, C. E., & Lynch, J. (2009). Health status of people undergoing foreclosure in the Philadelphia region. *American Journal of Public Health*, *99*(10), 1833.

Pollard, T. (2008). Fiscal fiasco: A time of reckoning for the NHS. *British Journal of Nursing (Mark Allen Publishing)*, *17*(22), 1379.

Pyle, S. A., Haddock, C. K., Poston, W. S. C., Bray, R. M., & Williams, J. (2007). Tobacco use and perceived financial strain among junior enlisted in the U.S. military in 2002. *Preventive Medicine*, *45*(6), 460–463. https://doi.org/10.1016/j.ypmed.2007.05.012

Raitt, J., & Arcaya, M. (2010). Foreclosure: Community impacts, prevention, and stabilization strategies. *PAS Memo*, September/October, 1–8.

RealtyTrac. (2011a, January 13). Record 2.9 million U.S. Properties Receive Foreclosure Filings in 2010 Despite 30-Month Low in December. Retrieved January 27, 2011, from http://www.realtytrac.com/content/press-releases/record-29-million-us-properties-receive-foreclosure-filings-in-2010-despite-30-month-low-in-december-6309

RealtyTrac. (2011b, February 3). Foreclosure Laws and Procedures By State. Retrieved February 8, 2011, from http://www.realtytrac.com/foreclosure-laws/foreclosure-laws-comparison.asp

RealtyTrac. (2011c, February 3). Property foreclosure overview and foreclosure process. Retrieved February 3, 2011, from http://www.realtytrac.com/foreclosure/overview.html

Reisen, W. K., Takahashi, R. M., Carroll, B. D., & Quiring, R. (2008). Delinquent mortgages, neglected swimming pools, and West Nile virus, California. *Emerging Infectious Diseases*, *14*(11), 1747.

Robertson, C. T., Egelhof, R., & Hoke, M. (2008). Get sick, get out: The medical causes of home mortgage foreclosures. *Health Matrix: Journal of Law-Medicine*, *18*(65).

Rogers, W., & Winter, W. (2009). The impact of foreclosures on neighboring housing sales. *Journal of Real Estate Research*, *31*(4), 455–479.

Rüger, H., Löffler, I., Ochsmann, E., Alsmann, C., Letzel, S., & Münster, E. (2010). Mental illness and over-indebtedness: Mental illness, social networks and financial strain in over-indebted persons. *Psychotherapie, Psychosomatik, Medizinische Psychologie*, *60*(7), 250–254. https://doi.org/10.1055/s-0029-1202364

Schootman, M., Deshpande, A. D., Pruitt, S. L., & Jeffe, D. B. (2012). Neighborhood foreclosures and self-rated health among breast cancer survivors. *Quality of Life Research: An International Journal of Quality of Life Aspects of Treatment, Care and Rehabilitation*, *21*(1), 133–141. https://doi.org/10.1007/s11136-011-9929-0

Schuetz, J., Been, V., & Ellen, I. G. (2008). Neighborhood effects of concentrated mortgage foreclosures. *Journal of Housing Economics*, *17*(4), 306–319.

Schulz, A. J., Israel, B. A., Zenk, S. N., Parker, E. A., Lichtenstein, R., Shellman-Weir, S., & Klem, A. B. L. (2006). Psychosocial stress and social support as mediators of relationships between income, length of residence and depressive symptoms among African American women on Detroit's eastside. *Social Science & Medicine (1982)*, *62*(2), 510–522. https://doi.org/10.1016/j.socscimed.2005.06.028

Steptoe, A., Brydon, L., & Kunz-Ebrecht, S. (2005). Changes in financial strain over three years, ambulatory blood pressure, and cortisol responses to awakening. *Psychosomatic Medicine*, *67*(2), 281–287. https://doi.org/10.1097/01.psy.0000156932.96261.d2

Steptoe, A., & Feldman, P. J. (2001). Neighborhood problems as sources of chronic stress: Development of a measure of neighborhood problems, and associations with socio-economic status and health. *Annals of Behavioral Medicine: A Publication of the Society of Behavioral Medicine*, *23*(3), 177–185.

Stoddard, J. L., Johnson, C. A., Sussman, S., Dent, C., & Boley-Cruz, T. (1998). Tailoring outdoor tobacco advertising to minorities in Los Angeles County. *Journal of Health Communication*, *3*(2), 137–146.

Stucky, T. D., Ottensmann, J. R., & Payton, S. B. (2012). The effect of foreclosures on crime in Indianapolis, 2003–2008. *Social Science Quarterly*, *93*(3), 602–624. https://doi.org/10.1111/j.1540-6237.2012.00890.x

Szanton, S. L., Thorpe, R. J., & Whitfield, K. (2010). Life-course financial strain and health in African-Americans. *Social Science & Medicine (1982)*, *71*(2), 259–265. https://doi.org/10.1016/j.socscimed.2010.04.001

Taylor, M. P., Pevalin, D. J., & Todd, J. (2007). The psychological costs of unsustainable housing commitments. *Psychological Medicine*, *37*(07), 1027–1036.

Tsai, A. C. (2015). Home foreclosure, health, and mental health: A systematic review of individual, aggregate, and contextual associations. *PLOS ONE*, *10*(4), e0123182. https://doi.org/10.1371/journal.pone.0123182

Tucker-Seeley, R. D., Harley, A. E., Stoddard, A. M., & Sorensen, G. G. (2013). Financial hardship and self-rated health among low-income housing residents. *Health Education & Behavior*, *40*(4), 442–448.

Vásquez-Vera, H., Rodríguez-Sanz, M., Palència, L., & Borrell, C. (2016). Foreclosure and health in Southern Europe: Results from the Platform for People Affected by Mortgages. *Journal of Urban Health: Bulletin of the New York Academy of Medicine*, *93*(2), 312–330. https://doi.org/10.1007/s11524-016-0030-4

West, J. H., Blumberg, E. J., Kelley, N. J., Hill, L., Sipan, C. L., Schmitz, K. E., . . . Hovell, M. F. (2010). Does proximity to retailers influence alcohol and tobacco use among Latino adolescents? *Journal of Immigrant and Minority Health/Center for Minority Public Health*, *12*(5), 626–633. https://doi.org/10.1007/s10903-009-9303-2

Wood, J. N., Medina, S. P., Feudtner, C., Luan, X., Localio, R., Fieldston, E. S., & Rubin, D. M. (2012). Local macroeconomic trends and hospital admissions for child abuse, 2000–2009. *Pediatrics*, *130*(2), e358–e364. https://doi.org/10.1542/peds.2011-3755

Yilmazer, T., Babiarz, P., & Liu, F. (2015). The impact of diminished housing wealth on health in the United States: Evidence from the Great Recession. *Social Science & Medicine*, *130*, 234–241. https://doi.org/10.1016/j.socscimed.2015.02.028

Zimmerman, F. J., & Katon, W. (2005). Socioeconomic status, depression disparities, and financial strain: What lies behind the income-depression relationship? *Health Economics*, *14*(12), 1197–1215. https://doi.org/10.1002/hec.1011

12

RESIDENTIAL SEGREGATION AND HEALTH

Michael R. Kramer

Segregation is the sorting and separation of individuals into groups based on their membership in, or assignment to, socially constructed categories such as race, ethnicity, gender, class, or religion. Because separate is rarely equal, segregation usually results in the explicit or implicit constraint or exclusion of some individuals or groups from particular services, places, or interactions with other groups. State-sponsored segregation of racial groups across multiple institutions—education, housing, public services, and marriage—was a prominent aspect of Apartheid policies in South Africa, and Jim Crow policies in the Southern United States. But segregation by religion (e.g., Protestants and Catholics in Northern Ireland; Maguire, French, & O'Reilly, 2016), gender (e.g., by occupation, or gender separation in some orthodox religious activities), and even ideological preference (e.g., segregation of social and information sharing networks; Gentzkow & Shapiro, 2011) is not an uncommon aspect of modern social life. *Residential segregation*, the focus of this chapter, is a specific type of social sorting that results in the spatial and physical separation of where individuals live in residential space. Because residential location anchors the life course geography of opportunity and exposure profile of individuals (e.g., the focus of much of this book), this class of segregation may have short- and long-term consequences for the life chances of individuals, and thus it has been referred to as a fundamental determinant of population health and health disparities (Williams & Collins, 2001).

Many observers struggle with defining exactly what constitutes segregation, falling back instead on Supreme Court Justice Potter Stewart's 1964 assertion in reference to obscene material not protected by free speech: "I know it when I see it" (Lattman, 2007). Residential segregation by race, ethnicity, and class is an apparent and ubiquitous aspect of the modern urban landscape across geographic locations (Lloyd, Shuttleworth, & Wong, 2014), but understanding how it originated, how it is maintained and reproduced, how it plausibly affects health and development, and even at a basic sense how to measure and quantify it is surprisingly challenging. In this chapter we consider conceptual, methodological, and empirical issues helpful for examining a segregation–health connection, divided into four sections.

In the first section, a conceptual understanding of residential segregation is developed. For example, segregation is an attribute of places at a point in time but also a historically contingent and temporally dynamic process. Additionally, to conceive of sorting individuals between neighborhoods implies that segregation involves at least two spatial scales simultaneously: local neighborhoods where a given individual resides, situated within a broader region or set of alternative neighborhoods where that individual does not live. Thus, conceptualizing segregation as a health-relevant process requires attention to both time and space. Translating these conceptual understandings of segregation for empirical research requires meaningful metrics for measurement. In the second section, approaches to the operationalization and measurement of segregation patterns are reviewed. Considering segregation as a topic of interest to public health begs the question of mechanisms linking residential sorting to health outcomes, and levers for intervention. Therefore, in the third section we briefly review theoretical and empirical evidence for a segregation–health association, including hypothesized mechanisms. Finally in the fourth section, possible future directions for segregation-health research are considered, including issues of study design, causal inference, and broadening conceptual framing of segregating processes in population health. Although residential segregation along one social dimension or another—ethnicity, race, class, religion—is present in most countries, the bulk of the literature on residential segregation and health has focused on racial and ethnic segregation, largely in the context of the United States. Many examples in this chapter reflect that fact, although the concepts addressed herein can be applied more broadly.

WHAT PRODUCES SEGREGATED RESIDENTIAL SPACE?

seg·re·gate

verb

/ˈsegrəˌgeɪt/

to set apart from the rest or from each other; isolate or divide.

seg·re·ga·tion

noun

/ˌsegrəˈgeɪʃ(ə)n/

the state of setting someone or something apart from other people or things or being set apart.

seg·re·gated

adjective
/ˈsegrəˌgeɪtəd/
set apart or separated from others of the same kind or group.

It seems sensible for investigations of the consequences of segregation to start at the beginning: How did people come to live in integrated or segregated places? Did they choose it, were they forced into the situation, or did it "just happen"? Fundamentally, segregation is about sorting or separating, suggesting the active *verb* form of the word would be important, whether the "action" is one of individual choice or structural constraint. However, conceptualization and measurement of residential segregation nearly universally attend to the *adjective* and *noun* forms of the word: Segregation scholars generally characterize the point-in-time spatial state of a population or monitor repeated cross-sectional snapshots across time (Reardon, 2006). This approach not only risks ignoring the process that produced—and may continue to reproduce—the spatial state of residential patterns but also presumes that all paths to segregation are equal in their dynamics and consequences. So is all segregation (e.g., all patterns of spatial separation) the same?

Social scientists detail several broad processes that could give rise to residential segregation and spatial concentration of specific racial or ethnic groups. *Spatial assimilation theory* describes the co-location of recent immigrants to a new destination or "port of entry" (Logan & Alba, 1993; Massey, 1985). For instance, waves of immigrants to the United States in the 19th and 20th centuries initially settled in ethnic enclaves (e.g., Little Italy, Little Havana, Chinatown), in part for the familiar cultural context of coethnics but also for the benefits of collective social capital of these communities. Accumulated knowledge and networks help newcomers navigate labor markets, interact with schools and government services, and aid in general assimilation (Logan, Alba, & Zhang, 2002). A notable characteristic of these immigrant enclaves is that they may be located in less desirable neighborhoods in part due to the group's initial limited material economic resources. These immigrant enclaves may therefore represent a form of temporary or transient segregation; as high-achieving members acquire material resources and become familiar with the destination culture, they translate those resources into "better" (and perhaps ethnically less distinct) neighborhoods. In other words, they are spatially assimilated over one or more generations. The full process of spatial assimilation is perhaps most evident in the experience of Irish, Italian, German, and other European immigrants to the United States in the past century. However, there is evidence for spatial assimilation in the late 20th and early 21st century among Hispanics (South, Crowder, & Pais, 2008) and Asians (Flippen & Kim, 2015), although in each case there is variation by country of origin. Although an important feature of spatial assimilation is the eventual conversion of newfound economic gains into better neighborhood environments, another version termed "ethnic communities" is represented by some recent immigrant waves with relatively high education and wealth upon arrival. These groups do not experience the same economic constraints on neighborhood selection but may still chose destinations with shared ethnic identity for other social and cultural benefits (Logan et al., 2002).

While spatial assimilation may be characterized by aspects of choice to reside with coethnics, possibly paired with the added constraint of limited economic resources, *spatial stratification* theory suggests that both places (e.g., neighborhoods) and social groups (e.g., racial or ethnic groups) are hierarchically ordered. Majority groups use political, economic, and social power to spatially separate themselves into "better" places and constrain nondominant groups in less desirable locations (Logan & Alba, 1993; Massey & Denton, 1998). A consequence of the imposed spatial constraints are that minority groups' acquisition of material wealth cannot be as readily translated into access to a wider range of neighborhoods nor to the opportunities and resources provided by those neighborhoods, thus impeding economic and social mobility. A potent example of the stratification of places and persons is the role taken by the US federal, state, and local governments in urban housing policy beginning in the 1920s and accelerating in the post–World War II era (Rothstein, 2017). During much of the 20th century, government enforced de jure or legally encoded and sanctioned racial discrimination in urban development and housing support. For instance, federal mortgage lending programs delineated predominantly Black neighborhoods with red lines on survey maps and disseminated these to lenders as indicative of areas of "high risk" for investment, presumably because the presence of Black homeowners reduced property values (thus the phrase "mortgage redlining"). Federal and state housing lending programs also utilized racial covenant laws that explicitly excluded sale of government-supported housing (e.g., supported by federal mortgage programs) to African Americans. Government investment in high-density public housing projects offered safety net housing but also racialized space in a way that persists to this day. The passage of the Civil Rights Act of 1968 outlawed much of this explicit housing segregation, but it gave way to persistent de facto exclusion or segregation through active and passive forms of racial or ethnic discrimination, including private mortgage redlining, real estate steering, and Whites' willingness to pay more to live separately (Cutler, Glaeser, & Vigdor, 1999). While de facto segregation may partially explain the persistence of Black–White segregation in US urban areas, Rothstein (2017) argues forcibly that the legacy of mid-century government-sanctioned and mandated racial stratification of residential space produced the persistently unequal geography of opportunity.

Spatial assimilation and stratification theories provide top-down descriptions of how and why segregation might be produced. Agent-based models (see Chapter 5) provide an alternative bottom-up generative look at the production of segregation. For example, Schelling (1971) demonstrated the power of individual and group-specific preference for or tolerance of neighborhood homogeneity and diversity in what was possibly the first agent-based model in the social sciences. In Schelling's model, members of each of two groups sharing residential space tolerated "neighborhood" diversity as long as their own group exceeded some fixed minimum threshold. If their own-group neighborhood composition slipped below that threshold, they would seek out a more desirable neighborhood. Interestingly, near complete segregation could be generated under a wide range of group preferences, including tolerance for 50-50 balance, and even with preference for some degree of integration. Subsequent and more sophisticated agent-based models further elaborate the interplay of individual choice, and economic or social exclusion. Varying combinations of social groups' preference for living with own-group (desire for ethnic communities), avoidance of other groups (discriminatory decision making), and the hierarchy or gradient of social groups and places can generate realistically complex residential segregation (Fossett, 2011).

An important conclusion from the rich theoretical and empirical literature on the generation and production of spatial separation is that "segregation" may not be a global or fixed exposure. Health inequities that arise out of dynamic population processes, such as residential mobility and constraint, and are active across the life course are historically contingent (Krieger, 2012b). Said another way, the race or ethnicity of one's neighbors is not inherently toxic or health protective; rather, the processes that gave rise to spatial separation or integration are interlinked with the allocation of health-relevant factors, and thus with population health itself. Therefore, interpretation of the health consequence of segregation must attend to the residential—and associated economic and social—dynamics which gave rise to the separation or the point-in-time "state of segregation."

MEASURING SEGREGATION

Saying segregation's effect on health is historically contingent suggests that macro and micro dynamics through time are important in understanding its health consequences. But a survey of the broad menu of available measures and indices of point-in-time segregation suggests that it is also multifaceted and spatially contingent. In other words, just as there is no single effect of spatial separation for all populations through all time, there is no single measure of segregation which captures all aspects of the population patterns which are derived from segregating dynamics. If residential segregation is defined as the spatial distribution of two or more groups defined by race, ethnicity, or class, then measures of point-in-time residential segregation can be described, compared, and implemented according to how they incorporate or address each of several questions about the nature of segregation.

Which Dimension of Segregation Is of Interest?

Early researchers of racial segregation in the United States produced a dizzying array of indices and measures of residential patterns. In an effort to bring a semblance of order to the variety of measures, Massey and Denton (1988) calculated values for 20 segregation indices previously used in the literature for each of the 50 largest metropolitan areas in 1980, and then summarized them with principal components analysis. From this process they proposed that segregation could be reduced to five distinct dimensions or patterns of residential distribution, and that each measure of segregation aligned more or less with one of these dimensions. The *evenness* dimension refers to how evenly or unevenly spread each social group is in a shared regional housing market. Unevenness exists when a group is overrepresented in some local neighborhoods and underrepresented in others relative to their proportion of the total regional population. The *exposure* dimension summarizes the likelihood for neighborhood-level interaction between members of two or more groups. In contrast to evenness, which is about the spatial distribution across neighborhoods, exposure (and its antonym, isolation) measures some aspect of the average experience of segregation in the form of the opportunity for local, intergroup contact. Because complete isolation requires residence in monolithic (e.g., monoracial) neighborhoods, this dimension and the related indices are sensitive to the absolute size of the social group population: It is more difficult to live in isolation from the majority group if the minority group in the larger region is small. The *concentration* dimension contrasts the relative density per areal unit of members of one group to other groups, and it arises from the observation that some patterns of segregation result in minority groups spatially concentrated in a small fraction of the region. The *centralization* dimension describes the extent to which a social group is predominantly located near the central urban core of a region. As with concentration, this dimension acknowledges a common pattern produced in many cities by White flight, resulting in predominantly poor and minority concentration is urban cores, and whiter and wealthier neighborhoods in suburbs and exurbs. Finally, the *clustering* dimension characterizes the degree to which neighborhoods predominated by a single social group tend to occur adjacent to one another, creating clusters of similarity in a subregion of the overall housing market.

Although these five dimensions are often referenced, more recently several scholars have suggested that Massey and Denton's five dimensions are reducible to two essential dimensions. Reardon and O'Sullivan (2004) argued that evenness and clustering are two extremes of a single continuum with populations evenly distributed through space or clustered in subareas; the distinction between evenness within areal units versus clustering among areal units is simply a function or the scale of aggregation, but not a distinct spatial pattern. Centralization and concentration are simply special cases of unevenly distributed populations; in the former, the minority group is unevenly located in the central urban area, and in the latter group they are unevenly concentrated in subregions of the total area. Thus, four of Massey and Denton's dimensions collapse into an evenness–clustering continuum. The second dimension in Reardon and O'Sullivan's schema is the same isolation/exposure dimension originally described by Massey and Denton. Johnston et al. (2007) revisited the principal components analysis of Massey and Denton with more recent data and arrived at a similar conclusion as Reardon and O'Sullivan, but termed the two dimensions *separation* (akin to exposure/isolation) and *location* (akin to centralization, unevenness, and concentration).

This refined and reduced two-dimensional framework for understanding residential spatial patterns can be more intuitively understood by observing the unique patterns produced by the cross-product of these two essential segregation dimensions (Figure 12-1). In this simplified scenario a hypothetical city is composed of neighborhoods surrounding a central business district. Black and White dots are distributed across the city in distinct patterns. In every case, the size of the total population is the same (N = 140), and the city-wide group composition is constant (35% Black dots, 65% White dots). In the left two panels (A and C), Black dots are more clustered in the southwest portion of the city, whereas in the right two panels (B and D) the Black dots are more evenly spread across the city. In contrast on the upper two panels (A and B), both Black and White dots tend to be isolated in relatively homogenous neighborhoods with little likelihood of intergroup exposure within the neighborhood. The lower two panels (C and D) represent patterns where Black dots have a higher degree of exposure to White dots within their neighborhoods.

Measuring Regional Segregation

So what are the options for quantitatively measuring these patterns? As mentioned earlier, there are numerous indices available, but we review a select subset and discuss the calculation and interpretation of each for the evenness/clustering and exposure/isolation dimensions. The first indices quantify the overall segregation for a given region often operationalized as a core-based statistical area (CBSA, including metropolitan and micropolitan statistical areas) or county or city. The choice of this regional unit should reflect understanding of the scale and extent of the housing and labor market in which residential sorting and stratification occur (Acevedo-Garcia & Osypuk, 2008). Indices of local rather than regional segregation patterns are discussed next. This first set of indices is further referred to as "aspatial" reflecting the dependence of each formula on data aggregated to possibly arbitrary areal

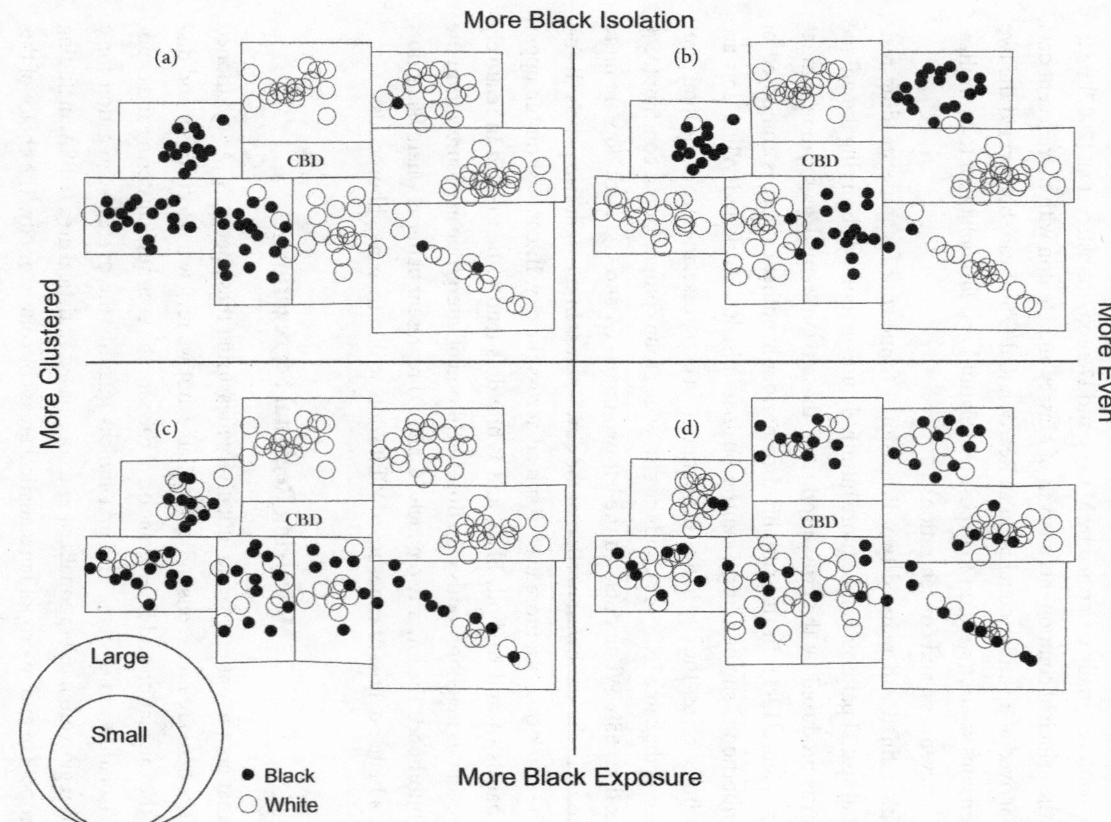

FIGURE 12-1 **Contrasting evenness–clustering and exposure–isolation dimensions of residential segregation. CBD, central business district. Figure adapted from Bell, et al., 2006.**

units such as census tracts; the distinction between aspatial and spatial is further developed next.

For measuring the *evenness* dimension, the dissimilarity index is perhaps the most widely used index in both health and social science research. Despite the common use of this measure, it has notable shortcomings in its adherence to common tests for the validity of segregation measures (Reardon & Firebaugh, 2002; Reardon & O'Sullivan, 2004; Roberto, 2015). Therefore, the dissimilarity index is not further discussed here. An increasingly used measure of evenness which overcomes many of the shortcomings of the dissimilarity index is Theil's Information Theory Index (H), which is derived from a class of entropy indices originally used in physics. Entropy quantifies randomness, chaos, or diversity in a system, and thus the use of entropy to quantify the even or uneven mixing of social groups is sensible. H, then, is a population-weighted average deviation of each local neighborhood's entropy (diversity) from the overall regional entropy; it ranges from 0 (every local area has the same group composition as the region overall and thus most even) to 1 (every local area is composed of only a single social group; e.g., monoracial and thus most clustered) (Table 12-1). Although much segregation research is limited to comparing the residential evenness of two social groups (e.g., White, Black), the H index readily accommodates greater than two categorical social groups such as race/ethnicity (Reardon & Firebaugh, 2002) and ordinal social groupings such as income or educational categories (Reardon, Firebaugh, O'Sullivan, & Matthews, 2006).

For measuring the regional exposure/isolation dimension of residential segregation the P* indices of exposure and isolation, which quantifies the average likelihood of local intergroup contact within neighborhoods, are most often used. The formula (Table 12-1, regional exposure index) is a population-weighted probability that any two randomly chosen individuals from a given neighborhood are of the same or different groups. The two versions of the index quantify the degree to which members of one group (e.g., Black) are exposed to or isolated from another group (e.g., White). The P* index is almost always used with two social groups, but extensions to multiple groups have been proposed (Reardon & Firebaugh, 2002).

Spatial Measures of Segregation

Segregation may be health relevant because of the way in which the dynamics of sorting, separation, and stratification affect the local context and environment of individuals. But how local is "local"? Is a neighborhood defined by cultural and historical boundaries? Or by physical barriers like railroad tracks and rivers? Or by the machinations that produce census geography? The same question of defining the bounds of neighborhood discussed elsewhere in this book (e.g., Chapter 2) are

Table 12-1 Measures of Residential Segregation

Dimension Local	*Index*	*Index Range and Interpretation*	*Aspatial*	*Spatial*
Evenness/ clustering	Regional Information theory index (H)	Range: 0 to 1 H = 0 Every local area has same intergroup diversity as region overall H = 1 each local area, *r*, is occupied by a single group (Reardon & O'Sullivan, 2004)	$H = \sum_{r \in R} \frac{t_r}{TE}(E - E_r)$ Where $E = -\sum_{m=1}^{M} \pi_m \log_M \pi_m$ $E_r = -\sum_{m=1}^{M} \pi_{mr} \log_M \pi_{mr}$	$\tilde{H} = 1 - \frac{1}{TE} \int_{q \in R} \tau_q \tilde{E}_q dq$ Where $\tilde{E}_q = -\sum_{m=1}^{M} \tilde{\pi}_{qm} \log_M \tilde{\pi}_{qm}$
	Local Divergence (D_r) index	Range: –1 to 1 $H_r < 0$ when area is more diverse than region overall ("hyperintegration") $H_r = 0$ when local group composition equals regional composition $H_r > 0$ when local area is less diverse than region overall $H_r = 1$ when any group is 100% of local composition (Reardon & O'Sullivan, 2004; Roberto, 2015)	$H_r = 1 - \frac{E_r}{E}$	$\tilde{H} = 1 - \frac{\tilde{E}_q}{E}$
	Local Divergence (D_r) index	Range: 0 to *max* (index can be normalized to 0,1 by dividing all local values by dataset specific maximum) $D_r = 0$ when local intergroup composition equals regional composition D_r is maximum when the regional *minority group* is 100% of the local population (Roberto, 2015)	$D_r = -\sum_{m=1}^{M} \pi_{mr} \log_M \frac{\pi_{mr}}{\pi_m}$	$\tilde{D}_q = -\sum_{m=1}^{M} \tilde{\pi}_{mq} \log_M \frac{\tilde{\pi}_{mq}}{\pi_m}$

Exposure/ isolation	Regional Exposure index (${}_mP_n^*$) Regional Isolation index (${}_mP_m^*$)	(${}_mP_n^*$) range: 0 to 1 0 = least exposure of group *m* to group *n* (most segregated) 1 = maximal exposure of group *m* to group *n* (least segregated) (${}_mP_m^*$) range: 0 to 1 0 = least exposure of group *m* to others of group *m* (least segregated/ isolated) 1 = maximal exposure of group *m* to others of their own group (maximally segregated/isolated) (Reardon & O'Sullivan, 2004)	${}_mP_n^* = \sum_{r \in R} \frac{t_{mr}}{T_m} \pi_{nr}$ ${}_mP_m^* = \sum_{r \in R} \frac{t_{mr}}{T_m} \pi_{mr}$	${}_m\tilde{P}_n^* = \int_{q \in R} \frac{\tau_{qm}}{T_m} \tilde{\pi}_{qn} dq$ ${}_m\tilde{P}_m^* = \int_{q \in R} \frac{\tau_{qm}}{T_m} \tilde{\pi}_{qm} dq$
Other local measures	Local Location Quotient (LQ_r)	Range: 0 to ∞ LQ < 1 Proportion of group underrepresented in local area *r* relative to their proportion in overall region LQ = 1 Group *t* proportion in local area *r* relative to their proportion in overall region LQ > 1 Group *t* is overrepresented in local area *r* relative to their proportion in overall region (Brown & Chung, 2006a)	$LQ_{rm} = \frac{\pi_{rm}}{\pi_m}$	$\widetilde{LQ}_{qm} = \frac{\tilde{\pi}_{qm}}{\pi_m}$

(*continued*)

Table 12-1 Continued

Dimension	*Index*	*Index Range and Interpretation*	*Aspatial*	*Spatial*
Local				
	Local Index of Concentration at Extremes (ICE_r)	Range: −1 to +1 ICE < 0 Population in region *r* has excess lower status as compared to higher status group members ICE = 0 Even distribution of high (*p*) and low (*a*) status groups in region *r* ICE > 0 Population in region *r* has excess higher status as compared to lower status group members (Krieger et al., 2017)	$ICE_r = \frac{(a_r - p_r)}{t_r}$	$I\tilde{C}E_q = \frac{(\tilde{\tau}_{aq} - \tilde{\tau}_{pq})}{\tilde{\tau}_q}$

Aspatial parameters

T = total population count in region (e.g., city, county, MSA)

t_r = population count in local area *r* (e.g., census tract)

t_{rm} = population count of group *m* in local area *r*

a_r = population count of affluent or privileged group, local area *r*

p_r = population count of poor or less privileged

π_{rm} = proportion group *m* in area *r* (e.g., % Black in tract *r*)

π_m = proportion group *m* in overall region (e.g., % Black in MSA)

Note: entropy formula's presented here use $\log_m$ rather than natural log to ensure maximum values are 1. If calculated with natural log, the maximum entropy would be ln(M) and thus would need to be normalized to scale from 0 to 1.

Spatial parameters

τ_q = population density at local point *q*

τ_{qm} = population density of group *m* at local point *q*

$\tilde{\tau}_{aq}, \tilde{\tau}_{pq}$ = population density of group *a*, *p* in local environment of *q*

$\tilde{\pi}_{qm}$ = proportion group *m* in local environment of point *q*

Source: Notation adapted from Reardon & O'Sullivan, 2004.

important for operationalizing segregation. In the United States the most common approach in segregation research—and indeed in neighborhood effects research more generally—is to adopt the geographic boundaries of the Census Bureau and to treat units such as the census block, block group, or tract as a proxy for local neighborhoods. Although census geographies can change over time (e.g., areal units might be split or merged as populations change), methods to create longitudinally harmonized boundaries permit the linkage of demographic, social, and economic data collected by the Census Bureau (Logan, Xu, & Stults, 2014). For instance, each of the segregation indices mentioned in the previous section can be readily calculated from Census data using block groups or tracts as the local areas, *r*, within counties or metropolitan regions, *R*. However, two problems arise from this practice, one methodological and the other potentially substantive.

The methodological concern comes from reliance on the possibly arbitrary boundary system for defining local neighborhoods. Individual members of social groups are distributed in a relatively continuous manner with persons and families occupying housing units at a given address or point in space. However, aspatial segregation indices require the aggregation of individuals into local neighborhood areas and broader regional areas. Aggregating population counts within areal units which do not have inherent substantive meaning can lead to biased and misleading estimates as a result of the modifiable areal unit problem (MAUP) (Openshaw, 1983). As discussed in Chapter 2, the MAUP results when arbitrary spatial scale and arbitrary boundaries or zoning of areal units provides misleading summaries of the distribution of populations through space. The spatial scale refers to the spatial extent or size of the areal units used for aggregating. For instance, local neighborhoods could be proxied by census blocks, block groups, or tracts. In the Atlanta metropolitan area, the average area of a census block is only 0.02 square miles, whereas the average area of a census tract is 2.1 square miles, a 100-fold difference. Thus, the granularity of population distribution within each "neighborhood" is quite different, and this difference in the scale of aggregation can lead to different segregation index values and even different rank-ordering of metropolitan areas by segregation (Reardon et al., 2008). In addition to the scale of aggregation, the reliance on census boundaries as distinguishing meaningful lived environments is questionable. For instance, members of a common "neighborhood" are presumed to share more environmental experience than members of other neighborhoods; but residents near boundaries may share more environmental experience with residents from adjacent neighborhoods than with some of their own. If the boundaries or scale is substantively relevant (e.g., using county boundaries to examine services provided by county governments or using school enrollment boundaries to examine differences in school performance), then MAUP may not be a concern. Similarly, there are instances where real boundaries (social and physical) exist, although they may not align with administrative units (Roberto & Hwang, 2015). But in many instances there is nothing but tradition to guide our reliance on convenient administrative boundaries such as census tracts.

The more substantive concern is the realization that for measuring segregation, space matters. Census boundaries constitute only a single, possibly arbitrary, representation of the local environmental experience of residents. Even if census boundaries capture some portion of the residential patterning, it is unlikely that every social and health consequence of segregation is equally conceptualized or experienced at that same scale. For example, relationships with neighbors, concerns about crime, and walkability might be relevant in the immediate vicinity of one's home, but few people work, buy groceries, or seek secondary or higher education on their own block. Instead, those activities occur at a larger scale; to be sure, there is a limit to how far one can or will travel for work, but it is plausibly a different spatial scale than one might walk his or her dog. Therefore, rather than there being a single "right" spatial scale, variation in patterns across scale could shed light on how the social or environmental process is structured. The possible dependence on scale of association is not only a concern for the measurement of segregation; associations between segregation and other place-based processes may also impact health differently as a function of the spatial scale of analysis (Kramer, 2016; Kramer, Cooper, Drews-Botsch, Waller, & Hogue, 2010a).

Several investigators have developed explicitly spatial versions of segregation indices in order to minimize reliance on administrative zoning systems, thereby maintaining the focus on the relative arrangement of populations in residential space (Reardon & O'Sullivan, 2004; Rey & Folch, 2011; Sullivan, Wong, O'Sullivan, & Wong, 2007; Wong, 2005). For example, Reardon et al.'s approach uses spatially continuous kernel density functions to create egocentric neighborhoods defined as the area around each point in space. In that way, every location (e.g., each house or street segment) has its own definition of the "local environment," with the spatial extent of "local" defined in a flexible manner (Reardon et al., 2009, 2008). Segregation can then be estimated under alternative definitions such as small walkable environments up to larger subregions of the city. Spatial version of both the regional H index and the P* indices are provided in Table 12-1, with the main distinction being a shift from mutually exclusive areal units, *r*, to spatially continuous summaries of local environments indicated by the superimposed tilde symbol.

Returning to the residential segregation patterns of four "cities" depicted in Figure 12-1, I have calculated both spatial and aspatial measures of evenness (H index) and exposure (Black isolation, ${}_{m}P_{m}^{*}$) (Table 12-2). The aspatial measures rely on the boundary system of local neighborhood illustrated on the figure. The

Table 12-2 Spatial and Aspatial Segregation Indices for Housing Regions in Figure 12-1

	City Representation From Figure 12-1			
	A.	*B.*	*C.*	*D.*
Evenness/clustering				
Aspatial H	0.72	0.88	0.48	0.28
Spatial H (small neighborhood)	0.61	0.45	0.28	0.05
Spatial H (large neighborhood)	0.51	0.18	0.19	0.03
Segregation granularity ratio (Spatial H large/small)	0.83	0.41	0.69	0.50
Exposure/isolation				
Aspatial Black isolation	0.86	0.89	0.57	0.41
Spatial Black isolation (small neighborhood)	0.80	0.67	0.54	0.39
Spatial Black isolation (large neighborhood)	0.73	0.49	0.50	0.36
Segregation granularity ratio (Spatial H large/small)	0.92	0.72	0.92	0.94

All "cities" have same total population and racial composition: 35% Black, 65% White.

Spatial measures calculated with egocentric kernel density definitions of "local neighborhood." See Figure 12-1 for size of "large" and "small."

spatial measures use a kernel density function to describe the egocentric local spatial environment across continuous space. Spatial measures are estimated at two scales: "large" and "small"; see legend on Figure 12-1 for proportionate size of these definitions.

Several points help illustrate the distinction between indices, and the importance of spatial scale in understanding and interpreting segregation indices. As reviewed earlier, cities B and D are presumed to be the "most even" (least segregated), whereas cities A and C are the "least even" (most clustered). For all three versions of the H index of evenness-clustering segregation, city D is in fact the least segregated (lowest H). However, not all measures agree with respect to city B, and in fact the aspatial H measure suggests that city B is the *most* segregated city! The explanation for this discrepancy is clear when we consider the reliance of the aspatial measure on aggregation to neighborhood boundaries. Clearly the bounded neighborhoods in city B are each quite monoracial, and thus at that particular scale, the population is unevenly distributed. However, both the small and large neighborhood versions of the spatial H suggest much less segregation. The difference is that the spatial measures consider the subregional density of populations without respect to the administrative neighborhood boundaries. Which index is more accurate depends on the social meaning of the boundaries. The Black isolation index is more consistent across spatial scale of aggregation, although it is worth noting that as the size of the neighborhood increases—in other words, as the spatial extent of hypothesized social interaction increases—isolation of Blacks from Whites decreases.

Another feature of the use of varying spatial scales in the calculation of residential segregation is the opportunity to describe a segregation profile across a range of scales to answer how much a given region has micro- versus macro-spatial patterns (Reardon et al., 2008). For instance, the ratio of segregation with large as compared to small spatial scales characterizes the *granularity* of segregation. The ratio ranges from 0 to 1, representing the proportion of the micro-segregation, which is explained by macro patterns. Returning to Table 12-2, in city B less than half (41%) of the small-scale H segregation is explained by larger scale patterns. In contrast, cities A and C have more of their micro-segregation explained by larger scale patterns (83% and 69%, respectively).

Local Measures of Segregation

Up to this point, the emphasis on measurement has been on characterizing segregation or sorting in a region such as a metropolitan statistical area, as a function of the distribution of social groups across the constituent neighborhoods within the region; in other words, there is a single index value for each region. This regional focus derives from the notion that the macrosocial process of residential stratification and sorting happens across neighborhoods. However, researchers are frequently interested in localizing the causes and consequences of segregation by characterizing the contribution of individual neighborhoods to overall segregation. Recent work has developed a number of segregation measures that characterize local aspects of evenness and isolation within the comparative context of regional expectations.

Two local measures of the evenness dimension of segregation are summarized in Table 12-1. The local H index (H_r for areal data and $\tilde{H}_q$ for spatially continuous representation) summarizes the degree to which the local diversity differs from the overall diversity of the region. Unlike the regional H, the local H can take on negative values when local areas are "hyperintegrated," meaning they are more diverse than the region overall (Reardon & O'Sullivan, 2004). A related but distinct local index has been termed the local Divergence index, D (not to be confused with the dissimilarity index sometimes also denoted D) (Roberto, 2015). The conceptual distinction between the local H and local D indices is that the former measures difference in local diversity, whereas the latter measures the difference from a reference pattern. One implication is that the maximal value of local H reflects no diversity (e.g., monoracial neighborhood), whereas the maximal value of local D reflects the greatest departure from the overall pattern, which is not only a monoracial neighborhood but one that is dominated by the regional minority group.

The local derivative of the exposure/isolation index is in fact the local racial composition of a given neighborhood. While potentially of interest to researchers, as already discussed the local racial composition in isolation is an inadequate proxy for the degree to which a given neighborhood is like or unlike another neighborhood with respect to the experience of isolation or exposure between groups. While not necessarily indicative of exposure/isolation, one measure increasingly used for quantifying local segregation patterns is the location quotient (LQ_r), which contrasts the proportion of a given group in the local area to their proportion in the region overall (Brown & Chung, 2006; Sudano, Perzynski, Wong, Colabianchi, & Litaker, 2013). The LQ takes a value of 1 for neighborhoods which reflect the regional social composition; values between 0 and 1 suggest the social group is underrepresented in the neighborhood relative to the region; and values greater than 1 suggest the group is overrepresented in the neighborhood relative to the region. An important consideration in use of this index is that as a ratio, it is asymmetric around the equality value of 1. In other words if a neighborhood has half the proportion Black as the region overall, the LQ would be 0.5 or 0.5 units from the equality value of 1; but if it had the inverse, or twice the proportion Black, the LQ would be 2 or 1 unit above the equality value of 1. Thus, investigators considering the LQ in statistical analysis (e.g., multivariable regression) might categorize or log-transform it to assure comparisons of over- and underrepresentation are fairly counted.

The final local measure does not actually meet the definition of comparing local social group patterns to a larger context. However, it does describe a consequence of segregation—the spatial concentration of socially privileged or less privileged groups in space. The index of concentration at the extremes (ICE_r) contrasts the number of individuals in a neighborhood who are at extremes of social privilege, either defined by income, racial hierarchy, or the combination (Kramer, 2016; Krieger et al., 2015). ICE ranges from −1 indicating concentrated deprivation to +1 indicating concentrated privilege. A novel extension of this measure is the construction of intersected social status groups, such as the contrasting of low-income Black and high-income White in a given area (Feldman, Waterman, Coull, & Krieger, 2015; Krieger et al., 2017).

Choosing and Calculating Indices

Selecting one or more measures of residential segregation for a given research question requires attention to the hypothesized segregation dynamics, mechanisms for social and health impact, and the importance of spatial scale. Collecting and formatting the data for calculation of the wide array of indices available to health researchers can be a formidable task. While formulas for these and other indices are widely available (e.g., Lloyd et al., 2014; Oka & Wong, 2016; Reardon, 2006; Reardon & Firebaugh, 2002; Reardon & O'Sullivan, 2004), open-source software platforms for automating calculation are increasingly available. An open-source, cross-platform, standalone application accepts geographic information system (GIS) shapefiles with census data as inputs and calculates each of 43 measures of local and regional segregation (Apparicio et al., 2013). The package "**seg**" in the open-source R environment has functions for calculating a variety of aspatial and spatial segregation indices (Hong et al., 2014).

SEGREGATION AND HEALTH: EVIDENCE AND MECHANISMS

Having gained some familiarity with the generating processes of segregation, and with the measurement of segregation patterns, it is finally time to more completely consider segregation as a process, exposure, and context that is relevant for population health. The empirical literature testing the association between local and regional segregation and health has grown rapidly over the past 20 years, primarily focusing on racial/ethnic segregation in US metropolitan areas. This literature will not be reviewed in detail here, pointing interested readers to the growing number of systematic reviews of residential segregation and obesity (Corral et al., 2015), cancer (Landrine et al., 2016), and pregnancy outcomes (Ncube, Enquobahrie, Albert, Herrick, & Burke, 2016), as well as reviews across health behaviors and other outcomes such as smoking, physical activity, injury, infection, and all-cause and cause-specific mortality (Kramer & Hogue, 2009; White & Borrell, 2011; White, Haas, & Williams, 2012). Several broad patterns emerge from this literature. In multilevel analyses, residence in a more versus less segregated region (e.g., metropolitan statistical area) is generally associated with poorer health outcomes for African Americans, although results vary to some degree depending on the dimension of segregation under consideration, as discussed next. The association between segregation and health for Hispanics is less consistent than for African Americans, with some studies finding null or even protective health effects (Kershaw & Albrecht, 2014; Kershaw, Albrecht, & Carnethon, 2013), and others finding deleterious effects on health behaviors (Corral, Landrine, & Zhao, 2014; Mellerson et al., 2010). Although many studies have examined the effects of income inequality on health, fewer have looked at the related but distinct patterns of spatial segregation by income (Waitzman & Smith, 1998).

These differences in findings among studies may reflect important interstudy differences in design, measurement, or outcome. Alternatively, different associations between segregation and health by outcome, race, and ethnicity may be indicative of the historically contingent nature of the segregation generating process reviewed earlier. The health consequences of segregation for African Americans must surely be understood in the historic context of the legacy of slavery, 20th-century government sanctioned housing and education discrimination, and the persistence of de facto segregation processes. In contrast, the processes producing segregation of Hispanics may vary by region of the country and by generational status. For instance, in the Southwestern United States, Hispanics have a longer history in some communities than Anglos, while Hispanic immigrant laborers in Georgia, North Carolina, and South Carolina arrived more recently and may experience the "port of entry" segregation posited by spatial assimilation. The point is that different histories may produce different social and economic dynamics and, consequently, different health consequences.

Figure 12-2 represents a simplified conceptual framework summarizing several leading hypotheses about the pathways connecting the macrosocial process of residential segregation to the inequitable production and distribution of disease in populations. Starting from the left-hand side of the figure, segregation is conceived as a spatiotemporally dynamic process of sorting, separation, and stratification of individuals based on race, ethnicity, and class, into residential environments. In broad terms, segregation affects health—and population health disparities—to the degree that segregation induces dependency between social groups and health-relevant exposures and experiences, including environmental and contextual exposures of place, and individual behaviors and socioeconomic trajectories. This is represented in the figure first by the arrow flowing from segregation to place-based opportunities and exposures, including socioeconomic, built, and social environments. Segregation may also directly affect individual health risk profiles, as suggested by

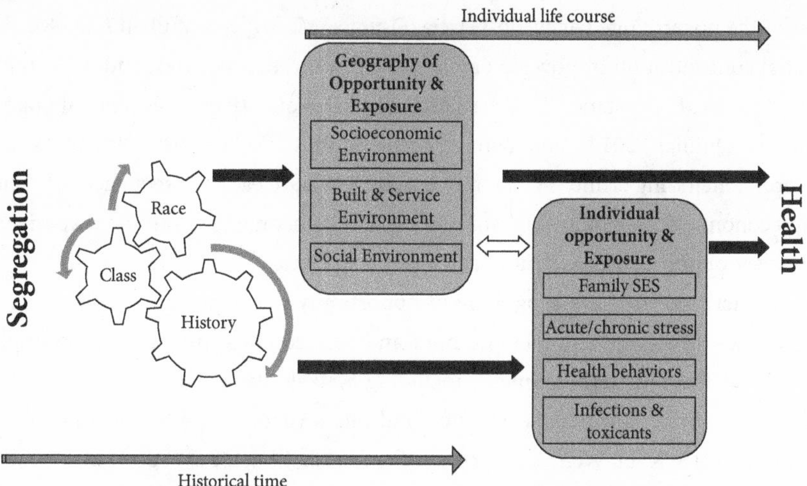

FIGURE 12-2 **Conceptual model for pathways connecting residential segregation and population health.**

the arrow flowing from segregation to individual-level factors, including socioeconomic status, experiences of psychosocial stress, health behaviors, and exposure to environmental toxicants. These associations are reviewed in more detail next. The bidirectional arrow between the boxes for area-level processes and individual-level factors recognizes that context affects individuals, but that individuals also dynamically interact with and create attributes of the places they inhabit (Cummins, Curtis, Diez-Roux, & Macintyre, 2007; Macintyre, Ellaway, & Cummins, 2002). A final feature of the conceptual model in Figure 12-2 is the two representations of time: on the top is the life course of individuals, recognizing that segregation may have different consequences at particular critical windows in development or aging (Osypuk, 2013); and on the bottom is the chronologic passing of historic time representing the changing dynamics of residential settlement, socioeconomic stratification, and the diffusion of health-relevant resources through populations.

Segregation and Neighborhood Context

The socioeconomic stratification of places is one of the hallmarks of racial segregation in the United States, and it results in the concentration of poverty and affluence in space, differentially by race (Intrator, Tannen, & Massey, 2016; Massey, 1996; Massey & Fischer, 2000). This spatial concentration of poverty produces distinct contextual environment for individuals, potentially independent of their individual socioeconomic position. For instance, in the 100 largest metropolitan areas in the United States, an average White child from a low-income family lives in a neighborhood with a 13.6% poverty rate, while the average Black or Hispanic child from similarly low-income families lives in neighborhoods with twice (29.2% and 26.2%, respectively) the poverty rate (Acevedo-Garcia, Osypuk, McArdle, & Williams, 2008). The spatial concentration of poverty patterns the resources, exposures, and opportunities of places. For instance, local variation in school quality and educational opportunities (Quillian, 2014), employment opportunities (Dickerson, 2009), and social disorder, including crime (Peterson & Krivo, 2010), are each consequences of racial and economic segregation, with minority and low-income communities experiencing fewer opportunities and more deleterious exposures.

Another aspect of the geography of opportunity that is influenced by regional segregation processes includes the built and service environments. For example, aspects of the built environment, including walkability, street connectivity, and green space, may vary with segregation and infrastructure investment (Kershaw & Albrecht, 2015; K. Li, Wen, & Henry, 2014) (also see Chapter 8). Food environment quantity and quality may also vary with segregation, with evidence that segregation promotes higher density of fast food restaurants in predominantly low-income and minority neighborhoods (Kwate, 2008; Kwate & Loh, 2010) (also see Chapter 9). The distribution of social and health services also varies in space. Blacks are more likely to be in neighborhoods with a shortage of primary care physicians and to utilize health services differently in low- versus high-segregation environments (Gaskin, Dinwiddie, Chan, & McCleary, 2012a, 2012b). White et al. (2012) developed a broader framework for understanding disparities in healthcare and services as a function of residential segregation.

Through the spatial concentration of both race/ethnicity and poverty, and increased social disorganization, residential segregation may also affect the social capital of communities situated in places (Kawachi, 1999; Kawachi, Kennedy, Lochner, & Prothrow-Stith, 1997). Social capital is a collective good developed through relationships in social networks that can provide social support, transmit and enforce social norms, and produce identity (Moore & Kawachi, 2017). If segregation promotes social disorganization and residential instability, social ties may be weakened, resulting in decreased collective efficacy (Sampson, Morenoff, & Earls, 2011). On the other hand, the concentration of members of minority groups in space may facilitate relationships built on shared cultural values and institutions, suggesting that some aspects of segregation could enhance rather than diminish social capital (Pickett, Shaw, Atkin, Kiernan, & Wilkinson, 2009).

Segregation and Individual-Level Health Determinants

Earlier in this chapter the health consequences of segregation were conceived of as mediated by the neighborhood environments produced by segregation. However, segregation may impact health above and beyond the built and social environments of the neighborhoods, by directly affecting individual-level health-relevant exposures, opportunities, and behaviors. First, as a result of segregation's influence on educational opportunities, individual-level life course socioeconomic trajectory can be established based on the segregation of the residential area in childhood and adolescence (Card & Rothstein, 2007; Quillian, 2014). Segregation-related variation in economic opportunities can further influence adult employment, income, and home ownership, shaping ongoing socioeconomic trajectories (Fullilove & Wallace, 2011; H. Li, Campbell, & Fernandez, 2013; Squires & Kubrin, 2005).

The experience of discrimination and chronic stress related to material deprivation and social status is an important theoretical link for explaining the biological embodiment of social experience (Geronimus et al., 2010; Krieger, 2012a). Segregation could either increase or decrease exposure to discrimination and stress. For instance, associations between segregation and violent crime would presumably increase experience of stress around safety (Krivo et al., 2015). However, there is also evidence that minority residence in minority-dominated neighborhoods reduces exposure to interpersonal discrimination, possibly reducing experiences of stress (Borrell, Kiefe, Diez-Roux, Williams, & Gordon-Larsen, 2013). In addition to the physiologic response to experienced discrimination or stress, these exposures can also produce stress-coping behavioral changes that are health relevant. For instance, smoking during pregnancy varies in complex ways by race and segregation, suggesting a mix of stress-smoking and changing smoking norms as neighborhood context changes (Bell, Zimmerman, Mayer, Almgren, & Huebner, 2007; Shaw, Pickett, & Wilkinson, 2010; Yang, Shoff, Noah, Black, & Sparks, 2014).

Finally, an individual's exposure to infectious and toxic agents can be systematically patterned by segregation. Regional and local segregation patterns are associated with concentrated transmission of sexually transmitted infections and tuberculosis through both spatial density mechanisms, as well as the connections between social and sexual networks and geographic constraints (D. Acevedo-Garcia, 2000, 2001; Adimora & Schoenbach, 2005). Environmental toxicants in air, water, and housing may also be inequitably distributed in space in ways that disproportionately burden minority and low-income communities (Gee, Payne-Sturges, 2004; Morello-Frosch & Lopez, 2006). For example, the extended exposure to dangerously high levels of lead from municipal water supply in Flint, Michigan, beginning in 2014 (Kennedy et al., 2016) was directly related to the economic and political status of the city. The slow governmental response to the emerging crisis has been attributed to the fact that Flint is predominantly Black and working class (Bellinger, 2016).

Integrating Social Theory, Spatial Patterns, and Mediating Pathways

Social theories of spatial stratification and spatial assimilation, spatial patterns of residential evenness or exposure, and mediating pathways are each toolsets for understanding the health consequences of residential segregation. These different tools do not map directly onto one another; there is not a one-to-one relationship between theory and pattern, or between pattern and pathway. However, because each toolset draws attention to a unique aspect of the segregation–health relationship, efforts to link the tools can lead to richer understanding and enhance potential for effective public health action. Two simple illustrations are provided next, although there is great potential for further work in this area.

First, assimilation theory suggests that the spatial separation of groups (e.g., by nativity, ethnicity, immigrant status) may be partly characterized by differences in individual socioeconomic status, but that net of this there may be collective social benefits for the minority group (Bécares et al., 2012). The literature studying "ethnic enclaves" often uses spatial concentration and clustering of groups as a measurement tool, suggesting that the evenness/clustering dimension of segregation may be particularly useful for study of spatial assimilation dynamics. While material deprivation may consistently mark higher health risk, conditional on absolute socioeconomic status, pathways commonly hypothesized to connect residence in ethnic enclaves to positive health effects include increased social support, collective efficacy, and social capital (Stroope, Martinez, Eschbach, Peek, & Markides, 2015; Viruell-Fuentes, Morenoff, Williams, & House, 2013).

On the other hand, spatial stratification theory focuses on the use of social, political, and economic power of socially dominant groups to spatially exclude and concentrate groups with lower social status. This pattern is more consistent with the history and persistence of Black–White segregation in the United States (Pais, South, & Crowder, 2012), and as noted, it is characterized by the spatial concentration of poverty, and more dramatic differentiation of neighborhood environments. While measures of Black–White segregation for both the evenness and exposure dimensions are high, the exposure/isolation dimension may be more strongly associated with some health outcomes, including preterm birth and low birthweight (Bell, Zimmerman, Almgren, Mayer, & Huebner, 2006; Kramer, Cooper, Drews-Botsch, Waller, & Hogue, 2010b). In each case Black women residing in metropolitan areas characterized by high-isolation segregation had poorer pregnancy outcomes than Black women in less segregated places. However, conditional on the degree of Black isolation, higher Black clustering (unevenness) was health protective. High Black isolation in metropolitan areas is more strongly tied to higher violent crime rates, concentrated poverty, and lower educational attainment, suggesting these mediators may be particularly important at least for some health outcomes. However, clustering segregation may provide—conditional on the social and economic consequences of high isolation—buffers against interpersonal stressors such as discrimination or offer collective social goods through social and political capital and social networks.

FUTURE DIRECTIONS

In the first edition of this book and elsewhere, Acevedo-Garcia and Lochner (2003; D. Acevedo-Garcia, Lochner, Osypuk, & Subramanian, 2003) identified future directions for segregation and health research. Since that time, important progress has been made in some areas, including a transition from primarily ecologic to multilevel study designs and statistical analyses, increased attention to conceptualizing and operationalizing the multiple dimensions of segregation, preliminary attention beyond Black–White segregation to include other racial/ethnic groups, and modest attention paid to the potentially health-protective aspects of segregation. These areas have been reviewed in this chapter, and much work remains for each of these topics. However, several topics identified by Acevedo-Garcia and Lochner 15 years ago remain substantially underdeveloped today. For instance, while there is now greater theory for understanding mediating pathways between segregation and health, very few empirical studies operationalize and quantify the role of competing mediating pathways. As reviewed here, there are numerous pathways hypothesized to connect segregation to health-relevant exposure, and ultimately to health outcomes, but their relative importance independently, jointly, or in complex dynamics is not clear. This is important because public health and social policy to address the health consequences of segregation will likely involve action on particular intermediate pathways, but evidence is lacking for optimal targets. There also remains a large gap in understanding economic segregation independently and as intersected by racial segregation in patterning population health and health disparities. This gap is particularly surprising given the importance sociologists and health researchers alike have put on the socioeconomic stratifying consequences of segregation. In the United States, racial segregation has declined modestly since 1970, but economic segregation overall, and within race, has been steadily increasing, making the separation of poor from affluent an increasingly important spatial pattern (Bischoff & Reardon, 2014; Reardon, Fox, & Townsend, 2015). To this list of persistent needs, I will add two broad topics for continued segregation-health research: fuller attention to time and temporal dynamics both of people and of places; and further grounding of segregation research in causal study design and in causal thinking about the health effects of place.

Attending to Time

Two scales of time were highlighted in the conceptual framework (Figure 12-2): the life course developmental time of individuals, and the historical, spatiotemporal dynamics of places. The shift in thinking in study designs of segregation and health from purely ecologic to multileveled since the first edition of this book reflected the important recognition that the impact of area-level segregation on individual-level health outcomes was in fact a cross-level phenomenon. Now researchers, policy makers, and practitioners need to appreciate that, with few exceptions, the reliance on cross-sectional study designs is inadequate for what is most plausibly a longitudinal exposure with consequences that may act differentially at different life stages and may be accumulated through time (Osypuk, 2013). For example, as already reviewed, a large body of empirical work has focused on the association between residential segregation and pregnancy outcomes, commonly finding that pregnancy outcomes are worse for African American women living in more versus less segregated metropolitan areas. What is often unaddressed in this research is the growing evidence for the long-lasting consequences on the offspring of epigenetic fetal programming; segregation's effects on pregnancy may be the end of the story for the mother, but it is only the beginning for the child whose adult health status may be impacted by these early intrauterine exposures (Kramer et al., 2017). Educational and employment consequences of segregation may also be more critical during specific life stages (childhood and working-age adult, respectively), whereas the health consequences of broader socioeconomic, built, and service environments may accumulate with increased years of exposure. More intentionally linking the social epidemiology of segregation to the rich conceptual and empirical toolbox of life course theory could prove insightful (Kuh, Ben-Shlomo, Lynch, Hallqvist, & Power, 2003).

The second time scale, that of spatiotemporal dynamics of residential sorting and stratification includes but is not limited to measuring segregation indices in repeated cross-sections to distinguish trends. Undoubtedly, this is important. However, recently a group of sociologists and demographers called for a more integrative approach to understanding the dynamic processes of residential stratification and inequality (Lee, Matthews, Iceland, & Firebaugh, 2015). They recognized that point-in-time residential segregation represents the consequences of spatial sorting, but they observed that three other bodies of sociological literature seek to characterize the individual and structural dynamics which give rise to patterns of segregation: residential mobility, locational attainment, and neighborhood change. While these three dynamic processes are tightly interlinked in the real world, they have historically been studied in separate literatures with little connection between them or with segregation; they have also been primarily studied with respect to social and economic outcomes but are only rarely considered in population health studies.

Residential mobility refers simply to the tendency for individuals or families to remain in a given location, to move of their own volition to a new location, or to be pushed out of a given location because of housing instability, changes in the economy, or perception of inhospitable neighborhood demographics. Residential mobility has only occasionally been examined as a social determinant of health (Jelleyman & Spencer, 2008), as well as a source of bias in cross-sectional analyses (Geronimus, Bound, & Ro, 2014). *Locational attainment* is a more broadly scaled version of residential mobility, examining the degree to which social groups (e.g., as characterized by race, ethnicity, class) can translate their human, material, and social capital into similarly salubrious neighborhood environments. For instance, there is substantial evidence that Blacks attain fewer neighborhood amenities than Whites at the same socioeconomic status (Pais et al., 2012). *Neighborhood change* refers to the dynamics of place, not just persons, and includes processes such as gentrification and suburbanization of the poor. A handful of studies have explored the health consequences of gentrification for either those displaced or those who remain in the face of change (Gibbons & Barton, 2016; Huynh & Maroko, 2014; Wolch, Byrne, & Newell, 2014).

Research approaches that intentionally link these dynamic processes with the production of segregation and health outcomes could enhance both etiologic understanding of the social determinants of health and identify possible levers for public health intervention.

Regional Segregation, Local Neighborhoods, and Causal Inference

Much has been written about the challenges of establishing causal evidence for the effects of neighborhoods on individual and population health (e.g., Kaufman & Cooper, 1999; Oakes, 2004b). Knowledge that establishing causal linkages in observational research is difficult is nothing new, but the rapid evolution of formal causal frameworks such as counterfactuals has permitted a new level of technically detailed awareness as to how difficult the task is. While space does not permit a comprehensive accounting of all the challenges of causal inference, two topics closely related to segregation are worth brief mention: structural confounding and neighborhood selection mechanisms. Structural confounding describes a severe form of confounding in which individuals in the "exposed" group (for example, a neighborhood with a high crime rate) had nearly zero probability of being in the unexposed group (for example, a neighborhood with a low crime rate). In other words, the problem is not just one of imbalance of important covariates but complete separation of social experience, making causally meaningful contrasts of health outcomes between places untenable (Schempf & Kaufman, 2012). Structural confounding can be produced in the presence of strong mechanisms selecting individuals into neighborhoods. Oakes (2004a, 2004b) argues that because investigators cannot randomly assign individuals to neighborhoods, their unique attributes—their cultural background, income, education, health status, and more—make up the selection mechanism that largely determines the neighborhood environment to which they will be exposed (reside in). When neighborhood stratification is strong—as is hypothesized in severe regional segregation—individual-level attributes may nearly fully determine neighborhood context. This is problematic for causal inference in neighborhood effects studies because there is no plausible counterfactual to the experience of being in one neighborhood or another.

Structural confounding and selection mechanisms are problematic, but it is worth emphasizing that it is the process of regional segregation that may be one of the main drivers of neighborhood-level structural confounding. In other words selection and structural confounding hinder inference about the independent effects of neighborhoods on individual health, but explicitly studying regional segregation could be a way to understand the health relevance of this selection and confounding. This approach implies a shift from the conventional two-level multilevel model to a richer three-level model. Most approaches to date have been limited to two levels because of data constraints. For instance, studies may either examine neighborhoods within a single metropolitan area (e.g., using local registry or cohort data) or examine individuals from multiple metropolitan areas (e.g., using national vital records), but without any neighborhood-level measures. Each of these approaches has limitations. In a study of a single city, there is only variation in local measures of segregation, but no variation in regional variation (e.g., there is only $n = 1$ region). Thus, the potential structural confounding produced by high segregation could make counterfactual contrasts of neighborhoods within the city inadvisable. However, in the second case with individual data spread across a range of metropolitan areas, regional segregation can be quantified and contrasted, but national data rarely include neighborhood or local measures of environment.

To advance understanding of both regional segregation and local neighborhood effects, identification of data sources including measures at three levels may be illuminating: individuals measured with their relevant socioeconomic, behavioral, and health outcome data nested within neighborhoods with measures of their relevant economic, physical, and social contextual processes nested within an adequate number of regional housing markets (e.g., metropolitan statistical areas) to provide heterogeneity in the degree of residential stratification. Such a design and corresponding data structure would permit examination and modeling of both the residential selection processes, which vary across regions, as well as the local neighborhood effects, which could vary within and between regions. Such an analysis is not readily performed in the commonly used vital statistics data (e.g., birth or death certificates), but it could be accomplished in any number of large, population-based cohort studies which are broadly sampled and include neighborhood geocodes such as the National Health Interview Study, Panel Study of Income Dynamics, Add Health, Early Childhood Longitudinal Study, National Longitudinal Study of Youth, and more. This approach does not fully resolve the problem of selection mechanisms and confounding, but it does make clear that a "problem" at one spatial scale (confounding at neighborhood scale) is in fact the question of interest at another spatial scale (regional segregation as a stratifying process).

CONCLUSION

The conceptualization, measurement, and empirical evidence detailing associations between residential segregation and health have advanced substantially in the 15 years since the first edition of this book. However, it could be argued that the segregation-health literature has reached a plateau of diminishing returns. It is true that more measures of association continue to be produced using varied segregation indices and health outcomes. What remains elusive is either enhanced etiologic and mechanistic clarity, or clear translatable and actionable evidence to inform policy makers, public health scholars, and practitioners in reducing segregation-related health disparities. Perhaps social epidemiologists have once again fallen into the trap of providing "all the right answers to all the wrong questions" (Harper & Strumpf, 2012). But if segregation is in fact a fundamental determinant of health disparities, efforts should be redoubled to provide more "consequentialist" evidence (Galea, 2013). This includes continued documentation of associations for a wider variety of health outcomes and among a larger set of social groups. However, it should also include fuller attention to the dynamic processes in the lives of individuals and the fabric of places which produce segregation and the health consequences of segregation. For example, connecting study of housing policy, zoning, and urban renewal to patterns of residential mobility, place stratification, and health disparities can help triangulate opportunities to more fully attend to the ways in which place gets under the skin. This renewed and recalibrated attention can take advantage of natural experiments to quantify external "interventions" and characterize the relative importance of competing social processes and intermediate pathways with respect to health (see also Chapter 6). In addition, development of health databases with adequate numbers and geographic resolution to simultaneously measure individual attributes, neighborhood attributes, and regional segregation across a wide range metropolitan areas will allow consideration of segregation as a causal factor but also as a source of selection bias in understanding more local processes.

REFERENCES

Acevedo-Garcia, D. (2000). Residential segregation and the epidemiology of infectious diseases. *Social Science & Medicine (1982)*, *51*(8), 1143–1161. Retrieved from http://www.ncbi.nlm.nih.gov/pubmed/11037206

Acevedo-Garcia, D. (2001). Zip code-level risk factors for tuberculosis: neighborhood environment and residential segregation in New Jersey, 1985–1992. *American Journal of Public Health*, *91*(5), 734–741. Retrieved from http://www.pubmedcentral.nih.gov/articlerender.fcgi?artid=1446660&tool=pmcentrez&rendertype=abstract

Acevedo-Garcia, D., & Lochner, K. (2003). Residential segregation and health. In I. Kawachi & L. F. Berkman (Eds.), *Neighborhoods and health* (pp. 265–287). New York, NY: Oxford University Press.

Acevedo-Garcia, D., Lochner, K. a, Osypuk, T. L., & Subramanian, S. V. (2003). Future directions in residential segregation and health research: A multilevel approach. *American Journal of Public Health*, *93*(2), 215–221. Retrieved from http://www.pubmedcentral.nih.gov/articlerender.fcgi?artid=1447719&tool=pmcentrez&rendertype=abstract

Acevedo-Garcia, D., & Osypuk, T. L. (2008). Invited commentary: Residential segregation and health—the complexity of modeling separate social contexts. *American Journal of Epidemiology*, *168*(11), 1255–1258. https://doi.org/10.1093/aje/kwn290

Acevedo-Garcia, D., Osypuk, T. L., McArdle, N., & Williams, D. R. (2008). Toward a policy-relevant analysis of geographic and racial/ethnic disparities in child health. *Health Affairs (Project Hope)*, *27*(2), 321–333. https://doi.org/10.1377/hlthaff.27.2.321

Adimora, A. A., & Schoenbach, V. J. (2005). Social context, sexual networks, and racial disparities in rates of sexually transmitted infections. *The Journal of Infectious Diseases*, *191 Suppl*, S115–S122. https://doi.org/10.1086/425280

Apparicio, P., Martori, J. C., Pearson, A. L., Fournier, É., Apparicio, D., Fournier, E., & Apparicio, D. (2013). An open-source software for calculating indices of urban residential segregation. *Social Science Computer Review*, *32*(1), 117–128. https://doi.org/10.1177/0894439313504539

Bécares, L., Shaw, R., Nazroo, J., Stafford, M., Albor, C., Atkin, K., . . . Pickett, K. (2012). Ethnic density effects on physical morbidity, mortality, and health behaviors: A systematic review of the literature. *American Journal of Public Health*, *102*(12), 1–34. https://doi.org/10.2105/AJPH.2012.300832

Bell, J. F., Zimmerman, F. J., Almgren, G. R., Mayer, J. D., & Huebner, C. E. (2006). Birth outcomes among urban African-American women: A multilevel analysis of the role of racial residential segregation. *Social Science & Medicine (1982)*, *63*(12), 3030–3045. https://doi.org/10.1016/j.socscimed.2006.08.011

Bell, J. F., Zimmerman, F. J., Mayer, J. D., Almgren, G. R., & Huebner, C. E. (2007). Associations between residential segregation and smoking during pregnancy among urban African-American women. *Journal of Urban Health : Bulletin of the New York Academy of Medicine*, *84*(3), 372–388. https://doi.org/10.1007/s11524-006-9152-4

Bellinger, D. C. (2016). Lead contamination in Flint—An abject failure to protect public health. *The New England Journal of Medicine*, *374*(12), 1101–1103. https://doi.org/10.1056/NEJMp1601013

Bischoff, K., & Reardon, S. F. (2014). Residential segregation by income, 1970–2009. In J. R. Logan (Ed.), *Diversity and disparities: America enters a new century* (pp. 208–232). New York, NY: Russell Sage Foundation.

Borrell, L. N., Kiefe, C. I., Diez-Roux, A. V., Williams, D. R., & Gordon-Larsen, P. (2013). Racial discrimination, racial/ethnic segregation, and health behaviors in the CARDIA study. *Ethnicity & Health*, *18*(3), 227–243. https://doi.org/10.1080/13557858.2012.713092

Brown, L. A., & Chung, S. (2006). Spatial segregation, segregation indices and the geographical perspective. *Population, Space and Place*, *12*(2), 125–143. https://doi.org/10.1002/psp.403

Card, D., & Rothstein, J. (2007). Racial segregation and the black–white test score gap. *Journal of Public Economics*, *91*(11–12), 2158–2184. https://doi.org/10.1016/j.jpubeco.2007.03.006

Corral, I., Landrine, H., Hall, M. B., Bess, J. J., Mills, K. R., & Efird, J. T. (2015). Residential segregation and overweight/obesity among African-American adults: A critical review. *Front Public Health*, *3*(July), 169. https://doi.org/10.3389/fpubh.2015.00169

Corral, I., Landrine, H., & Zhao, L. (2014). Residential segregation and obesity among a national sample of Hispanic adults. *Journal of Health Psychology*, *19*(4), 503–8. https://doi.org/10.1177/1359105312474912

Cummins, S., Curtis, S., Diez-Roux, A. V, & Macintyre, S. (2007). Understanding and representing "place" in health research: A relational approach. *Social Science & Medicine (1982)*, *65*(9), 1825–1838. https://doi.org/10.1016/j.socscimed.2007.05.036

Cutler, D. M., Glaeser, E. L., & Vigdor, J. L. (1999). The rise and decline of the American ghetto. *Journal of Political Economy*, *107*(3), 455. https://doi.org/10.1086/250069

Dickerson, N. T. (2009). Black employment, segregation, and the social organization of metropolitan labor markets. *Economic Geography*, *83*(3), 283–307. https://doi.org/10.1111/j.1944-8287.2007.tb00355.x

Feldman, J. M., Waterman, P. D., Coull, B. A., & Krieger, N. (2015). Spatial social polarisation: Using the Index of Concentration at the Extremes jointly for income and race/ethnicity to analyse risk of hypertension. *Journal of Epidemiology and Community Health*, jech-2015-205728. https://doi.org/10.1136/jech-2015-205728

Flippen, C., & Kim, E. (2015). Immigrant context and opportunity: New destinations and socioeconomic attainment among Asians in the United States. *The ANNALS of the American Academy of Political and Social Science*, *660*(1), 175–198. https://doi.org/10.1177/0002716215577611

Fossett, M. (2011). Generative models of segregation: Investigating model-generated patterns of residential segregation by ethnicity and socioeconomic status. *The Journal of Mathematical Sociology*, *35*(1–3), 114–145. https://doi.org/10.1080/0022250X.2010.532367

Fullilove, M. T., & Wallace, R. (2011). Serial forced displacement in American cities, 1916–2010. *Journal of Urban Health : Bulletin of the New York Academy of Medicine*, *88*(3), 381–389. https://doi.org/10.1007/s11524-011-9585-2

Galea, S. (2013). An argument for a consequentialist epidemiology. *American Journal of Epidemiology*, *178*(8), 1185–1191. https://doi.org/10.1093/aje/kwt172

Gaskin, D. J., Dinwiddie, G. Y., Chan, K. S., & McCleary, R. (2012a). Residential segregation and disparities in health care services utilization. *Medical Care Research and Review: MCRR*, *69*(2), 158–175. https://doi.org/10.1177/1077558711420263

Gaskin, D. J., Dinwiddie, G. Y., Chan, K. S., & McCleary, R. R. (2012b). Residential segregation and the availability of primary care physicians. *Health Services Research*, *47*(6), 2353–2376. https://doi.org/10.1111/j.1475-6773.2012.01417.x

Gee, G. C., Payne-sturges, D. C. (2004). Environmental health disparities: A framework integrating psychosocial and environmental concepts and environmental health disparities. *Environmental Health Perspectives*, *112*(17), 1645–1653.

Gentzkow, M., & Shapiro, J. M. (2011). Ideological segregation online and offline. *Quarterly Journal of Economics*, *126*(4), 1799–1839. https://doi.org/10.1093/qje/qjr044

Geronimus, A. T., Bound, J., & Ro, A. (2014). Residential mobility across local areas in the United States and the geographic distribution of the healthy population. *Demography*, *51*(3), 777–809. https://doi.org/10.1007/s13524-014-0299-4

Geronimus, A. T., Hicken, M. T., Pearson, J. A., Seashols, S. J., Brown, K. L., & Cruz, T. D. (2010). Do US black women experience stress-related accelerated biological aging?: A novel theory and first population-based test of Black-White differences in telomere length. *Human Nature (Hawthorne, N.Y.)*, *21*(1), 19–38. https://doi.org/10.1007/s12110-010-9078-0

Gibbons, J., & Barton, M. S. (2016). The association of minority self-rated health with Black versus White gentrification. *Journal of Urban Health, 93*(6), 909–922. https://doi.org/10.1007/s11524-016-0087-0

Harper, S., & Strumpf, E. C. (2012). Social epidemiology: Questionable answers and answerable questions. *Epidemiology (Cambridge, Mass.), 23*(6), 795–798. https://doi.org/10.1097/EDE.0b013e31826d078d

Hong, S.-Y., O'Sullivan, D., Sadahiro, Y., Johnston, R., Poulsen, M., Forrest, J., . . . Shaw, S. (2014). Implementing spatial segregation measures in R. *PLoS ONE, 9*(11), e113767. https://doi.org/10.1371/journal.pone.0113767

Huynh, M., & Maroko, a R. (2014). Gentrification and preterm birth in New York City, 2008–2010. *Journal of Urban Health : Bulletin of the New York Academy of Medicine, 91*(1), 211–220. https://doi.org/10.1007/s11524-013-9823-x

Intrator, J., Tannen, J., & Massey, D. S. (2016). Segregation by race and income in the United States, 1970–2010. *Social Science Research, 60*, 45–60. https://doi.org/10.1016/j.ssresearch.2016.08.003

Jelleyman, T., & Spencer, N. (2008). Residential mobility in childhood and health outcomes: A systematic review. *Journal of Epidemiology and Community Health, 62*(7), 584–592. https://doi.org/10.1136/jech.2007.060103

Johnston, R., Poulsen, M., & Forrest, J. (2007). Ethnic and racial segregation in U.S. metropolitan areas, 1980–2000: The dimensions of segregation revisited. *Urban Affairs Review, 42*(4), 479–504. https://doi.org/10.1177/1078087406292701

Kaufman, J. S., & Cooper, R. S. (1999). Seeking causal explanations in social epidemiology. *American Journal of Epidemiology, 150*(2), 113–120. Retrieved from http://www.ncbi.nlm.nih.gov/pubmed/10412955

Kawachi, I. (1999). Social capital and community effects on population and individual health. *Annals of the New York Academy of Sciences, 896*, 120–130. Retrieved from http://www.ncbi.nlm.nih.gov/pubmed/10681893

Kawachi, I., Kennedy, B. P., Lochner, K., & Prothrow-Stith, D. (1997). Social capital, income inequality, and mortality. *American Journal of Public Health, 87*(9), 1491–1498. Retrieved from http://www.pubmedcentral.nih.gov/articlerender.fcgi?artid=1380975&tool=pmcentrez&rendertype=abstract

Kennedy, C., Yard, E., Dignam, T., Buchanan, S., Condon, S., Brown, M. J., . . . Breysse, P. (2016). Blood lead levels among children aged <6 years—Flint, Michigan, 2013–2016. *MMWR. Morbidity and Mortality Weekly Report, 65*(25), 650–654. https://doi.org/10.15585/mmwr.mm6525e1

Kershaw, K. N., & Albrecht, S. S. (2014). Metropolitan-level ethnic residential segregation, racial identity, and body mass index among U.S. Hispanic adults: A multilevel cross-sectional study. *BMC Public Health, 14*, 283. https://doi.org/10.1186/1471-2458-14-283

Kershaw, K. N., & Albrecht, S. S. (2015). Racial/ethnic residential segregation and cardiovascular disease risk. *Current Cardiovascular Risk Reports, 9*(3). https://doi.org/10.1007/s12170-015-0436-7

Kershaw, K. N., Albrecht, S. S., & Carnethon, M. R. (2013). Racial and ethnic residential segregation, the neighborhood socioeconomic environment, and obesity among blacks and Mexican Americans. *American Journal of Epidemiology, 177*(4). https://doi.org/10.1093/aje/kws372

Kramer, M. R. (2016). Race, place, and space: Ecosocial theory and spatiotemporal patterns of pregnancy outcomes. In F. M. Howell, J. R. Porter, & S. A. Matthews (Eds.),

Recapturing space: New middle-range theory in spatial demography (pp. 275–299). Cham, Switzerland: Springer. https://doi.org/10.1007/978-3-319-22810-5

Kramer, M. R., Cooper, H. L., Drews-Botsch, C. D., Waller, L. A., & Hogue, C. R. (2010a). Do measures matter? Comparing surface-density-derived and census-tract-derived measures of racial residential segregation. *International Journal of Health Geographics*, *9*(1), 29. https://doi.org/10.1186/1476-072X-9-29

Kramer, M. R., Cooper, H. L., Drews-Botsch, C. D., Waller, L. A., & Hogue, C. R. (2010b). Metropolitan isolation segregation and Black-White disparities in very preterm birth: A test of mediating pathways and variance explained. *Social Science & Medicine (1982)*, *71*(12), 2108–2116. https://doi.org/10.1016/j.socscimed.2010.09.011

Kramer, M. R., & Hogue, C. R. (2009). Is segregation bad for your health? *Epidemiologic Reviews*, *31*(1), 178–194. https://doi.org/10.1093/epirev/mxp001

Kramer, M. R., Schneider, E. B., Kane, J. B., Margerison-Zilko, C., Jones-Smith, J., King, K., . . . Grzywacz, J. G. (2017). Getting under the skin: Children's health disparities as embodiment of social class. *Population Research and Policy Review*. https://doi.org/10.1007/s11113-017-9431-7

Krieger, N. (2012a). Methods for the scientific study of discrimination and health: An ecosocial approach. *American Journal of Public Health*, *102*(5), 936–945. https://doi.org/10.2105/AJPH.2011.300544

Krieger, N. (2012b). Who and what is a "population"? Historical debates, current controversies, and implications for understanding "population health" and rectifying health inequities. *Milbank Quarterly*, *90*(4), 634–681. https://doi.org/10.1111/j.1468-0009.2012.00678.x

Krieger, N., Feldman, J. M., Waterman, P. D., Chen, J. T., Coull, B. A., & Hemenway, D. (2017). Local residential segregation matters: Stronger association of census tract compared to conventional city-level measures with fatal and non-fatal assaults (total and firearm related), using the Index of Concentration at the Extremes (ICE) for Racial, Econ. *Journal of Urban Health: Bulletin of the New York Academy of Medicine*. https://doi.org/10.1007/s11524-016-0116-z

Krieger, N., Waterman, P. D., Spasojevic, J., Li, W., Maduro, G., & Van Wye, G. (2015). Public health monitoring of privilege and deprivation with the Index of Concentration at the Extremes. *American Journal of Public Health*, e1–e8. https://doi.org/10.2105/AJPH.2015.302955

Krivo, L. J., Byron, R. A., Calder, C. A., Peterson, R. D., Browning, C. R., Kwan, M.-P., & Lee, J. Y. (2015). Patterns of local segregation: Do they matter for neighborhood crime? *Social Science Research*, *54*, 303–318. https://doi.org/10.1016/j.ssresearch.2015.08.005

Kuh, D., Ben-Shlomo, Y., Lynch, J., Hallqvist, J., & Power, C. (2003). Life course epidemiology. *Journal of Epidemiology and Community Health*, *57*(10), 778–783. https://doi.org/10.1136/jech.57.10.778

Kwate, N. O. A. (2008). Fried chicken and fresh apples: Racial segregation as a fundamental cause of fast food density in black neighborhoods. *Health & Place*, *14*(1), 32–44. https://doi.org/10.1016/j.healthplace.2007.04.001

Kwate, N. O. A., & Loh, J. M. (2010). Separate and unequal: The influence of neighborhood and school characteristics on spatial proximity between fast food and schools. *Preventive Medicine*, *51*(2), 153–156. https://doi.org/10.1016/j.ypmed.2010.04.020

Landrine, H., Corral, I., Lee, J. G. L., Efird, J. T., Hall, M. B., & Bess, J. J. (2016). Residential segregation and racial cancer disparities: A systematic review. *Journal of Racial and Ethnic Health Disparities*. https://doi.org/10.1007/s40615-016-0326-9

Lattman, P. (2007, September 27). The origins of Justice Stewart's "I Know It When I See It." *Wall Street Journal.* Retrieved from http://blogs.wsj.com/law/2007/09/27/the-origins-of-justice-stewarts-i-know-it-when-i-see-it/

Lee, B., Matthews, S., Iceland, J., & Firebaugh, G. (2015). Residential inequality: Orientation and overview. *The ANNALS of the American Academy of Political and Social Science, 660*(1), 8–16. https://doi.org/10.1177/0002716215579832

Li, H., Campbell, H., & Fernandez, S. (2013). Residential segregation, spatial mismatch and economic growth across US metropolitan areas. *Urban Studies, 50*(13). https://doi.org/10.1177/0042098013477697

Li, K., Wen, M., & Henry, K. A. (2014). Residential racial composition and black-white obesity risks: Differential effects of neighborhood social and built environment. *International Journal of Environmental Research and Public Health, 11*(1), 626–642. https://doi.org/10.3390/ijerph110100626

Lloyd, C. D., Shuttleworth, I., & Wong, D. W. S. (2014). *Social-spatial segregation concepts, processes and outcomes.* Bristol, UK: Policy Press.

Logan, J. R., & Alba, R. D. (1993). Locational returns to human capital: Minority access to suburban community resources. *Demography, 30*(2), 243–68. Retrieved from http://www.ncbi.nlm.nih.gov/pubmed/8500639

Logan, J. R., Alba, R. D., & Zhang, W. (2002). Immigrant enclaves and ethnic communities in New York and Los Angeles. *American Sociological Review, 67*(2), 299–322.

Logan, J. R., Xu, Z., & Stults, B. J. (2014). Interpolating U.S. decennial census tract data from as early as 1970 to 2010: A longitudinal tract database. *The Professional Geographer, 66*(3). https://doi.org/10.1080/00330124.2014.905156

Macintyre, S., Ellaway, A., & Cummins, S. (2002). Place effects on health: How can we conceptualise, operationalise and measure them? *Social Science & Medicine (1982), 55*(1), 125–39. https://doi.org/10.1016/S0277-9536(01)00214-3

Maguire, A., French, D., & O'Reilly, D. (2016). Residential segregation, dividing walls and mental health: A population-based record linkage study. *Journal of Epidemiology and Community Health, 70*(9), 845–854. https://doi.org/10.1136/jech-2015-206888

Massey, D. S. (1985). Ethnic residential segregation: A theoretical synthesis and empirical review. *Sociology and Social Research, 69*(3), 315–350. Retrieved from http://cat.inist.fr/?aModele=afficheN&cpsidt=11964438

Massey, D. S. (1996). The age of extremes: Concentrated affluence and poverty in the twenty-first century. *Demography, 33*(4), 395–412. Retrieved from http://link.springer.com/article/10.2307/2061773

Massey, D. S., & Denton, N. A. (1988). The dimensions of residential segregation. *Social Forces, 67*(2), 281–315. https://doi.org/10.1093/sf/67.2.281

Massey, D. S., & Denton, N. A. (1998). *American apartheid: Segregation and the making of the underclass.* Cambridge, MA: Harvard University Press.

Massey, D. S., & Fischer, M. (2000). How segregation concentrates poverty. *Ethnic and Racial Studies.* Retrieved from http://www.tandfonline.com/doi/abs/10.1080/01419870050033676

Mellerson, J., Landrine, H., Hao, Y., Corral, I., Zhao, L., & Cooper, D. L. (2010). Residential segregation and exercise among a national sample of Hispanic adults. *Health and Place, 16*(3), 613–615. https://doi.org/10.1016/j.healthplace.2009.12.013

Moore, S., & Kawachi, I. (2017). Twenty years of social capital and health research: A glossary. *Journal of Epidemiology and Community Health*, jech-2016-208313. https://doi.org/10.1136/jech-2016-208313

Morello-Frosch, R., & Lopez, R. (2006). The riskscape and the color line: Examining the role of segregation in environmental health disparities. *Environmental Research*, *102*(2), 181–96. https://doi.org/10.1016/j.envres.2006.05.007

Ncube, C. N., Enquobahrie, D. A., Albert, S. M., Herrick, A. L., & Burke, J. G. (2016). Association of neighborhood context with offspring risk of preterm birth and low birthweight: A systematic review and meta-analysis of population-based studies. *Social Science & Medicine (1982)*, *153*, 156–164. https://doi.org/10.1016/j.socscimed.2016.02.014

Oakes, J. M. (2004a). Causal inference and the relevance of social epidemiology. *Social Science & Medicine (1982)*, *58*(10), 1969–71. https://doi.org/10.1016/j.socscimed.2003.05.001

Oakes, J. M. (2004b). The (mis)estimation of neighborhood effects: Causal inference for a practicable social epidemiology. *Social Science & Medicine (1982)*, *58*(10), 1929–52. https://doi.org/10.1016/j.socscimed.2003.08.004

Oka, M., & Wong, D. W. S. (2016). Spatializing area-based measures of neighborhood characteristics for multilevel regression analyses: An areal median filtering approach. *Journal of Urban Health*. https://doi.org/10.1007/s11524-016-0051-z

Openshaw, S. (1983). The modifiable areal unit problem. *Concepts and Techniques in Modern Geography*, *38*.

Osypuk, T. L. (2013). Invited commentary: Integrating a life-course perspective and social theory to advance research on residential segregation and health. *American Journal of Epidemiology*, *177*(4), 310–315. https://doi.org/10.1093/aje/kws371

Pais, J., South, S. J., & Crowder, K. (2012). Metropolitan heterogeneity and minority neighborhood attainment: Spatial assimilation or place stratification? *Social Problems*, *59*(2), 258–281. https://doi.org/10.1525/sp.2012.59.2.258

Peterson, R., & Krivo, L. (2010). *Divergent social worlds: Neighborhood crime and the racial-spatial divide*. New York, NY: Russell Sage Foundation. Retrieved from https://books.google.com/books?hl=en&lr=&id=XgMFEHKNi-IC&oi=fnd&pg=PR13&dq=Divergent+Social+Worlds:+Neighborhood+Crime+and+the+Racial-Spatial+Divide&ots=g5f4ovagmF&sig=0G4uy6S54qRzcJit8hgVEyuB2D0

Pickett, K. E., Shaw, R. J., Atkin, K., Kiernan, K. E., & Wilkinson, R. G. (2009). Ethnic density effects on maternal and infant health in the Millennium Cohort Study. *Social Science & Medicine (1982)*, *69*(10), 1476–1483. https://doi.org/10.1016/j.socscimed.2009.08.031

Quillian, L. (2014). Does segregation create winners and losers? Residential segregation and inequality in educational attainment. *Social Problems*, *61*(3), 402–426. https://doi.org/10.1525/sp.2014.12193.This

Reardon, S. F. (2006). A conceptual framework for measuring segregation and its association with population outcomes. In J. M. Oakes & J. S. Kaufman (Eds.), *Methods in social epidemiology* (pp. 169–192). San Francisco, CA: Jossey-Bass.

Reardon, S. F., Farrell, C. R., Matthews, S., Sullivan, D. O., Bischoff, K., & Lee, B. A. (2009). Race and space in the 1990s: Changes in the geographic scale of racial residential segregation, 1990–2000. *Social Science Research*, *38*(1), 55–70.

Reardon, S. F., & Firebaugh, G. (2002). Measures of multigroup segregation. *Sociological Methodology*, *32*(1), 33–67. https://doi.org/10.1111/1467-9531.00110

Reardon, S. F., Firebaugh, G., O'Sullivan, D., & Matthews, S. (2006). A new approach to measuring socio-spatial economic segregation. In *International Association for Research in Income and Wealth*. Finland: Joensuu. Available at http://www.iariw.org/papers/2006/reardon.pdf

Reardon, S. F., Fox, L., & Townsend, J. (2015). Neighborhood income composition by household race and income, 1990–2009. *The ANNALS of the American Academy of Political and Social Science*, *660*(1), 78–97. https://doi.org/10.1177/0002716215576104

Reardon, S. F., Matthews, S. A., Sullivan, D. O., Lee, B. A., Firebaugh, G., & Farrell, C. R. (2008). The Geographic Scale of Metropolitan Racial Segregation. *Demography*, *45*(3), 489–514. https://doi.org/10.1353/dem.0.0019

Reardon, S. F., & O'Sullivan, D. (2004). Measures of spatial segregation. *Sociological Methodology*, *34*(1), 121–162. https://doi.org/10.1111/j.0081-1750.2004.00150.x

Rey, S. J., & Folch, D. C. (2011). Impact of spatial effects on income segregation indices. *Computers, Environment and Urban Systems*, *35*(6), 431–441. https://doi.org/10.1016/j.compenvurbsys.2011.07.008

Roberto, E. (2015). The Divergence Index: A decomposable measure of segregation and inequality. Retrieved from http://arxiv.org/abs/1508.01167

Roberto, E., & Hwang, J. (2015). Barriers to integration: Institutionalized boundaries and the spatial structure of residential segregation. Retrieved from http://arxiv.org/abs/1509.02574

Rothstein, R. (2017). *The color of law: A forgotten history of how our government segregated America*. New York, NY: Liverwright.

Sampson, R. J., Morenoff, J. D., & Earls, F. (2011). Beyond social capital: Spatial dynamics of collective efficacy for children. *American Sociological Review*, *64*(5), 633–660.

Schelling, T. C. (1971). Dynamic model of segregation. *Journal of Mathematical Sociology*, *1*, 143–186.

Schempf, A. H., & Kaufman, J. S. (2012). Accounting for context in studies of health inequalities: A review and comparison of analytic approaches. *Annals of Epidemiology*, *22*(10), 683–690. https://doi.org/10.1016/j.annepidem.2012.06.105

Shaw, R. J., Pickett, K. E., & Wilkinson, R. G. (2010). Ethnic density effects on birth outcomes and maternal smoking during pregnancy in the US linked birth and infant death data set. *American Journal of Public Health*, *100*(4), 707–713. https://doi.org/10.2105/AJPH.2009.167114

South, S. J., Crowder, K., & Pais, J. (2008). Inter-neighborhood migration and spatial assimilation in a multi-ethnic world: Comparing Latinos, Blacks, and Anglos. *Social Forces; a Scientific Medium of Social Study and Interpretation*, *87*(1), 415–444. https://doi.org/10.1353/sof.0.0116

Squires, G., & Kubrin, C. (2005). Privileged places: race, uneven development and the geography of opportunity in urban America. *Urban Studies*, *42*(1), 47–68. https://doi.org/10.1080/0042098042000309694

Stroope, S., Martinez, B. C., Eschbach, K., Peek, M. K., & Markides, K. S. (2015). Neighborhood ethnic composition and problem drinking among older Mexican American men: Results from the Hispanic established populations for the epidemiologic study of the elderly. *Journal of Immigrant and Minority Health*, *17*(4), 1055–1060. https://doi.org/10.1007/s10903-014-0033-8

Sudano, J. J., Perzynski, A., Wong, D. W., Colabianchi, N., & Litaker, D. (2013). Neighborhood racial residential segregation and changes in health or death among older adults. *Health & Place*, *19*, 80–88. https://doi.org/10.1016/j.healthplace.2012.09.015

Sullivan, D. O., Wong, D. W. S., O'Sullivan, D., & Wong, D. W. S. (2007). A surface-based approach to measuring spatial segregation. *Geographical Analysis*, *39*(2), 147–168. https://doi.org/10.1111/j.1538-4632.2007.00699.x

Viruell-Fuentes, E. A., Morenoff, J. D., Williams, D. R., & House, J. S. (2013). Contextualizing nativity status, social ties, and ethnic enclaves: Implications for understanding immigrant and Latino health paradoxes. *Ethnicity & Health*, *18*(6), 586–609. https://doi.org/10.1080/13557858.2013.814763

Waitzman, N. J., & Smith, K. R. (1998). Separate but lethal: The effects of economic segregation on mortality in metropolitan America. *The Milbank Quarterly*, *76*(3), 341–373, 304. https://doi.org/10.2307/3350468

White, K., & Borrell, L. N. (2011). Racial/ethnic residential segregation: Framing the context of health risk and health disparities. *Health & Place*, *17*(2), 438–448. https://doi.org/10.1016/j.healthplace.2010.12.002

White, K., Haas, J. S., & Williams, D. R. (2012). Elucidating the role of place in health care disparities: The example of racial/ethnic residential segregation. *Health Service Research*, *47*(3 pt 2), 1278–1299. https://doi.org/10.1111/j.1475-6773.2012.01410.x

Williams, D. R., & Collins, C. (2001). Racial residential segregation: A fundamental cause of racial disparities in health. *Public Health Reports*, *116*(5), 404–416. https://doi.org/10.1093/phr/116.5.404

Wolch, J. R., Byrne, J., & Newell, J. P. (2014). Urban green space, public health, and environmental justice: The challenge of making cities "just green enough." *Landscape and Urban Planning*, *125*, 234–244. https://doi.org/10.1016/j.landurbplan.2014.01.017

Wong, D. W. (2005). Formulating a general spatial segregation measure. *The Professional Geographer*, *57*(2), 285–294.

Yang, T., Shoff, C., Noah, A. J., Black, N., & Sparks, C. S. (2014). Racial segregation and maternal smoking during pregnancy: A multilevel analysis using the racial segregation interaction index. *Social Science & Medicine (1982)*, *107*, 26–36. https://doi.org/10.1016/j.socscimed.2014.01.030

INDEX

Tables, figures, and boxes are indicated by an italic *t*, *f*, and *b* following the page number.